MILADY'S STANDARD TEXTBOOK OF PROFESSIONAL BARBER-STYLING

REVISED EDITION

Revised by

Maura T. Scali-Sheahan

Milady Publishing Company
(A Division of Delmar Publishers Inc.)

NOTICE TO READER

CREDITS:
Senior Administrative Editor: Catherine Frangie
Developmental Editor: Joseph Miranda
Senior Project Editor: Laura Gulotty
Production Manager: John Mickelbank
Art Coordinator: John Lent
Design Coordinator: Karen Kunz Kemp

Artists: Shizuko Horii, Judy Francis, Robert Richards, Cynthia Saniewski, CEM, Ron Young, Nelva Richardson
PHOTOGRAPHER: Michael A. Gallitelli on location at The Rielm Salon, Latham, NY and at the Austin Beauty School, with Dino Petrocelli
MEDICAL PHOTOGRAPHER: (Nail Disorders): Elvin G. Zook, M.D., Division of Plastic Surgery, Southern Illinois University School of Medicine (Photographs of onycholysis and onycholysis caused by trauma courtesy of Orville J. Stone, M.D., Dermatology Medical Group, Huntington Beach, California and *NAILS* Magazine)

Copyright © 1984, 1993
Milady Publishing Company
(A Division of Delmar Publishers Inc.)
3 Columbia Circle, Box 12519
Albany, NY 12212–2519

Printed in the United States of America

2 3 4 5 6 7 8 9 10 XXX 99 98 97 96 95 94 93

Library of Congress Cataloging-in-Publication Data

Scali-Sheahan, Maura T.
    Milady's standard textbook of professional barber-styling / Maura T.
Scali-Sheahan. —Rev. ed.
        p. cm.
    Includes index.
    ISBN 1–56253–104–2
    1. Barbering.   I. Title.
TT957.S33   1993
646.7'24—dc20   92–20470
                                CIP

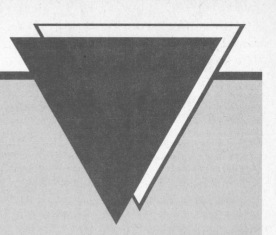

Contents

18—Electricity and Light Therapy 482

19—Chemistry 498

20—Anatomy and Physiology 519

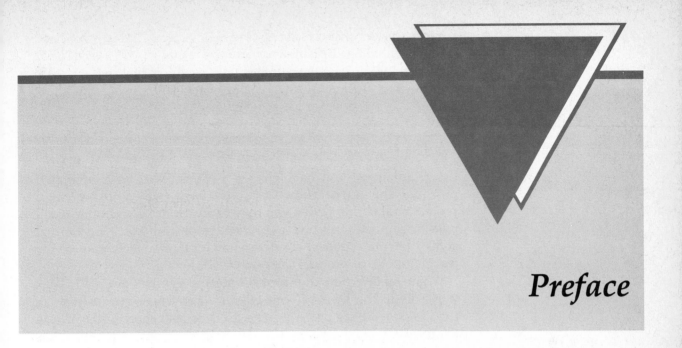

Preface

The material contained in this new edition of *Milady's Standard Textbook of Professional Barber-Styling* has been completely revised and brought up-to-date with respect to both the theory and the practice of barber-styling.

The theory of barber-styling denotes the great fund of knowledge available in this field, and has been developed into a systematic and coherent body of related barber-styling information.

The practice deals with the skill and dexterity demonstrated by the professional practitioner in the performance of the various barber-styling services.

The information contained in this text has been prepared to allow great flexibility and adaptability to whatever system or routine is followed in either school or shop. The materials presented are not designed or intended to standardize all barber-styling practice. They are not designed or intended to in any way stifle initiative in barber-styling education or method. Rather, they are presented in such a manner as to encourage teachers to be flexible, modern, and alert to change and improvements.

The text clearly presents the step-by-step instructions in the art and practice of basic services. Many illustrations, charts, review examination questions, and a glossary/index have been included to facilitate teaching and learning. Phonetic pronunciations also have been provided for difficult and technical terms.

Barber-styling school graduates who used this text in their studies have found themselves better prepared to cope with the great demands of the practice of barber-styling.

To the Student

Congratulations! You have chosen a career filled with unlimited potential and opportunity. Once you have trained to become a professional barber-stylist you may choose to open a shop, participate in competitions, and platform demonstrations. As a barber-stylist, you may opt to specialize in hair replacement techniques, the teaching field, or product sales.

Whatever direction your professional career takes, you will play a vital role in the lives of your clients. They will come to you for professional advice and expertise that you will share with them in the forms of creativity and technical skill. As a professional barber-stylist you will have the ability to provide a rewarding personal service to your clients that will be recognized and appreciated.

This textbook provides you with basic techniques and methods that, with practice, you will gradually master. You will be introduced to a whole new world of creative expression, technical skills, and human relation techniques that will be enhanced continually as you spend time working in the profession.

You will learn from gifted and giving instructors who will share their skills and experiences with you. You will meet other industry professionals at seminars, workshops, and conventions where you'll learn the latest techniques, specific product knowledge, and management procedures. All of the experiences in which you have the opportunity to participate will provide you with additional insights into the profession you have chosen. You will build a network of professionals to turn to for career advice, opportunity, and direction.

Whatever direction you choose, we wish you a successful and enjoyable journey.

To the Instructor

This edition of *Milady's Standard Textbook of Professional Barber-Styling* represents the most recently updated revision of content and appearance presentation in the long history of this best-selling text.

Our entire staff of editors, designers, and artists have worked closely with the revision author in the development of this book. We hope that we have made the subjects easier for you to teach and that this text will please and help to motivate your students.

If you have used *Milady's Standard Textbook of Professional Barber-Styling* in the past, you will note the following exciting changes:

- Chapter presentation in the sequence most used and preferred by instructors.
- A two-color design with a variety of new illustrations and photographs.
- Up-to-date methods and information.
- A streamlined re-organization of chapters which ties theory and practice together more closely.
- Illustrations of women and men from diverse cultural backgrounds and of varying ages.
- Detailed, step-by-step procedures.
- Highlighted safety cautions, particularly for the chemical services.
- Key terms in boldface type with their pronunciations.
- Learning Objectives that are explained in the major topics of each chapter and then reinforced by the Review Questions.
- A comprehensive Glossary/Index, combined to provide concise definitions of key terms along with pertinent page references so the student can find detailed explanations within the text.
- A wide selection of supplementary materials for the student and for the teacher.

Acknowledgments

My sincere thanks to Milady Publishing Company for giving me the opportunity to service the barber-styling profession in the thrilling capacity of revision author.

A special thank-you to Catherine Frangie, senior administrative editor, for her enthusiasm and confidence in my efforts. It has been a pleasure working with you!

In loving memory of my father for encouraging creative thought, inspiration and expression; to my mother for sharing her no-nonsense approach to life and all its challenges, and to my family for their love and support. Thank you everyone.

Maura T. Scali-Sheahan
Jacksonville, Florida

The author and publisher would also like to thank the following barber-styling professionals for their assistance and expertise in reviewing this book.

- Denise L. Dennis
  Atlanta Area Technical School
  Atlanta, GA
- Camille Mariani Ferrari
  Pittsburgh Beauty Academy
  Pittsburgh, PA
- Forrest F. Green, Jr.
  Michigan Barber School, Inc.
  Detroit, MI
- Michaelene Heskett
  Detroit Barber College, Inc.
  Roseville, MI
- Lloyd Le Jeune
  Lloyd's of Lafayette
  Lafayette, LA
- Phillip S. Mazza
  Gambrills, MD
- Francis G. Mielkey, I
  Jacksonville, FL
- Jayne Morehouse
  Cleveland, OH
- Joseph Pasquale
  Buena Vista Correctional Facility
  Salida, CO

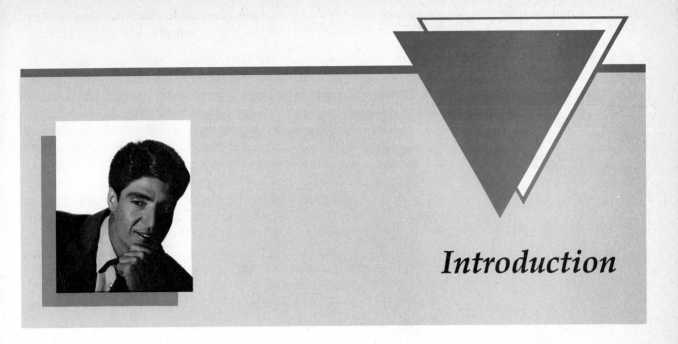

Introduction

Courtesy of: The National Cosmetology Association's Ice Cream Collection. Danny Ewert, Design Team Director. Jim Douglass, photographer.

▼ WELCOME TO THE PROFESSION OF BARBER-STYLING

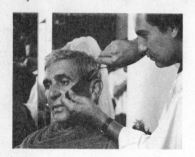

Congratulations on taking the first step down the path to an exciting professional career choice—barber-styling. An ambitious man or woman can look forward to a lucrative and growth-filled career, offering opportunities for artistic and creative expression, personal satisfaction, and the mastery of a technical skill. Your success will depend upon talent, dedication, interest, goals, and ambition. Opportunities in the field of barber-styling are unlimited. The path you have chosen can lead into an exciting new world . . . .

The practice of modern barber-styling combines scientific knowledge and artistic ability. Science deals with the knowing, art with the doing. The science of barber-styling consists of knowledge essential to the performance of professional hair and skin services; the art requires that manual skill and dexterity be applied in order to produce professional results.

Barbering refers to the performance of those techniques and arts, such as haircutting, shaving, massaging, facial treatments, and the trimming and styling of facial hair, which make up the major services performed by a barber-stylist. The premises where the art of barber-styling is practiced is known by various titles. The most popular are barber shop, barber-styling shop, hairstyling shop, barber-stylist's, or unisex salon (a shop or salon where barbers and cosmetologists perform hair care services for both male and female clients). The titles are used interchangeably, as are the words shop and salon, to indicate the premises where the professional services are offered.

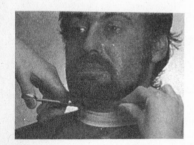 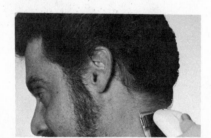 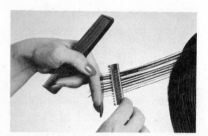

▼ CAREER OPPORTUNITIES FOR BARBER-STYLISTS

Many career opportunities exist in the field of barber-styling for the well-trained individual. A review of the following career specialties will present some options within this dynamic and fascinating field.

Barber-Stylist

After successfully completing your education and passing the state examination, you will be ready to practice barber-styling services in your state. A barber-stylist's first position allows for the opportunity to enhance and expand basic skills, provides experience in day-to-day shop operations, perfects communication skills and offers an in-depth view of the industry. The experience of watching your clientele grow will be exciting. For every satisfied customer that leaves your styling chair, several more will seek you out as their stylist. The day that the appointment book shows that you are booked solid, you will have achieved an important step in professional growth followed by a real sense of emotional gratification. The fact that this level of performance was achieved through your own efforts will provide inspiration, and the financial rewards will provide a clear indication of your potential.

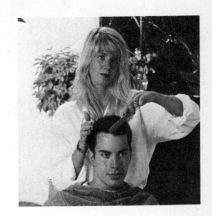

Barber-Stylist Shop Manager

In addition to the qualifications needed as a barber-stylist, becoming a successful shop manager requires many of the same qualities as does ownership of a shop. However, the financial responsibilities, policy-making, and liabilities sometimes associated with ownership are limited. Shop management provides experience in staff supervision, purchasing, quality control, and many other aspects of operations. Managing a shop or salon provides the best preparation and background for shop ownership.

Shop Owner

If you have clear ideas about methods of operations and enjoy varied responsibilities, challenges, and the business aspects of barber-styling, then shop ownership may be a good choice. An owner sets the standards for the quality of service in the shop. As the owner, you will choose the products and services to be offered, and establish the level of skill expected from the staff. Ownership requires the ability to make decisions, take risks, and a commitment to long hours. It also offers creativity, versatility, and independence in shop management and operations.

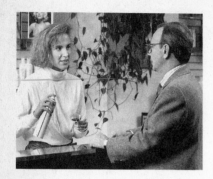

Sales and Marketing

This career choice may be one to explore if you have a flair for selling, communicate well, and enjoy working with a variety of people in various locations. Sales and marketing specialists work with manufacturers, distributors, and shops or salons. Requirements include a solid scientific base, technical and practical application skills, and basic sales techniques. Such experience allows a sales or marketing representative to promote specific products, provide training seminars, or service accounts including schools and shops. Sales in the barber-styling industry can be both lucrative and rewarding.

Competition and Platform Specialist

Perfectionism and competitiveness are qualities that make for success in this specialty. Competition stylists compete for prizes and prestige in both national and international hairstyling championships. Champions often own shops or salons, work as trainers, or perform platform work at industry shows and seminars. A competition champion's reputation as a distinguished artist increases prosperity in all business endeavors.

Education

The field of education offers a broad spectrum of choices, from instructor, to product researcher, to trade journal writer. Just as industry trends are constantly changing because of new techniques and products, opportunities and demands in education change to meet these needs.

State Licensing Member

Members of state licensing organizations must be highly qualified and experienced in their specific professions. They conduct examinations, grant licenses, and inspect schools to see that certain physical standards, such as space and equipment, are maintained. In addition, they see that educational materials meet certain specifications. This is a career area that allows you to be part of a group of people who structure and change the profession of barber-styling, today and tomorrow.

A VARIETY OF CAREER CHOICES

Professionals in the field will agree that there is always something new to learn or a new approach to master in the barber-styling industry. It is because of the ever-changing nature of the profession that it is an exciting, challenging, and rewarding career choice. The list of career opportunities is endless. Everything that you learn can be of value. To illustrate this important lesson, it may be helpful to follow the careers of two individuals.

As can be seen from these charts, both barber-stylists used their experience and success as a foundation for the next opportunity. Their extra efforts (attending trade shows and seminars, association participation and demonstration work) influenced their future success, and their careers evolved naturally, based upon their individual interests, talents, and dedication. Clearly it is beneficial to leave open as many options as possible. Within the barber-styling field there is ample opportunity for a wide range of interests and forms of expression. The choice is up to the individual, and whatever that choice may be for you, we hope that you will find that the profession of barber-styling lives up to your expectations.

John Doe

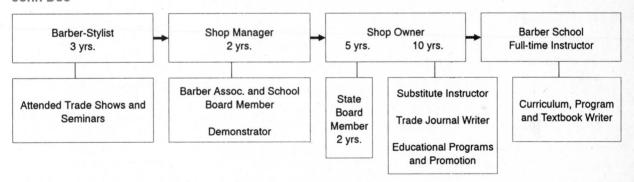

Jane Doe

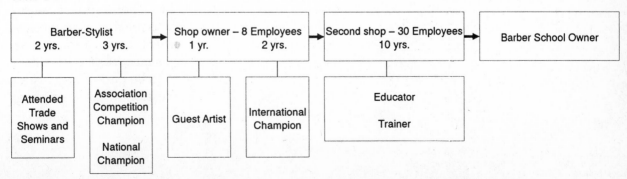

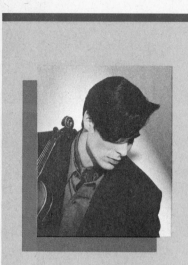

The History of Barber-Styling

Learning Objectives

After completing this chapter, you should be able to:

1. *Demonstrate an understanding of the evolution of barbering from ancient times to the present.*
2. *Define the origin of the word barber.*
3. *Be able to describe and discuss barber-surgeons.*
4. *Explain the origin of the barber pole.*
5. *Identify and describe the organizations responsible for the upgrading of the barbering profession.*
6. *Describe the importance and functions of state boards.*
7. *List the factors that have improved barber-styling in recent years.*

Barbering and hairstyling is one of the oldest professions in the world. With the advance of civilization, barbering and hairstyling developed from insignificant beginnings into a recognized profession.

The study of this progression leads to an appreciation of the accomplishments, evolution, and position of high esteem attained by the early practitioners. The cultural, esthetic, and technical heritage they developed provides the basis for the prestige and respect of the profession and its services today.

ORIGIN OF THE BARBER

The word *barber* is derived from the Latin word *barba*, meaning beard. (Fig. 1.1) Another Latin word, *tonsorial* meaning the cutting, clipping, or trimming of hair with shears or a razor, is often used in conjunction with barbering. (Fig. 1.2) Hence, barbers are sometimes referred to as tonsorial artists.

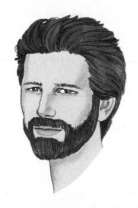

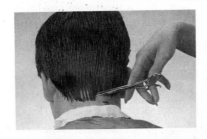

1.1 – The word *barber* is derived from the Latin word *barba* meaning beard.

1.2 – Trimming the hair with shears.

Archeological studies reveal that haircutting and hairstyling were practiced in some form as early as the glacial age. The simple but effective implements used were shaped from sharpened flints, oyster shells, or bone. Animal sinew or strips of hide were used to tie the hair back, or as adornment.

The Egyptians were the first to cultivate beauty in an extravagant fashion. Excavations from tombs have revealed such relics as combs, brushes, mirrors, cosmetics, and razors made of tempered copper and bronze. Although eye paint was the most popular of all cosmetics, henna was used extensively to produce a reddish tint to the hair, and is still used to some extent today. Written records have been found that substantiate the use of barbers by the nobility and priesthood of Egypt, some 6,000 years ago. (Fig. 1.3)

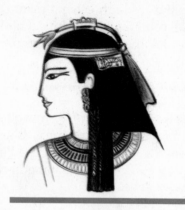 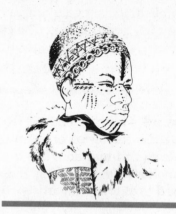

1.4 – African

At approximately the same point in history, in Africa hair was groomed with intricately carved combs and ornamented with beads, clay, and colored bands. (Fig. 1.4)

However, it wasn't until the time of Moses (1450–2400 B.C.) that barber services were available to the general population of that culture. During the Golden Age of Greece (500 B.C.), almost a thousand years later, barbering and hairstyling became highly developed arts. Barbers' services were eventually introduced in Rome in 296 B.C. It was there that the concept of barbering was further expanded to include what became famous as the Roman baths.

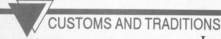

CUSTOMS AND TRADITIONS

In almost every early culture hairstyles indicated social status.

Noblemen of ancient Gaul indicated their rank by wearing their hair long until Caesar made them cut it after he conquered them, as a sign of submission.

In ancient Greece, boys would cut their hair upon reaching adolescence, while their Hindu counterparts would shave their heads.

Following the invasion of China by the Manchus, Chinese men adopted the queue as a mark of dignity and manhood.

In Africa, Masai warriors wove their front hair into three sections of tiny braids and the rest of the hair into a queue down the back. Braiding was used extensively, with the intricate patterns frequently denoting status within the tribe.

The ancient Britons were extremely proud of their long hair. Blond hair was brightened with washes composed of tallow, lime, and the extracts of certain vegetables. Darker hair was treated with dyes extracted and processed from plants, trees, and various soils. The Danes, Angles, and Normans (early invaders of ancient Briton) dressed their hair not only for beautification and adornment, but also for ornamentation during battle. Glittering hair ornaments reflected the sunlight, blinding and intimidating the Britons, while headdresses of metal or leather and horn created the illusion of half-beast, half-human warriors with an equally intimidating effect.

In ancient Rome, the color of a woman's hair indicated her class or rank. Noblewomen tinted their hair red; those of the middle class colored their hair blond; and poor women were compelled to dye their hair black.

Religion, occupation, and politics also influenced the length and style of hair.

Clergymen were distinguished by the tonsure—a shaved patch on the head. During the 7th century, Celtic and Roman church leaders disagreed on the exact shape the tonsure should take. Eventually, it was decided that the Roman tradition of shaving the whole crown would constitute the official tonsure.

British barristers indicated their occupation by wearing grey wigs, while the various branches of the law and military wore specific styles according to their military corps.

By the 17th century in England, political affiliation and religion were indicated by the long, curling locks of the Royalist Anglican Cavaliers and the cropped hair of the Parliamentarian Puritan Roundheads.

Most rulers and monarchs became trend setters by virtue of their position and power in society. Personal whim, taste, and even physical limitations could become the basis for changes in hairstyles and fashion. In the 16th century when Francis I of France accidentally burned his hair with a torch, his loyal subjects had their hair, beards, and mustaches cut short.

During the reign of Louis XIV in the 17th century, noblemen wore wigs because the king, who was balding, did so. During the 19th century in France, men and women showed appreciation

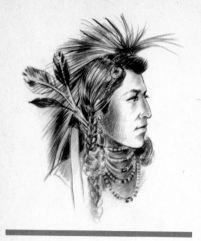

1.5 – Native American

for antiquity by cutting their hair in the style of the early Roman emperors.

The beliefs, rituals, and superstitions of early civilizations varied from one ethnic group to another, depending upon the region and social interaction with other groups. There was a general belief among many tribes that people could be bewitched by hair clippings. Hence, the privilege of haircutting was reserved for the priest, medicine man, or other spiritual leader of the tribe. According to the Greek, Pythagoras, the hair was the source of the brain's inspiration and cutting it decreased an individual's intellectual capacity. The Irish peasantry believed that if hair cuttings were burned or buried with the dead, no evil spirits would haunt the individual. Among some American Indian tribes it was believed that the hair and the body were so linked that anyone possessing a lock of hair of another might work his will on the individual. The Indian custom of scalping had its origin in this belief. (Fig. 1.5)

▼ SIGNIFICANCE OF THE BEARD

The importance of the beard lies more in the past than the present. Nonetheless, it is interesting to note the various fashions and customs associated with it.

In early times in most nations, the beard was considered to be a sign of wisdom, strength, and manhood. In some cultures, it was thought of as almost sacred. Among Orthodox Jews, the beard was a symbol of religious devotion. To cut off the beard was contrary to Mosaic law.

As long ago as 400 B.C., shaving was introduced by the Macedonians. Later, it spread to Egypt and the Eastern countries including China. In Greece and Rome, the wealthy and free men were shaved by their valets, while the so-called common classes patronized the barber shops. Such shops became the gathering places where news was shared and comraderie was found. Slaves were forced to wear beards. The first shave on a young Roman's twenty-second birthday constituted a rite of passage from boyhood to manhood, and was celebrated with great festivity.

Certain rulers required that beards be removed. Alexander the Great ordered his soldiers to shave so that their enemies could not seize their beards during battle. Peter the Great encouraged shaving by imposing a tax on beards.

During the spread of Christianity, long hair came to be considered sinful and the clergy were directed to shave their beards. Although the shaving of the beard was still forbidden among Orthodox Jews, the use of scissors to remove excess growth was permitted. The Moslems took great care in trimming the beard after prayer. The hair that was removed was preserved, to be buried with the owner.

In the Middle Ages three hairs from the king's beard were imbedded in the wax of the royal seal. During the reign of Queen Elizabeth in England, it became fashionable to dye the beard and cut it into a variety of shapes.

THE RISE OF THE BARBER-SURGEONS

During the Middle Ages, barbers not only practiced shaving, haircutting, and hairstyling, but also entered the world of medicine, where they figured prominently in the development of surgery as a recognized branch of medical practice.

When Pope Alexander III forbade the clergy to shed blood, barbers assisted monks and priests during surgery. Barbers performed blood-letting and minor surgery, administered herbs, and later pulled teeth. For centuries, dentistry was performed only by barbers and for more than a thousand years they were known as barber-surgeons.

The symbol of the barber-surgeon evolved from the technical aspects of blood-letting. The white cloth bandages used to stop the bleeding were washed and hung out to dry. The stained bandages would then twist together in the breeze, forming a red and white pattern.

The original symbol of barber-surgeons consisted of a striped pole from which a basin was suspended. The fillet around the pole represented the bandage that was wrapped around the arm, and the basin was the vessel used for receiving the blood. One interpretation of the colors of the barbers' pole was that red represented the blood, blue the veins, and white the bandage. This sign, without the basin, has been retained by the modern barber-stylist.

The barber-surgeons formed their first organization in France in 1096 A.D. Soon after, the first school of surgery was established in Paris. During the 1100s, a guild of surgeons was organized from the barber-surgeon group which specialized in the study of medicine. To protect themselves, the Barbers' Company of London was formed during the 13th century with the objective of regulating the profession. The Barbers' Company was ruled by a master and consisted of two classes of barbers—those who practiced barbering and those who specialized in surgery.

Aside from the Barbers' Company, there was also a surgeon's guild in England. Although there is reason to believe that competition and antagonism existed between the two organizations, a law uniting the two groups was passed in 1450 for the purpose of fostering the science of surgery. A law was enacted separating the practices of barbering and surgery—barbers could perform no surgery except dentistry, and surgeons were forbidden to act as barbers.

With the advancement of medicine, the ancient practice of bloodletting became all but obsolete. Although the barber-surgeons' medical practice dwindled in importance, they were still relied upon for dispensing medicinal herbs and pulling teeth. Finally, in 1745, a law was passed separating the barbers from the surgeons and the alliance was completely dissolved.

Barber-surgeons also flourished in France and Germany. In 1371, a corporation was organized by the French barber-surgeons under the rule of the king's barber, but with the advent of the French Revolution the corporation was dissolved. In the 19th century, wigs became so elaborate and fashionable that a separate corporation of barbers was founded in France. Not until 1779 was a corporation formed in Prussia, and this was disbanded in 1809 when new unions were started.

Many Europeans had become so dependent upon the services of the barber-surgeons that Dutch and Swedish settlers brought barber-surgeons with them to America to look after the well-being of the colonists.

▼ MODERN BARBERS AND BARBERING

By the 19th century, barbering was completely separated from religion and medicine and began to emerge as an independent profession. During the late 1800s, the profession's structure changed and it began to follow new directions. Employer organizations known as **master barber groups,** and employee organizations known as **journeymen barber groups,** were the first step toward upgrading and regulating the profession. During this era, precedents were set in the history of barbering, in part due to the emergence and growth of these organizations.

The Journeymen Barbers' Union was formed at its first convention in Buffalo, New York, in 1887 and was affiliated with the American Federation of Labor. In 1893, A.B. Moler established America's first barber school in Chicago, Illinois, and published the first barbering textbook, *The Moler Manual of Barbering*, in the same year.

Minnesota was the first state to pass a barber licensing law. This legislation, passed in 1897, set standards for sanitation, minimum education and technical requirements for barbers in that state.

In 1924, the Associated Master Barbers of America was organized in Chicago, Illinois. The name was changed in 1941 to the Associated Master Barbers and Beauticians of America. This association represented shop and salon owners and managers.

By 1925, the Associated Master Barbers of America established the National Educational Council, the purposes of which were to standardize and upgrade barber training. The council was successful in standardizing barber schools, the training of barber instructors, the establishment of a curriculum, and the legislation required for the passage of state licensing laws.

The National Association of Barber Schools was formed in 1927. In cooperation with the Associated Master Barbers of America, it worked to develop a program standardizing the operation of barber schools.

By 1929, the National Association of State Board of Barber Examiners was organized in St. Paul, Minnesota. Its purpose was to standardize the qualifications required for barber examination applicants and the methods of evaluation to be used. The Associated Master Barbers of America also adopted a Barber Code of Ethics, to promote professionalism and responsibility in the trade.

Since 1929, all states, with the exception of several counties in Alabama, have passed laws regulating the practice of barbering and hairstyling. The state boards are primarily concerned with the maintenance of high educational standards in order to assure competent and skillful service. Schools, unions, and associations have cooperated in the enforcement of state laws, and in the protection of members' rights, privileges, and public health and welfare.

In addition to establishing legal regulatory guidelines, barbering also has advanced technologically. Since the invention of electricity, rapid strides have been made in the development of barbering and hairstyling tools and appliances, with updated designs becoming available each year. Moreover, greater emphasis on hygiene and sanitation, and an increased knowledge of products and the art of haircutting has improved the quality of contemporary barber skills and services.

Some important factors that recently have improved the practice of barbering and hairstyling include:

1. Implementation of regulatory and educational standards
2. Improved practice of sanitation in the shop

3. Use of better implements and tools
4. Use of electrical appliances in the shop
5. Study of anatomy dealing with those parts of the body (head, face, and neck) that are serviced by the barber-stylist
6. Study of products and preparations used in connection with facial, scalp, and hair treatments

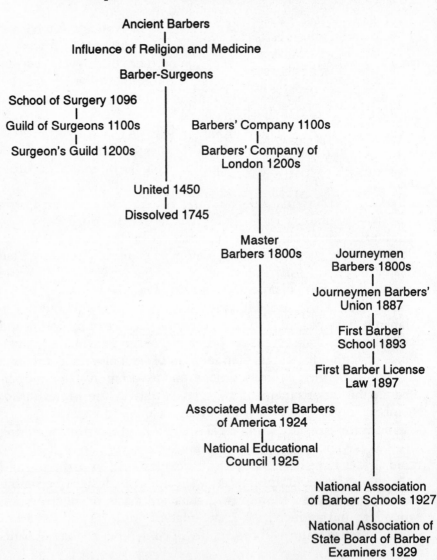

Ancient Barbers

Influence of Religion and Medicine

Barber-Surgeons

School of Surgery 1096

Guild of Surgeons 1100s

Surgeon's Guild 1200s

Barbers' Company 1100s

Barbers' Company of London 1200s

United 1450

Dissolved 1745

Master Barbers 1800s

Journeymen Barbers 1800s

Journeymen Barbers' Union 1887

First Barber School 1893

First Barber License Law 1897

Associated Master Barbers of America 1924

National Educational Council 1925

National Association of Barber Schools 1927

National Association of State Board of Barber Examiners 1929

1.6 – An Illustrated History of Barber–Styling

1. What is the origin of the word *barber*?
2. Why did men wear beards in ancient times?
3. Name two ancient nations which practiced barbering.
4. When did the Macedonians introduce the practice of shaving?
5. In what year did barbers become known in Rome?
6. When did barbers become popular in Greece?
7. Who were the barber-surgeons?
8. When did the barber-surgeons start their practice?
9. What were the duties of the barber-surgeons?
10. Describe the barber's sign used by the barber-surgeons.
11. What was the origin of the modern barber pole?
12. What kind of organization was the Barbers' Company of London?
13. When was the Barbers' Company organized in London?
14. When was the first corporation for barber-surgeons organized in France?
15. Who brought the barber-surgeons to America?
16. What were the employer organizations called?
17. What were the employee organizations called?
18. In what year was the Journeymen Barbers' Union formed?
19. In what year did A. B. Moler open the first barber school in America?
20. In what year did the state of Minnesota pass the first barber license law?
21. Who was represented by the Associated Master Barbers of America?
22. What was the purpose of the National Educational Council?
23. What was the purpose of the National Association of Barber Schools?
24. What was the purpose of the National Association of State Board of Barber Examiners?
25. In what year did the Associated Master Barbers of America adopt a code of ethics?
26. In what are the state boards primarily interested?
27. What are three important advantages of having barber-styling licensing laws?
28. What important factors have improved the practice of barber-styling in recent years?

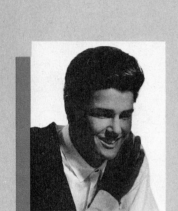

2

Your Professional Image

Learning Objectives

After completing this chapter, you should be able to:

1. *List guidelines to maintain a healthy body and mind.*
2. *Demonstrate communication and human relation skills.*
3. *List the qualities of professional ethics.*

Professional image is a reflection of the individual. Personality, personal hygiene and good grooming, general health, posture, attitude, moral character, professional ethics, and technical ability are all components of the total professional image in the field of barber-styling. It is this image that will be projected to the people with whom you come in contact. It is wise to consider the importance and influence that professional image has on present and future success.

PERSONAL AND PROFESSIONAL HEALTH

In accordance with the general concepts of the profession, the barber-stylist should be a personal representation of good health. To achieve success, it is helpful to follow a set of guidelines that help maintain both a healthy body and mind.

Hygiene

Hygiene is the branch of applied science concerned with healthful living; its main purpose is to preserve health.

Personal Hygiene

Personal hygiene is the daily maintenance of cleanliness and healthfulness which includes daily washing, use of deodorant, brushing teeth, using mouthwash, and having clean and well-groomed hair and nails.

Rest

Adequate sleep is essential for good health because without it you cannot function efficiently. The body should be allowed to recover from the fatigue of the day's activities and should be replenished with a good night's sleep. The amount of sleep needed to feel refreshed varies from person to person. Some people function well with six hours of sleep; others need eight hours.

Exercise

Exercise and recreation in the form of walking, dancing, sports, and gym activities tend to develop the muscles and help to keep the body fit. A few of the benefits resulting from regular and non-stren-uous exercises are:

1. An improvement in the proper functioning of organs
2. An improvement in blood circulation
3. The body is supplied with more life-giving oxygen due to the increased action of the lungs.

Relaxation

Relaxation is important as a change of pace from day-to-day rou-tine. Going to a movie or a museum, reading a book, watching television, or dancing are ways to "get away from it all." When you return to work, you will feel refreshed and eager to attend to your duties.

Nutrition

What you eat affects your health, appearance, personality, and per-formance on the job. The nutrients in food supply the body with energy and ensure that the body functions properly. A balanced diet should include foods containing a variety of important vitamins and minerals. Drink plenty of water daily. Try to avoid sugar, salt, caffeine, and fatty or highly refined and processed foods.

Healthy Lifestyle

You should practice stress management through a combination of relaxation, rest, and exercise, and avoid substances that can have a negative effect on health, such as cigarettes, alcohol, and drugs.

Healthy Thoughts

The body and mind operate as a unit; thoughts and emotions can influence the body's activities. A thought may either stimulate or depress the way the body functions. Strong emotions such as worry and fear have a harmful effect on the heart, arteries, and glands. Depression weakens the functioning of the body's organs, thereby lowering resistance to disease.

Good Posture

Good posture not only presents personal appearance to its best advantage; it also creates an image of confidence, and helps to lessen fatigue and the possibility of other physical problems. (Fig. 2.1) Barber-stylists spend most of their time at work standing;

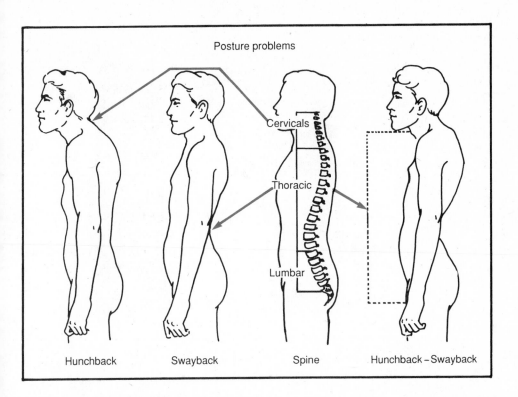

Posture problems

Cervicals

Thoracic

Lumbar

Hunchback   Swayback   Spine   Hunchback – Swayback

2.1 – Posture problems

therefore, good posture should be developed through regular exercise and self-discipline for both professional and health-related reasons. (Fig. 2.2)

Correct Sitting Posture

Just as there is a mechanically correct posture for standing, so is there one for sitting. It is extremely important to sit correctly, or **in balance.**

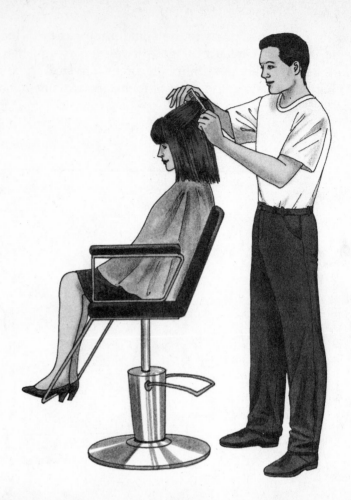

2.2 – Good posture is essential when spending a great deal of time on your feet.

1. Place your feet on the floor directly under your knees.
2. Have the seat of the chair even with your knees. This will allow the upper and lower legs to form a 90–degree angle at the knees.
3. Allow your feet to carry the weight of your thighs.
4. Rest the weight of your torso on the thigh bones, not on the end of your spine.
5. Keep your torso erect.
6. Make sure your desk is at the correct height so that the upper and lower parts of your arm form a right angle when you are writing. (Figs. 2.3, 2.4)

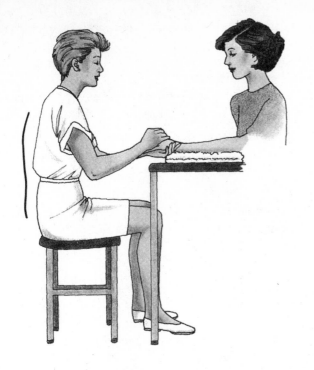

2.3 – Good sitting posture

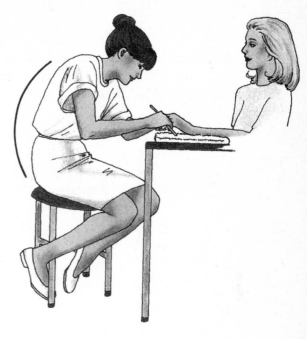

2.4 – Poor sitting posture

Personal Grooming

Personal grooming is an extension of personal hygiene. A well-groomed barber-stylist is one of the best advertisements for a salon. If you present a poised and attractive image, your client will have confidence in you as a professional. Many shop owners and managers consider appearance, personality, and poise to be as important as technical knowledge and manual skills. Some barber shops do not require standard uniforms, but they may have a specific dress code. For example, some shops require that all personnel wear the same color clothing. Select your outfits so that you reflect the image of the shop. Although excessive jewelry should be avoided, a wristwatch will help you to maintain your schedule.

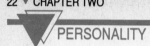
PERSONALITY

Personality plays an important role in both your personal and professional life. Personality can be defined as the outward reflection of inner feelings, thoughts, attitudes, and values. Your personality is expressed through your voice, speech, and choice of words, as well as through your facial expressions, gestures, actions, posture, clothing, grooming, and environment. Since your personality has an important effect on other people, it is the largest factor in your professional image.

Desirable Qualities for Effective Client Relations

Emotional Control

Learn to control your emotions. Do not reveal negative emotions such as anger, envy, and dislike. An even-tempered person is usually treated with respect.

Positive Approach

Be pleasant and gracious. Be ready with a smile of greeting and a word of welcome for each client and co-worker. A good sense of humor is also important in maintaining a positive attitude. A sense of humor enriches your life and cushions the disappointments. When you are able to laugh at yourself, you will have gained the ability to accept and deal positively with difficult situations.

Good Manners

Good manners reflect your thoughtfulness of others. Treating others with respect, exercising care of other people's property, being tolerant and understanding of their shortcomings and efforts, and being considerate of those with whom you work, all express good manners. Courtesy is one of the most important keys to a successful career.

Mannerisms

Gum-chewing and nervous habits, such as tapping your foot or playing with your hair, detract from the effectiveness of your image. Yawning, coughing, and sneezing should be concealed when in the presence of others. Control negative body language—sarcastic or disapproving facial grimaces, for example. Pleasant mannerisms and attractive gestures and actions should be your goal at all times.

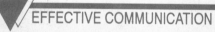
EFFECTIVE COMMUNICATION

Communication includes listening skills, voice, speech, and conversational ability. The manner in which you communicate will have a great influence on your effectiveness as a barber-stylist. A stylist needs good communication skills for the following reasons:

- To make contacts
- To meet and greet clients
- To understand a client's needs, likes, dislikes, and desires
- To be self-promoting
- To sell services and products
- To build business
- To talk on the telephone
- To carry on a pleasant conversation
- To interact with the shop/salon staff

HUMAN RELATIONS AND PROFESSIONAL ATTITUDE

Human relations is the psychology of getting along well with others. Your professional attitude is expressed by your own self-esteem, confidence in your profession, and by the respect you show others.

Good habits and practices acquired during your education lay the foundation for a successful career in barber-styling. The following guidelines for good human relations will help you gain confidence and deal comparably with others, and become successful professionally.

1. Always greet a client by name, using a pleasant tone of voice. Address a client by his or her last name unless the client prefers first names or it is customary to use first names in your salon.
2. Be alert to the client's mood. Some clients prefer quiet and relaxation; others like to talk. Be a good listener and confine conversation to the client's needs. Never gossip or tell off-color stories. (Fig. 2.5)
3. Topics of conversation should be carefully chosen. Friendly relations are achieved through pleasant conversations. Let the client guide the topic of conversation. In a business setting it is best to avoid such controversial topics as religion and politics, personal problems, or subjects relating to other people. Never discuss other clients or fellow workers, and always maintain confidentiality.
4. Make a good impression by looking the part of the successful barber-stylist, and by speaking and acting in a professional manner at all times.
5. Cultivate self-confidence, and project a pleasing personality.

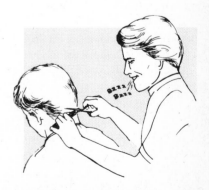

2.5 – When conversing with a client take your cue from the client's mood.

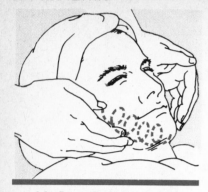

2.6 – Be gentle, and clients will remember you. Harsh, rough treatment chases clients away.

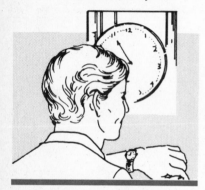

2.7 – Be punctual. Get to work on time and you won't miss any clients. Tardiness never pays.

6. Show interest in the client's personal preferences and give the client undivided attention. (Fig. 2.6)
7. Use tact and diplomacy when dealing with problems you may encounter. Deal with all disputes and differences in private. Take care of all problems promptly, and to the customer's satisfaction.
8. Be capable and efficient.
9. Be punctual. Arrive at work on time and keep appointments on schedule. Plan each day's schedule so that you manage your time effectively. (Fig. 2.7)
10. Develop your business and sales abilities. Use tact when suggesting additional services or products to clients.
11. Avoid saying anything that sounds critical, condemning, or demeaning of a client's opinions.
12. Keep informed of new products and services so you can answer clients' questions intelligently.
13. Continue to add to your knowledge and skills.
14. Be ethical in all dealings with clients and others with whom you come in contact.
15. Always let the client see that you practice the highest standards of sanitation.
16. Use tact when educating clients about the styles, services, or products best suited to them.

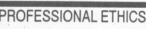

▼ PROFESSIONAL ETHICS

Ethics include standards of conduct and moral judgment. Codes of ethics are established for professions by their respective boards or commissions that directly relate to the occupation and its characteristics. In barber-styling, state boards set the standards that all the barbers and stylists who work in that state must follow.

Ethics, however, goes beyond a set of rules and regulations. In barber-styling, ethics is also a code of conduct, which is expressed through your personality, human relation skills, and professional image.

Ethical conduct helps to build the client's confidence in you. Having clients speak well of you is the best form of advertising and helps to build a successful business. The following rules of ethics should be practiced by all professional barber-stylists.

1. Give courteous and friendly service to all clients. Treat everyone honestly and fairly; do not show favoritism.

2. Be courteous and show respect for the feelings, beliefs, and rights of others.

3. Keep your word. Be responsible and fulfill your obligations.

4. Build your reputation by setting an example of good conduct and behavior.

5. Be loyal to your employer, managers, and associates.

6. Obey all provisions of the state laws relating to barber-stylists.

7. Practice the highest standards of sanitation to protect your health and the health of your co-workers and clients.

8. Believe in your chosen profession. Practice it faithfully and sincerely.

9. Do not try to sell clients a product or service they do not need or want.

10. As a student:

- Be loyal to, and cooperate with, school personnel and fellow students.
- Comply with school and clinic rules and regulations.

Questionable practices, extravagant claims, and unfulfilled promises violate the rules of ethical conduct and cast an unfavorable light on barber-stylists. Unethical practices affect the student, the barber-stylist, the school or salon, and the entire industry.

GUIDES FOR STUDENT SUCCESS

1. Participate in the classroom in a courteous manner.
2. School regulations are important—obey them all.
3. Personal calls interfere with teaching and learning.
4. Be careful with all school equipment and supplies.
5. Be clean and well-groomed at all times. (Fig. 2.8)
6. Cooperation with teachers is essential for effective learning.
7. Notebooks and workbooks are important review aids.
8. Loafing or loitering makes a poor impression on others.
9. Be courteous and considerate at all times.
10. Be tactful and polite to clients.
11. Observe safety rules and prevent accidents.
12. Develop a pleasing personality.
13. Think and act positively.
14. Attend trade shows and conventions to increase knowledge.
15. Carefully complete all homework assignments.
16. Keep clothes and uniform spotlessly clean.

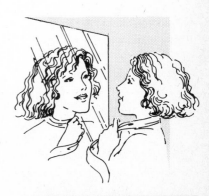

2.8 – Be neat, clean, attractive, and free from body odors and bad breath.

17. Follow teachers instructions and techniques.
18. Show clients that you are interested and sincere.
19. Maintain good attendance.
20. Ask for clarification of anything you do not understand.
21. Bathe daily and use a body deodorant.
22. Develop and exhibit good manners at all times.
23. Be respectful to teachers and supervisors.
24. Develop good work habits as essential to success.

To be successful, you should extend courtesy to all with whom you come in contact. This includes state board members and inspectors who are contributing to the higher standards of the profession.

State Laws

The successful barber-stylist must know the laws, rules, and regulations governing the profession and must comply with them. They are designed to contribute to the health, welfare, and safety of the community.

REVIEW QUESTIONS

Your Professional Image

1. Of what personal details does professional image consist?
2. Define hygiene; personal hygiene.
3. List eight basic requirements for good health.
4. Define personality; communication; human relations.
5. How is your professional attitude expressed?
6. What is professional ethics?

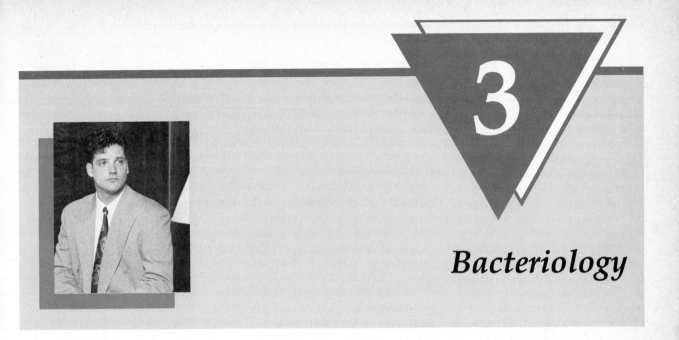

3

Bacteriology

Learning Objectives

After completing this chapter, you should be able to:

1. List the types and classifications of bacteria.
2. Describe the growth and reproduction of bacteria.
3. Describe the relationship of bacteria to the spread of disease.

Courtesy of: Hair: Geno Levi, ABBA Senior Affiliate. Photo: Jack Cutler.

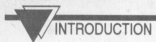

INTRODUCTION

Barber-stylists must understand how the spread of disease can be prevented and become familiar with the precautions necessary to safeguard their own health and that of their clients. An understanding of the relationship between bacteria and disease underscores the need for cleanliness and sanitation. State barber boards and health departments require that sanitary measures be applied while serving the public. Contagious diseases, skin infections, and blood poisoning can be caused either by the transmission of infectious material from one individual to another, or by the use of unsanitized implements such as combs, brushes, clippers, shears, and razors.

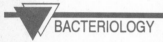

BACTERIOLOGY

Bacteriology (bak-teer-i-**OL**-o-jee) is that science which deals with the study of the **microorganisms** (meye-kroh-**OR**-gah-niz-ems) called bacteria.

Bacteria (bak-**TEER**-i-ah) are minute, one-celled microorganisms found nearly everywhere. They are especially numerous in dust, dirt, refuse, and diseased tissue. Bacteria are also known as **germs** (**JURMS**) or **microbes** (**MEYE**-krohbs).

Bacteria exist everywhere, particularly on the skin, in water, air, decayed matter, bodily secretions, on the clothing, and beneath the nails.

Bacteria are not visible without the aid of a **microscope** (**MEYE**-kroh-skohp). They are so minute in size that 1,500 rod-shaped bacteria barely reach across the head of a pin.

Types of Bacteria

There are hundreds of different kinds of bacteria. However, bacteria are classified into two types, depending on their **beneficial** (harmless) or **harmful** (disease-producing) qualities.

1. **Non-pathogenic** (non-path-o-**JEN**-ik) **organisms**, which are beneficial or harmless, make up the majority of bacteria. They perform many useful functions, such as decomposing refuse and improving the fertility of the soil. To this group belong the **saprophytes** (sap-**RO**-fyts) which live on dead matter and do not produce disease.
2. **Pathogenic** (path-o-**JEN**-ik) **organisms**, although in the minority, are harmful and cause considerable damage by invading plant or human tissues. Pathogenic bacteria

produce disease. To this group belong the **parasites** (PAR-ah-syts) which require living matter for their survival.

It is because of the possibility of poisoning due to pathogenic bacteria, **sepsis** (SEP-sis), that barber-styling schools and shops must maintain certain standards of cleanliness and sanitation in order to achieve an environment free of disease germs, **asepsis** (A-sep-sis).

Pronunciation of Terms Relating to Pathogenic Bacteria

Singular	**Plural**
coccus (**KOK**-us)	cocci (**KOK**-si)
bacillus (bah-**SIL**-us)	bacilli (ba-**SIL**-i)
spirillum (speye-**RIL**-um)	spirilla (speye-**RIL**-a)
staphylococcus (staf-i-lo-**KOK**-us)	staphylococci (staf-il-lo-**KOK**-si)
streptococcus (strep-to-**KOK**-us)	streptococci (strep-to-**KOK**-si)
diplococcus (dip-loh-**KOK**-us)	diplococci (dip-loh-**KOK**-si)

Classifications of Pathogenic Bacteria

Bacteria have distinct shapes that help to identify them. Pathogenic (harmful) bacteria are classified as **cocci, bacilli,** or **spirilla** (Fig. 3.1).

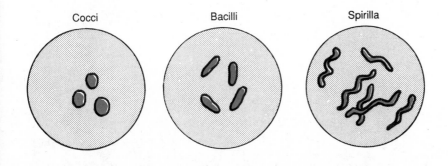

Cocci   Bacilli   Spirilla

3.1 — Pathogenic forms of bacteria

1. **Cocci** are round-shaped organisms that appear singly or in the following groups (Fig. 3.2.):

    a) **Staphylococci:** Pus-forming organisms that grow in bunches or clusters. They cause abscesses, pustules, and boils.

    b) **Streptococci:** Pus-forming organisms that grow in chains. They cause infections such as strep throat.

    c) **Diplococci:** They grow in pairs and cause pneumonia.

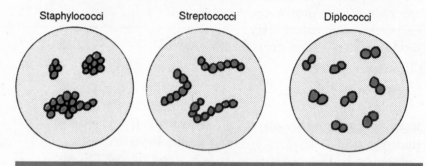

3.2 — Groupings of bacteria

2. **Bacilli** are short, rod-shaped organisms. They are the most common bacteria and produce disease such as tetanus (lockjaw), influenza, typhoid fever, tuberculosis, and diphtheria. (Fig. 3.3)

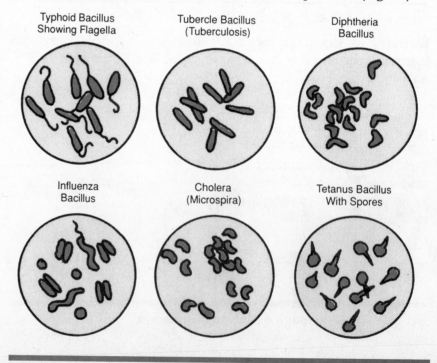

3.3 — Disease-producing bacteria

3. **Spirilla** are curved or corkscrew-shaped organisms. They are subdivided into several groups. Of chief importance to us is the **treponema pallida** (trep-o-NE-mah PAL-i-dah), which causes **syphilis** (SIF-i-lis).

Movement of Bacteria

Cocci rarely show active **motility** (self-movement). They are transmitted by air, dust, or the substance in which they settle. Bacilli and spirilla are both motile and use hairlike projections, known as **flagella** (flah-JEL-ah) or **cilia** (SIL-ee-a), to move about. A whiplike motion of these hairs propels bacteria in liquid.

BACTERIAL GROWTH AND REPRODUCTION

Bacteria generally consist of an outer cell wall and internal **protoplasm** (PROH-toh-plaz-em), material needed to sustain life. They manufacture their own food from the surrounding environment, give off waste products, and grow and reproduce. Bacteria have two distinct phases in their life cycle: the **active** or **spore-forming stage**, and the **inactive** or **vegetative stage**.

Active or Vegetative Stage

During the active stage, bacteria grow and reproduce. These microorganisms multiply best in warm, dark, damp, and dirty places where sufficient food is present.

When conditions are favorable, bacteria grow and reproduce. As food is absorbed, the bacterial cells grow in size. When the maximum growth is reached, the cells divide into two new cells. This division is called **mitosis** (my-TOH-sis) and the cells that are formed are called **daughter cells**. As many as sixteen million germs may develop in half a day from one bacterium. (See chapter on cells, anatomy, and physiology.) When favorable conditions cease to exist, bacteria either die or become inactive.

Inactive or Spore-Forming Stage

Certain bacteria, such as the anthrax and tetanus bacilli, form spherical spores having tough outer coverings during their inactive stage, in order to withstand periods of famine, dryness, and unsuitable temperature. In this stage, spores can be blown about in the dust and are not harmed by disinfectants, heat, or cold.

When favorable conditions are restored, the spores change into the **active** or **spore-forming stage** and again start to grow and reproduce.

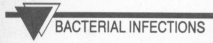

BACTERIAL INFECTIONS

Pathogenic bacteria become a menace to health when they invade the body. An **infection** occurs if the body is unable to cope with the bacteria and their harmful toxins. A **local infection** is indicated by a boil or a pimple that contains **pus**. The presence of pus is a sign of infection. **Staphylococci** are the most common pus-forming bacteria. Bacteria, waste matter, decayed tissue, body cells and blood cells, both living and dead, are all found in pus. A **general infection** results when the bloodstream carries the bacteria and their toxins to all parts of the body, as in blood poisoning or syphilis.

A disease becomes **contagious** (kon-**TAY**-jus) or **communicable** (ko-**MU**-ni-kah-bil) when it spreads from one person to another. Some of the more contagious diseases which would prevent a barber-stylist from working are tuberculosis, common cold, ringworm, scabies, head lice, and viral infections.

The chief sources of contagion are unclean hands or implements, open sores, pus, oral or nasal discharges, and the common use of drinking cups and towels. Uncovered coughing or sneezing and spitting in public also spread germs.

There can be no infection without the presence of pathogenic bacteria, which may enter the body by way of:

1. A break in the skin, such as a cut, pimple, or scratch
2. Breathing or swallowing
3. The eyes or ears

The body fights infection by means of its defensive forces:

1. The unbroken skin, the body's first line of defense
2. Body secretions such as perspiration and digestive juices
3. White blood cells, which destroy bacteria
4. Antitoxins which counteract the toxins produced by bacteria

Infections can be prevented and controlled through personal hygiene and public sanitation.

Other Infectious Agents

Filterable viruses (FIL-ter-a-bil VI-rus-es) are living organisms so small that they can pass through a porcelain filter. They cause the common cold and other **respiratory** (RES-pi-roh-torh-ee) and **gastrointestinal** (GAS-troh-in-**tes**-ti-nal) infections.

Parasites are plants or animals that live on another living organism without giving anything in return.

Plant parasites or **fungi** (FUN-ji) such as molds, mildews, and yeasts, can produce such contagious diseases as ringworm or **favus** (FA-vus).

Animal parasites such as certain insects are responsible for such contagious diseases as **scabies** (SKAY-beez), caused by the itch mite, and **pediculosis** (pe-dik-yoo-**LOH**-sis), caused by lice.

> CAUTION: Contagious diseases caused by parasites should never be treated in a barber-styling shop. Clients should be referred to their physicians.

Immunity (i-**MYOO**-ni-tee) is the ability of the body to resist invasion by, and destroy bacteria once they have entered the body. Immunity against disease may be either natural or acquired. **Natural immunity** means natural resistance to disease. It is partially inherited and partially developed. **Acquired immunity** is developed after the body has overcome a disease or through inoculations.

A **human disease carrier** is a person who is immune to a disease, but harbors germs that can infect other people. **Typhoid** (TI-foid) **fever** and **diphtheria** (dif-**THEER**-i-a) may be transmitted in this manner.

The destruction of bacteria may be accomplished by the use of disinfectants; intense heat such as boiling, steaming, baking, or burning; and ultraviolet rays.

> CAUTION: To avoid the spread of disease keep yourself, your surroundings, everything with which you come in contact, and everything you use, clean.

Acquired Immune Deficiency Syndrome (AIDS)

Acquired Immune Deficiency Syndrome (AIDS) is caused by the HIV virus. AIDS attacks and eventually destroys the body's immune system. The disease may lie dormant in an infected person's system for up to ten years, but it can mature into a fatal disease in two to ten years.

Unlike most other viruses, HIV cannot be transferred through casual contact with an infected person, sneezing, or coughing. AIDS is passed from one person to another through the transfer of bodily fluids such as semen and blood. The most common methods of transferring AIDS are through: sexual contact with an infected person, the use of or sharing of dirty hypodermic needles for intravenous drug use, the transfusion of infected blood. AIDS can also be transferred from mother to child during pregnancy and birth.

It is possible to transfer AIDS in the salon through the use of unsanitized implements. If you were to cut a client infected with AIDS you might transfer blood to a haircutting implement, razor, manicuring implement, etc. Then if you cut another client and transferred the AIDS infected blood to the second client, that client might get AIDS.

REVIEW QUESTIONS

Bacteriology

1. Why is a knowledge of bacteriology necessary for the barber-stylist?
2. Define bacteriology.
3. What are bacteria?
4. Where can bacteria exist? Give examples.
5. Define two types of bacteria.
6. What are parasites and saprophytes?
7. Name and define three forms of bacteria.
8. Name and define three types of cocci bacteria.
9. How do bacteria multiply?
10. Describe the active and inactive stages of bacteria.
11. How does bacteria move about?
12. Name two types of infection and define each.
13. What is a contagious or communicable disease?
14. How can infections be controlled or prevented?
15. Name two diseases produced by a) plant parasites and b) animal parasites.
16. Define immunity. Name two types.
17. How can bacteria be destroyed?

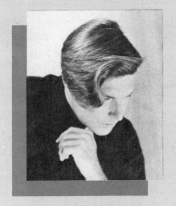

Sterilization, Sanitation and Safe Work Practices

Learning Objectives

After completing this chapter, you should be able to:

1. *Describe the various methods of sterilization.*

2. *Explain why sterilization and sanitation are important to barber-stylists.*

3. *Describe how the spread of disease can be prevented.*

4. *Identify the methods of sanitation used in the barber-styling shop.*

5. *List safety precautions for chemical sanitizing solutions.*

6. *Discuss the Rules of Sanitation.*

7. *Describe the responsibilities of safe work practices in the barber-styling shop.*

Courtesy of: Hair: Xenon, Attractions International Creative Director. Photo: Gina Uhlmann. Makeup: James of che Sequiro. Fashion Styling: Donna Forst.

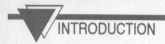

INTRODUCTION

Sterilization (ster-i-li-**ZAY**-shun) and **sanitation** (san-i-**TAY**-shun) are subjects of practical importance to barber-stylists because they protect individual and public health. Barber-stylists should know when, why, and how to use sterilization and sanitation techniques in order to maintain public health and a healthy environment.

Safe work practices deal with the day-to-day use of sanitation, efficiency, and safety by the barber-stylist in the shop or salon.

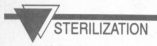

STERILIZATION

Sterilization is the process of rendering an object germ-free by destroying all bacteria, whether beneficial or harmful.

Health departments and state barber boards recognize that it is impossible to completely sterilize implements and equipment in the barber-stylist school and shop. Therefore, it is generally recognized that implements and equipment are sanitized rather than sterilized.

Throughout the entire text the term **sanitize** will be used to indicate all forms of sanitation.

Sterilization and sanitation are of practical importance to the barber-stylist since they deal either with methods for the prevention of the growth of germs or the destruction of them, particularly those that are responsible for infections and communicable diseases.

Methods of Sterilization and Sanitation

There are five well-known methods of sterilization and sanitation. These may be grouped under two main headings:

1. **Physical agents:**
   a) **Moist heat.**
      1. **Boiling water** at 212° fahrenheit (**FAR**-un-hite) for twenty minutes. (This method is no longer used in barber-styling shops.)
      2. **Steaming**—requires a steam pressure sterilizer. It is used in the medical field to kill bacteria and spores.
   b) **Dry heat** is used to sterilize sheets, towels, gauze, cotton, and similar materials.
   c) **Ultraviolet rays** may be used in an electric sanitizer in a barber-styling shop to keep sanitized implements sanitary.
2. **Chemical agents:**
   a) **Antiseptics** (an-ti-**SEP**-ticks) and **disinfectants** (dis-in-**FECK**-tants) are used in barber-styling shops.

b) **Vapors** (fumigants) in a cabinet sanitizer are used to keep sanitized implements sanitary.

Chemicals are the most effective sanitizing agents used in barber-styling shops to destroy or check bacteria. Chemical agents used for sanitizing purposes are antiseptics and disinfectants.

1. An **antiseptic** is a substance that may kill or retard the growth of bacteria without killing them. Antiseptics generally can be used safely on the skin.
2. A **disinfectant** destroys bacteria and is used to sanitize implements.

Several chemicals can be classed under both heads: a strong solution may be used as a disinfectant, and a weak solution as an antiseptic.

Requirements for a good disinfectant:

1. Convenient to prepare
2. Quick acting
3. Preferably odorless
4. Non-corrosive
5. Economical
6. Non-irritating to skin

Sanitizers

A **wet sanitizer** is a covered receptacle large enough to hold a disinfectant solution in which objects can be completely immersed. (Fig. 4.1) Wet sanitizers come in various sizes and shapes. Before immersing objects in a wet sanitizer containing a disinfectant solution, be sure to:

1. Remove hair from combs and brushes.
2. Wash them thoroughly with hot water and soap.
3. Rinse them thoroughly.

This procedure prevents contamination of the solution. Further, soap and hot water remove most of the bacteria.

After the implements are removed from the disinfectant solution they must be rinsed in clean water, wiped dry with a clean towel, and stored in a dry cabinet sanitizer until needed.

A **dry** or **cabinet sanitizer** is an air-tight cabinet containing an active **fumigant** (**FYOO**-mi-gant). A fumigant is a vapor that is used to keep clean objects sanitary. The sanitized implements are kept clean by storing them in the cabinet until they are needed.

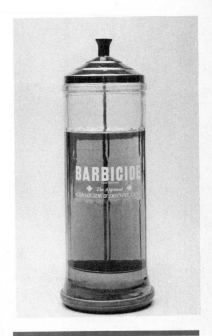

4.1 – Wet sanitizer

How to prepare a fumigant. Place 1 tablespoonful (15 ml) of borax and 1 tablespoonful (15 ml) of formalin on a small tray on the bottom of the cabinet. This will form formaldehyde vapors. Replace chemicals regularly. They lose their strength, depending on how often the cabinet door is opened and closed.

Formalin is also available in tablet form. Follow the manufacturer's directions.

Ultraviolet ray electric sanitizers are effective for keeping combs, brushes, and implements clean until they are ready for use.

Combs, brushes, and implements must be sanitized before they are placed in the ultraviolet sanitizer. Follow the manufacturer's directions for proper use.

Chemical Sanitizing Agents

There are many prepared chemical disinfectant agents on the market. Consult your state board of barber-styling or health department for a list of approved disinfectants. Chemicals commonly used in barber-styling shops include:

1. **Sodium hypochlorite** (SOH-di-um HY-po-chlor-it) to sanitize implements.
2. **Quaternary ammonium compounds** (quats) (KWAH-ter-nah-ree ah-MOH-nee-um KOM-pownds [KWATS]) to sanitize implements.
3. **Formaldehyde** (for-MAL-de-heyed) to sanitize implements.
4. **Alcohol** (AL-ko-hawl) to sanitize sharp cutting instruments and electrodes.
5. **Prepared commercial products** that clean floors, sinks, and toilet bowls.

Sodium Hypochlorite

Sodium hypochlorite (common household bleach) compounds are frequently used to provide the sanitizing agent, chlorine.

One of the key advantages of chlorine is its ability to destroy viruses. A 10 percent solution is recommended with an immersion time of ten minutes. Many prepared disinfectants contain sodium hypochlorite. Follow the manufacturer's directions for mixing and immersion time.

Quaternary Ammonium Compounds (QUATS)

These compounds are effective as disinfectants. They are available under different trade and chemical names.

Their advantages are: short disinfection time, odorless and color-less, non-toxic and stable. A 1:1000 solution is commonly used to sanitize implements. Immersion time ranges from one to five min-utes, depending upon the strength of the solution used.

CAUTION: Before using any quat, read and follow the manufacturer's directions on label and accompanying literature. Find out if the product can be used in naturally soft or hard water, or water that has been soft-ened. Inquire whether it contains a rust inhibitor. Should the product lack a rust inhibitor, the addition of ½% of **sodium nitrite** (SO-dee-um NIGH-trite) to the solution prevents the rusting of metallic implements.

How to Prepare a 1:1000 Strength Solution of a Quaternary Ammonium Compound

- 10 percent active ingredient, add 1¼ oz. quat solution to 1 gallon of water.
- 12½ percent active ingredient, add 1 oz. quat solution to 1 gallon of water.
- 15 percent active ingredient, add ¾ oz. quat solution to 1 gallon of water.

Formalin

Formalin (FOHR-mah-lin) acts as a sanitizing agent and can be used either as an antiseptic or a disinfectant, depending on the strength of the solution. As purchased, formalin is approximately 37 to 40 percent formaldehyde gas in water. Because formaldehyde is a controversial substance, check with your state board before using it.

Formalin may be used in various strengths, as follows:

- **25 percent solution** (equivalent to 10 percent formaldehyde gas)—used to sanitize implements. Immerse them in the solu-tion for at least ten minutes. (Preparation: two parts formalin, five parts water, one part glycerine.)
- **10 percent solution** (equivalent to 4 percent formaldehyde gas)—used to sanitize combs and brushes. Immerse them for at least twenty minutes. (Preparation: one part formalin, nine parts water.)
- **5 percent solution** (equivalent to 2 percent formaldehyde gas)—used to cleanse the hands after they have been in contact with wounds, skin eruptions, etc. Also used to sanitize shampoo

bowls and chairs. (Preparation: one part formalin, 19 parts water.)

Sanitizing with Chemical Disinfectants

1. Wash implements thoroughly with soap and hot water.
2. Rinse with plain water to remove all traces of soap.
3. Immerse implements in a wet sanitizer (containing approved disinfectant) for the required time.
4. Remove implements from wet sanitizer, rinse in water, and wipe dry with clean towel.
5. Store sanitized implements in individually wrapped cellophane envelopes, or keep in a cabinet sanitizer or in an ultraviolet ray cabinet until ready for use.

Sanitizing with Alcohol

Implements having a fine cutting edge are best sanitized by rubbing the surface with a cotton pad dampened with 70 percent alcohol. This method prevents the cutting edges from becoming dull.

Electrodes (ee-**LEK**-trohds) may be safely sanitized by gently rubbing the exposed surface with a cotton pad dampened with 70 percent alcohol.

After sanitizing, place implements into a dry sanitizer until ready for use.

Sanitizing Floors, Sinks, and Toilet Bowls

The disinfection of floors, sinks, and toilet bowls in barber-styling shops calls for the use of such commercial products as Lysol, CN, pine needle oil, or similar disinfectants. Deodorants are also useful to offset unpleasant smells and for replacing them with a fresh odor.

Whatever disinfectant is used, be sure to follow the manufacturer's instructions.

Safety Precautions

1. Purchase chemicals in small quantities and store them in a cool, dry place; they can deteriorate when exposed to air, light, and heat.
2. Carefully weigh and measure chemicals.
3. Keep all containers labeled, covered, and under lock and key.
4. Do not smell chemicals or solutions. Some have pungent odors and can irritate the nasal membranes.
5. Avoid spilling chemicals when diluting them.
6. Prevent burns by using forceps to insert or remove objects from the source of heat.
7. Keep a complete first aid kit on hand.

Sanitizing Rules

Chemical solutions in sanitizers should be changed regularly (according to state board of barbering regulations in your state).

Manicuring implements must be kept in a disinfectant solution (70 percent alcohol) at all times when not being used.

All articles must be clean and free from hair before being sanitized.

Sanitize electrical appliances by rubbing their surfaces with a cotton pad dampened with 70 percent alcohol.

All cups, finger bowls, or similar objects must be sanitized prior to being used for another client.

NOTE: Immersing implements in a chemical solution must conform to state board of barbering regulations in your state.

DISINFECTANTS COMMONLY USED IN BARBER-STYLING SHOPS

NAME	FORM	STRENGTH	USES
Quaternary Ammonium Compounds (Quats)	Liquid or tablet	1:1000 solution	Immerse implements into solution for 20 minutes or more.
Formalin	Liquid	25% solution	Immerse implements into solution for 10 minutes or more.
Formalin	Liquid	10% solution	Immerse implements into solution for 20 minutes or more.
Ethyl or Grain Alcohol	Liquid	70% solution	Sanitize sharp cutting implements and electrodes for 10 minutes or more.
Cresol (Lysol)	Liquid	10% soap solution	Cleanse floors, sinks, and toilets.
Sodium Hypochlorite	Liquid	10% solution	Immerse implements into solution for 10 minutes or more.

ANTISEPTICS COMMONLY USED IN BARBER-STYLING SHOPS

NAME	FORM	STRENGTH	USES
Boric Acid	White crystals	2–5% solution	Cleanse the eyes.
Hydrogen Peroxide	Liquid	3–5% solution	Cleanse skin and minor cuts.
Formalin	Liquid	5% solution	Cleanse hands, shampoo bowl, cabinet, etc.
Chloramine-T (Chlorazene; Chlorozol)	White crystals	½% solution	Cleanse skin and hands and for general use.
Sodium Hypochlorite (Javelle water; Zonite)	White crystals	½% solution	Rinse the hands.

CAUTION: It is advisable to check the above and other approved disinfectants and antiseptics that are being used in barber-styling shops with your State Board or Health Department.

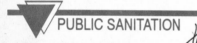

PUBLIC SANITATION

Public sanitation is the application of measures to promote public health and prevent the spread of infectious diseases.

The importance of sanitation cannot be over-emphasized. The barber-styling profession requires direct contact with clients' skin, scalp, and hair. Understanding sanitary measures insures the protection of the clients' health as well as your own.

Various government agencies protect community health by insuring that food is wholesome, the water supply untainted, and the refuse is disposed of properly.

In addition, barber boards and boards of health in each state have formulated sanitary regulations governing barber-styling shops. Every barber-stylist must obey these regulations.

The air within a barber-styling shop should be moist and fresh. Room temperature should be about 70 degrees fahrenheit. The shop should be equipped with an exhaust fan or an air conditioning unit. Air conditioning is an advantage since it permits changes in the quality and quantity of air in the shop. The temperature and humidity of the air may also be regulated by means of air conditioning.

A person ill with an infectious disease puts other people's health at risk. A barber-stylist having a cold or any other contagious disease should not serve clients. Likewise, clients suffering from infectious diseases must not be served until they are well. In this way, the best interests of other clients may be served.

Water should be pure. Be aware that crystal clear water still may be unsanitary if it contains pathogenic bacteria, which cannot be seen with the naked eye. Many municipal governments require water coolers in establishments that serve the general public.

Rules of Sanitation

The following rules of sanitation are intended to create a cleaner environment for the public.

1. Every barber-styling shop must be well lit, heated, and ventilated, in order to keep it clean and sanitary.
2. The walls, floors, and windows in the shop must be kept clean.
3. All barber-styling establishments must have hot and cold running water.
4. All plumbing fixtures should be properly installed.
5. The premises should be kept free of rodents, flies, or other insects.
6. Dogs, cats, birds, and other pets must not be permitted in a shop.
7. The barber-styling shop should not be used for eating, or sleeping, or as living quarters. If square footage is sufficient, a small room at the back of the shop may be used by staff during their breaks. State boards and local building inspectors can provide standards and codes.
8. Clean and sanitize all implements as they are used and return them to their proper place.
9. Clean work benches, chairs, and mirrors.
10. Remove all hair and waste materials from the floor.
11. The rest rooms must be kept in a sanitary condition.
12. Each barber-stylist must wear a clean uniform while working on clients.
13. Barber-stylists must cleanse their hands thoroughly before and after serving a client.
14. Barber-stylists must wash their hands after leaving the bathroom.

15. A freshly laundered towel or fresh paper towel must be used for each client. Towels ready for use must be stored in a clean, closed cabinet. All soiled linen towels and used paper towels must be disposed of properly. Keep dirty towels separate from clean towels.

16. Headrest coverings and neck strips or towels must be changed for each client.

17. Use a neckstrip to prevent the chair cloth from coming in contact with the client's skin.

18. The common use of hair brushes is prohibited unless sanitized after each client.

19. The common use of drinking cups, styptic pencils, or shaving mugs is prohibited.

20. Lotions, ointments, creams, and powders must be kept in clean, closed containers. Use a sanitized spatula to remove creams or ointments from jars. Use sterile cotton pledgets to apply lotions and powders. Re-cover containers after each use.

21. Combs and other implements must not be carried in the pockets of uniforms.

22. Combs, shears, and razors must be sanitized after each use.

23. All used instruments and articles must be sanitized before placing them in a dustproof or airtight container or a cabinet sanitizer.

24. Objects dropped on the floor should not be used until they are sanitized.

The public is increasingly aware of the importance of sanitation and therefore demands that every possible sanitary measure be used in the barber-styling shop. Adherence to the above rules of sanitation will result in cleaner and better service to the public.

The responsibility for maintaining good sanitation rests with each student in the school and each barber-stylist in the shop. The manager must provide the necessities for school and shop sanitation.

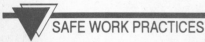

SAFE WORK PRACTICES

Safe work practices include a number of issues of which barber-stylists should be aware and for which they are responsible in the workplace. These include the maintenance of sanitation and safety. Although the overall responsibility for maintaining safety standards in the salon belongs to the owner or manager, it is up to the barber-stylist to comply with those standards. Be observant and recognize safety hazards, especially in areas where electricity and water are in close proximity to one another or where chemicals are stored. Learn to handle tools and implements with care and thus avoid unnecessary injuries. Try to prevent accidents before they happen. Assist clients who need help. In general, by using common sense and being alert, many accidents can be avoided.

Many products used in barber-styling can be dangerous if used incorrectly or without sufficient caution. The conscientious barber-stylist is careful to insure the safety and well-being of clients by acquiring thorough technical knowledge of products, adhering to safe work practices, and using common sense. In the case of injury to a client—minor or otherwise—always inform the client of the situation. Some implements are so sharp that the client may not immediately feel the nick of a trimmer, razor, or shears. Redness, irritation, or swelling of the skin due to a reaction to certain chemicals also may be unnoticed at first, but will intensify over time, resulting in a more severe reaction, if it is not rinsed and cared for immediately. Remember that honesty will protect you, your reputation, and the client's health.

OSHA

The Occupational Safety and Health Administration (OSHA) was created as part of the U.S. Department of Labor to regulate and enforce safety and health standards. Regulating employee exposure to toxic substances and informing employees of the dangers of the materials used in the workplace are key functions of the Occupational Safety and Health Act of 1970. This act established the Hazard Communication Rule, which requires that chemical manufacturers and importers assess the hazards associated with their products. Material safety data sheets (MSDS) and labeling are two important results of this law.

Material safety data sheets provide all pertinent information on products, ranging from content and associated hazards, to combustion levels and storage requirements. Material safety data sheets should be available for every product used in the barber-styling school or shop, and may be obtained from the product's distributor.

The standards set by OSHA are important to the barber-styling industry because of the nature of the chemicals used; for instance, the mixing, storing, and disposal of chemicals; the general safety of the workplace; and, most important, the right of the barber-stylist to know what is contained in the products he or she uses.

First Aid

Emergencies arise in every business. A knowledge of first aid is invaluable to the shop manager and staff.

A physician (or emergency ambulance) should be called as soon as possible after any serious accident for the safety and protection of both the victim and the shop owner. There are certain first aid measures, however, that the layman can use while awaiting medical assistance.

Keep a well-equipped first aid kit within easy access. As many staff members as possible should learn first aid and CPR techniques. For more information about emergency care, consult the latest edition of the First Aid Manual published by the American Red Cross.

Keep emergency information posted in plain view near all telephones, including telephone numbers for the fire and police departments, ambulance, hospital emergency room, doctors, taxis, telephone company, and telephone numbers of persons and organizations that provide service. Utility service companies such as electric, water, air conditioning, etc., also should be posted. Additional information might include the names and telephone numbers of the owner or manager, custodian, and building owner.

The shop owner or manager should have the names, addresses, and telephone numbers of employees on file in case of emergency. The file that is kept for regular clients also should include emergency information.

Each employee should know where exits are located and how to evacuate the building quickly. Fire extinguishers should be placed where they can be reached easily, and employees should know how to use them.

REVIEW QUESTIONS

Sterilization and Sanitation

1. What is sterilization?
2. Sanitization involves the use of agents that are both physical and _____.
3. Name two methods of keeping objects clean after sanitation has taken place.

4. What type of bacteria makes necessary the practice of sanitation in the barber-styling shop?
5. What are the dangers of using unsanitary implements and linens on clients?
6. Distinguish between asepsis, sterile, and sepsis.
7. Wash implements thoroughly with soap and _____ water.
8. Formaldehyde is the active gas found in _____.
9. What is an antiseptic?
10. What is a disinfectant?
11. What is a fumigant?
12. About how long does it take to sanitize implements when using: a) quats; b) 25 percent formalin; c) 10 percent formalin?
13. What is a wet sanitizer; how is it best used?
14. When using a disinfectant how are objects sanitized?
15. List six requirements of a good disinfectant.
16. What should be done with implements after sanitation in a disinfectant solution?
17. How should combs and brushes be kept after sanitation?
18. What is a dry or cabinet sanitizer?
19. What is the proper way to produce formaldehyde vapors in a cabinet sanitizer?
20. What is the composition of formalin?
21. What is the best way to sanitize sharp implements and prevent their dulling?
22. What is a safe way to sanitize electrodes?
23. Effective sanitation in the barber-styling shop prevents the spread of _____.
24. What strengths formalin solution are recommended to: a) sanitize implements; b) cleanse hands?
25. a) What are four advantages of using quats as a sanitizer?
    b) In what strength are quats commonly used?
26. List five safety precautions when using chemical agents.

1. Define sanitation.
2. Which unsanitary practices may spread disease in the barber-styling shop?
3. How should the hands be treated after touching a client suspected of having a skin or scalp infection?
4. What are five sanitary requirements in a barber-styling shop?
5. Which rule of sanitation should be observed regarding the use of headrests?
6. Why are neck strips or towels required?

Public Sanitation

7. What is the sanitary way to keep lotions, ointments, creams, and powders?
8. What is the sanitary way to remove creams and ointments from their containers?
9. Where should towels be kept after laundering?
10. Where should dirty towels be kept?
11. Which supplies must be changed for each client?
12. Why should styptic pencils never be used in common?
13. If a towel or an implement is accidentally dropped on the floor, how should it be treated?
14. Why is it important to have a pure water supply?
15. How should loose hair and other waste material be disposed of?
16. What is the objection to the use of the common towel?

Safe Work Practices and First Aid

1. What are the responsibilities of the barber-stylist regarding safe work practices?
2. List four ways in which the barber-stylist can practice safe work habits.
3. List three precautionary measures that the barber-stylist can take to insure the safety and well-being of clients.
4. In the case of injury to the client, what should the barber-stylist do?
5. The barber-stylist should always be _____ and _____.

5

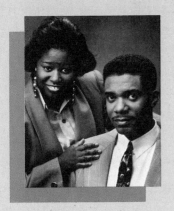

Implements, Tools, and Equipment

Learning Objectives

After completing this chapter, you should be able to:

1. *Identify barber-styling implements, tools, and equipment.*
2. *Identify the parts of the shears, clippers, and razors.*
3. *Demonstrate the correct techniques of holding combs, shears, clippers, trimmers, razors, and thermal hairstyling tools.*
4. *Discuss the care and sanitation procedures for implements.*
5. *Demonstrate honing and stropping techniques.*

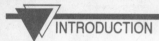 INTRODUCTION

All of the instruments and accessories used in barber-styling may be termed the implements, tools, or equipment of the barber-styling profession.

The barber-stylist should use superior implements. A myriad of choices are available and may be confusing to the student. Your instructor or a professional stylist should be able to assist you in appropriate selections.

Although all of the implements and tools associated with barber-styling will be used at some time, the seven principal implements used are combs, shears, clippers, trimmers, razors, brushes, and blow-dryers.

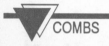 COMBS

Combs are available in a variety of styles and sizes. The correct comb to use depends on the type of service to be performed and individual preference. Combs can be made of hard rubber, bone, or plastic. Because of the cost, combs made from bone are not very popular. Plastic combs are not as durable as those made from either bone or rubber. Hard rubber combs are, therefore, the most popular.

> HINT: Barber-stylists can simplify their work by using light-colored combs on dark hair, and dark-colored combs on light hair.

The teeth of a comb may be fine (close together) or coarse (far apart). It is important that the teeth have rounded ends to avoid scratching or irritating a client's scalp.

Some comb styles are:

- All-purpose comb that may be used for general hair cutting and styling. A popular size is 7 ¾ inches long. (Fig. 5.1)

5.1 – All-purpose comb

- All-purpose comb with curved interior. Curved ends and interior assist in lifting subsections and partings of hair while cutting. The usual size is 7 ½ inches long. (Fig. 5.2)

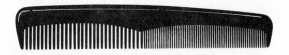

5.2 – All-purpose comb with curved interior

- Tapered haircutting comb used for cutting or trimming. The tapered end is especially useful for mustache trims, for tapering, and for blending around the ear areas. (Fig. 5.3)

5.3 – Tapered haircutting comb

- Wide tooth comb for flat tops. This comb is best used with the widest clippers. (Fig. 5.4)

5.4 – Wide tooth comb

- Handle comb with wide teeth. This comb can be used to spread relaxer in chemical hair straightening or for detangling. It is also available in a curved style. (Fig. 5.5)

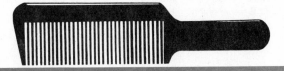

5.5 – Handle comb

- Tail comb. Best choice for sectioning long hair or when taking partings to wrap on perm rods. (Fig. 5.6)

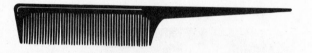

5.6 – Tail comb

Holding the Comb

The correct manner in which to hold the comb will be dictated by the type of comb, the service being performed, and the dexterity and comfort of the stylist. Figs. 5.7 to 5.11 show some holding positions that are often used for an all-purpose comb.

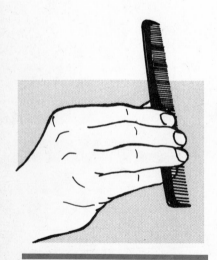

5.7 – Holding the comb by placing the three middle fingers on one side. Notice the fingers are placed close together and gripping the widest teeth of the comb.

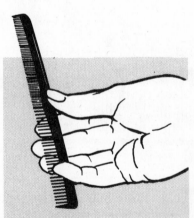

5.8 – The reverse side of holding position in Fig. 5.7 showing the position of the little finger and thumb.

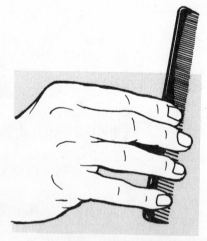

5.9 – Holding the comb by placing four fingers on one side. Notice the fingers are spread a little wider than in Fig. 5.7.

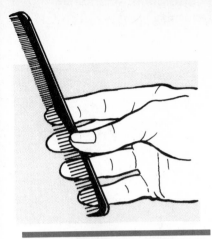

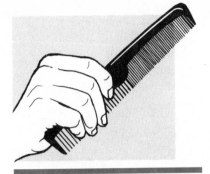

5.10 – The reverse side of holding position in Fig. 5.9 showing the position of the thumb.

5.11 – Holding the comb by placing four fingers on one side of the comb and the thumb on the other side. Notice the fingers are close together, slightly bent, and grip the widest teeth of the comb firmly.

Care of Combs

To keep combs in good condition, avoid exposing them to excessive or prolonged heat. **Combs must be sanitized after each client has been served.**

1. Remove loose hairs from the comb.
2. Wash it thoroughly with hot water and soap.
3. Rinse it thoroughly.
4. Place it in a wet sanitizer with disinfectant for at least 20 minutes.
5. Rinse it, wipe it dry, and place it in a dry or cabinet sanitizer with an active fumigant or, if available, an ultraviolet ray sanitizer, until needed.

HAIRCUTTING SHEARS

The two kinds of shears generally used by barber-stylists are the German type, without a finger brace, and the French type, with a brace for the small finger. The French type is used more frequently than the German type.

The main parts. These shears are composed of two blades, one movable and the other stationary, fastened with a screw that acts as a pivot. Other parts of the shears are the cutting edges of the blades, two shanks, finger grip, finger brace, and thumb grip. (Fig. 5.12)

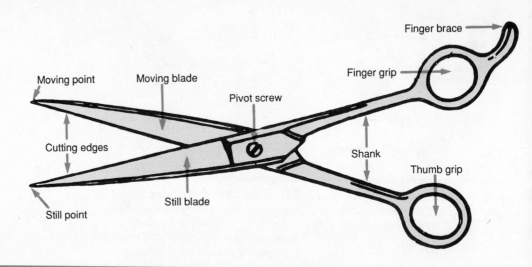

5.12 – The main parts of haircutting shears

Size. Shears are available in a variety of lengths which are measured in inches and half inches. Most barber-stylists prefer the 6½ to 7 ½ inch shears.

> HINT: The most comfortable and balanced length of shear can usually be determined by measuring the length of the hand from the base of the palm to the tip of the middle finger.

Grinds. There are two types of shear grinds, plain and corrugated. The plain grind is used most frequently. Its finish may be smooth (knife edge), medium, or coarse.

Set. The correct set of the shears is just as important as the grind of the blades. Even shears with the finest cutting edges can be poor cutting implements if the blades are not set properly.

Haircutting shears with detachable blades have become very popular. With these shears, old blades can be removed and replaced with new ones. This does away with the need to send shears out to be sharpened. (Fig. 5.13)

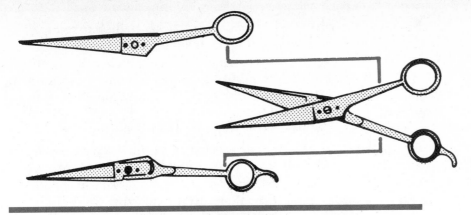

5.13 – Detachable blade shears

CAUTION: Shears must be sharpened by a reputable professional to prevent improper sharpening or damage.

How to Hold Haircutting Shears

Place the tip of the thumb in the thumb grip of the moving blade. Insert the ring finger into the finger grip of the still blade with the little finger resting on the finger brace. To ensure proper balance, brace the index finger on the shank of the still blade, approximately one-half inch from the pivot screw. (Figs. 5.14–5.16)

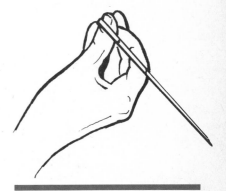

5.16 – Holding position for reverse-hand cutting for around and behind the ear areas or in the temple-to-sideburn areas. The shears are held the same as in Fig. 5.15 except the wrist is turned so the palm is facing up. This technique is most applicable on the left side of the client's head for the right-handed stylist and vice-versa for the left-handed stylist.

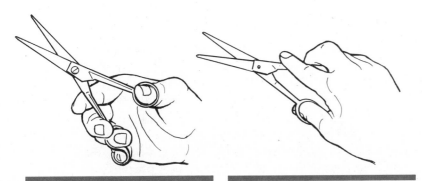

5.14 – Holding position used when cutting against the skin or perimeter of a haircut or during finger and shear cutting technique.

5.15 – Holding position used horizontally when tapering and blending and vertically when cutting interior hair sections.

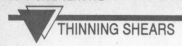

▼ THINNING SHEARS

Thinning or serrated shears are used by barber-stylists to reduce hair thickness or to create special texturizing effects. They may also be called texturizing shears. The first type has notched teeth on the cutting edge of one blade, while the other blade has a straight cutting edge. (Fig. 5.17) The second type has overlapping notched teeth on the cutting edges of both blades. (Fig. 5.18)

Thinning shears also differ in respect to the number of notched teeth on the cutting blade. The greater the number of notched teeth, the finer the hair strands can be cut. Recent designs include a wider notching pattern, with indentations slightly recessed in the notching teeth in order to perform alternative texturizing techniques.

The most common type used is the single serrated blade having 30 to 32 notched teeth. (Thinning shears are also available with detachable blades.)

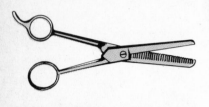

5.17 – Thinning shears with one blade notched

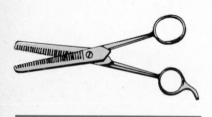

5.18 – Thinning shears with both blades notched

How to Hold Thinning Shears

Thinning or texturizing shears should be held in the same manner as haircutting shears.

Shears and comb should be held at all times during haircutting. For safety, shears need to be closed and resting in the palm while combing through the hair. This is called **palming** the shears and is achieved by slipping the thumb out of the thumb grip and simply pivoting the shear into the palm of the hand. With practice, palming will become a very natural motion. (Figs. 5.19, 5.20)

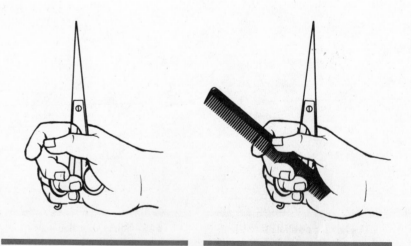

5.19 – Palming the shears   **5.20 – Palmed shears with comb**

Care of Haircutting and Thinning Shears

1. Avoid dropping shears.
2. Protect shears in a leather sheath or holder when carrying them in a kit, bag, or case.
3. Never cut anything but hair with haircutting shears.
4. Sanitize shears after each use with 70 percent ethyl alcohol or 90 percent isopropyl alcohol.
5. Place them in a dry or ultraviolet sanitizer until the next time they are used.

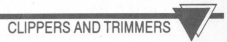

CLIPPERS AND TRIMMERS

Clippers and trimmers are two of the most important tools used in barber-styling. They can be used for a variety of cutting techniques, from blending to texturizing. Trimmers (also referred to as edgers or outliners) are essential for finish and detail work.

There are two types of clippers available—hand clippers, which are seldom used today, and electric clippers, which are used almost exclusively in barber-styling shops.

Electric Clippers

The two basic types of electric clippers are the motor-driven clipper and the vibratory, or magnetic, clipper. Both are available with detachable or non-detachable cutting heads. The visible parts of an electric clipper are the: cutting blade, still blade, heel, switch, set screw, and conducting cord. Clippers with a single cutting head will have a blade adjustment lever on the side of the unit. (Fig. 5.21)

Motor-Driven Clippers

Motor-driven clippers operate by means of a rotary motor which is capable of producing a powerful cutting action. Motor clippers usually have detachable cutting heads (clipper blades) that must be changed to achieve various hair lengths. They can be used for many years and generally require little or no repair. (Fig. 5.22)

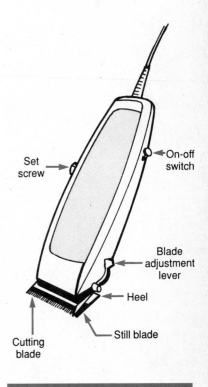

5.21 – Electric clipper

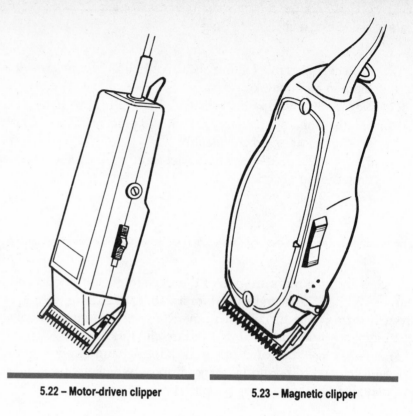

5.22 – Motor-driven clipper

5.23 – Magnetic clipper

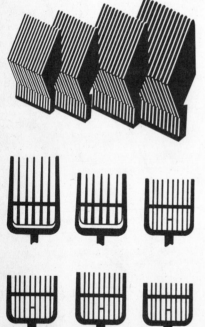

5.24 – Snap-on blade attachment combs (1/16" to 1") are available for most clipper styles.

Magnetic Clipper

Vibratory or magnetic clippers operate by means of an alternating spring and magnet mechanism. These clippers run faster than the motor-driven type and usually have a single cutting head that is adjustable for cutting a variety of hair lengths. Comb attachments that leave the hair longer than the original cutting head snap on for easy cutting versatility. (Figs. 5.23, 5.24)

The **outliner**, also known as a **trimmer** or **edger**, is a magnetic clipper. It has a very fine cutting head for outlining, arching, and design work. The cutting blade is usually available in two styles: a straight trimmer blade and a T-shaped blade. The versatility and utility of the T-blade when trimming rounded or difficult areas makes it the number one choice of many barber-stylists. The outliner is a very valuable implement for detail, precision design, and fine finish work. (Figs. 5.25, 5.26)

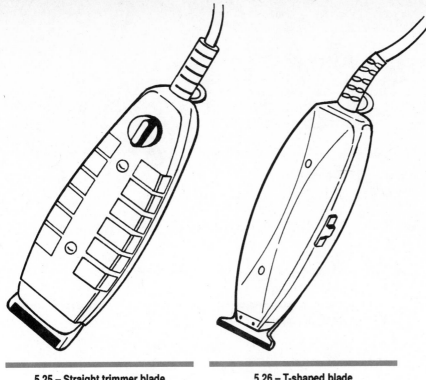

5.25 – Straight trimmer blade

5.26 – T-shaped blade

Cordless Clippers

A number of manufacturers have produced clippers and outliners that do not require an electric cord. These tools are designed to rest in a special unit that recharges their power. Cordless clippers are a very important innovation for barber-stylists. They are easily maneuverable and portable, both important advantages. (Fig. 5.27)

Blade Sizes

Illustrated in Fig. 5.28 are various clipper blades. (Each manufacturer has a different method of blade identification so that a distinguishing number for a particular brand does not mean necessarily that the same number on another brand represents the same cutting size. Care must be taken when ordering.)

Manufacturers are constantly improving their clipper blades to permit faster and better haircutting. Always be on the lookout for the newest developments in haircutting implements.

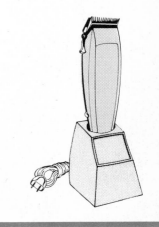

5.27 – Cordless clipper

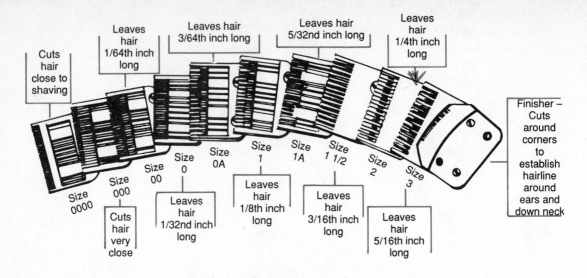

5.28 – A variety of clipper blade sizes

How to Hold Clippers

Clippers should be held in the right hand with the thumb placed on the left side of the unit and the fingers on the right side, with the blades pointing up. An alternative method is to place the thumb on top of the clipper with the fingers supporting it from the underside. The clipper should be held in a way that permits freedom of wrist movement. The left hand holds the comb and is used to steady the clipper while cutting hair.

Care of Electric Clippers

Magnetic clippers do not require frequent greasing. On occasion one or two drops of oil may be applied between the blades. If vibratory clippers seem to be cutting exceptionally slowly or are pulling the hair, immerse the blades into clipper oil or a prepared clipper cleaner and then turn the clippers on and off. This will clean the blades and oil them at the same time. Clippers may also be immersed in a cleaning solvent and then a few drops of oil added to the blades.

  Motor-driven clippers. To detach the cutting blade from the still blade, slide the still blade out from under the compression spring. The blades may be washed with hot water, reassembled, and a drop of oil placed in the two holes in the compression plate. Remove the name plate and check the grease. The grease chamber should be kept about two-thirds full. If the gears should come out, be careful to reassemble them the same way as they were originally. Remove the carbon brush knobs and check the carbon brushes. If they are worn down, replace them with new brushes. Add a few drops of oil weekly to the oiler at the rear of the clippers. Clean the hair from the oil vents surrounding the switch to ensure proper ventilation.

> CAUTION: If electric clippers are running incorrectly do not attempt to repair them. This may nullify your guarantee. Return the clippers to the manufacturer for professional, guaranteed service.

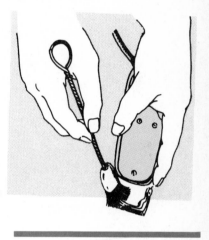

Whenever clipper blades are oiled, remove the excess oil with a dry cloth. Remember, even a little oil on the blades will reduce the cutting ability. Clipper blades are difficult to sharpen. Therefore, it is advisable that this be done by an expert. Keep in mind that repeated sharpenings will lessen the cutting thickness of the blade.

Properly cared for, electric clippers can last several years. Manufacturer's directions should be followed carefully, to assure optimal performance and to maintain the validity of the warranty.

The **clipper brush** has stiff bristles. It is used to remove loose hair clippings, keeping the clippers clean and sanitary. (Fig. 5.29)

5.29 – Cleaning clipper with a clipper brush

Hand Clipper

While hand clippers are rarely used in the modern barber-stylist shop, they should be available for use in case the electric clippers malfunction. (Fig. 5.30)

These clippers are equipped with cutting blades that range from #0000 (the shortest) to #3 (the longest). Because of the time required to change blades, barber-stylists usually use two pairs. The #000 and the #1 cutting blades are the most commonly used.

Care of Hand Clippers

The thumb screw must be adjusted to maintain proper tension between the blades. If this is not done, hair will get caught between the two sets of blades and cause hair to pull. Should this occur,

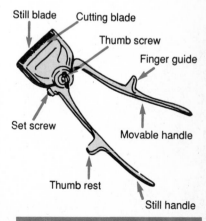

5.30 – Hand clipper

remove the thumb screw, the spring washer, the compression plate, and the cutting blade. Wash both blades with hot water, dry them thoroughly, and reassemble the clippers. A drop of oil may be applied toward the heel of the blades on the still blade. Bear in mind that over-oiling will also allow the hair to enter between the blades. The set screw must be altered to adjust the tension between the two blades. If the set screw is too tight, hand muscles will tire quickly. If the set screw is too loose, the moving handle will not return, causing the clipper to jam in the hair. Should this occur, the movable handle must be forced back to its original position. The hand clipper would then have to be disassembled, cleaned, and reassembled as in Fig. 5.30.

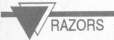

RAZORS

Razors are the sharpest and most delicate cutting implement. They are used by barber-stylists for facial shaves, neck shaves, finish work, and haircutting.

Straight Razors

There are two types of straight razors: the conventional straight razor which requires honing and stropping to maintain its cutting edge; and the changeable blade straight razor, with a razor guard. The changeable blade razor looks the same and is used in the same manner as the conventional razor. However, when the blade becomes dull, it is discarded and replaced with a new one.

Selecting the right kind of razor is a matter of personal choice. The best guides for buying high-quality razors are:

1. Consult with a reliable company or salesman who can recommend the type of razor best suited to your work.
2. Consult with more experienced practitioners about which razors they have found best for shaving and haircutting.

To judge the quality of a razor in any other way can be misleading. Neither the color nor design of a razor nor its ring gives any true indication of its caliber as an implement.

NOTE: For sanitary reasons, a new blade should be used for each client.

Structural Parts of a Razor

The structural parts of both conventional and changeable blade straight razors are the head, back, shoulder, tang, shank, heel, edge, point, blade, pivot, and handle. (Fig. 5.31)

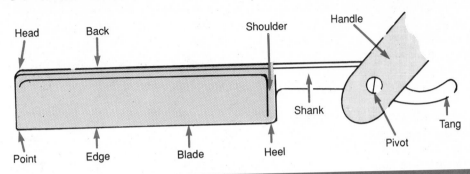

5.31 – Conventional straight razor

Changeable Blade Straight Razor

The changeable blade razor is the most popular type since it eliminates honing and stropping, saves time, and is usually lighter. The razor may be used without the guard for shaving, and with the guard for razor-cutting. Blades are available with a square point, a rounded point, or a combination, with one end rounded and the other end squared. (Fig. 5.32)

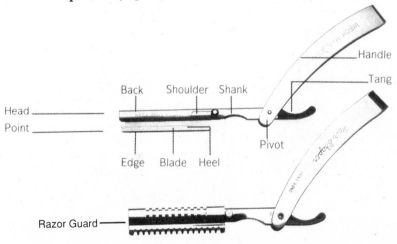

5.32 – Changeable blade straight razor

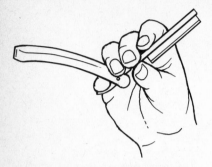

Basic Holding Positions of the Changeable Blade Razor

There are several methods of holding the razor, depending on the service being performed. Specific techniques will be covered in the Shaving and Haircutting chapters. However, it is advisable for the student to practice the following basic holding positions. (Figs. 5.33–5.37)

5.33 – The ball of the thumb supports the razor at the bottom of the shank between the blade and the pivot. The handle is angled up, allowing the little finger to rest on the tang. Place the index finger along the back of the razor for control. The two middle fingers should rest comfortably along the top of the shank.

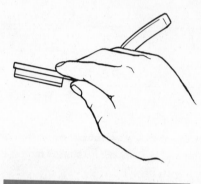

5.34 – Turning the wrist will position the razor for shaving and haircutting.

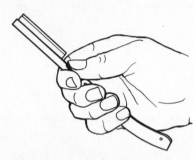

5.35 – Razor is straightened with the fingers wrapped around it as shown.

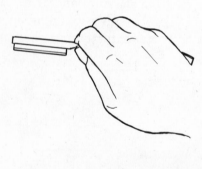

5.36 – The razor should be held more firmly in this position for shaving and haircutting.

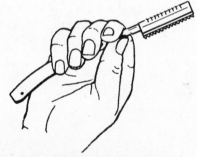

5.37 – Razor with guard. Notice the guard is toward you.

Changing the Blade

Follow the manufacturer's directions for inserting a new blade or removing an old blade from this type of razor. (Figs. 5.38–5.40)

The Conventional Straight Razor

Only the highest quality conventional straight razor should be used. In order to determine the quality of the razor, the barber-stylist must consider the following factors: razor balance, temper, grind, finish, size, and style. In addition, the barber-stylist must master the techniques of honing and stropping in order to produce a fine cutting edge.

The straight razor is comprised of a hardened steel blade attached to a handle by means of a pivot. The handle is made of either hard rubber, plastic, or bone.

Razor Balance

Razor balance refers to the weight and length of the blade relative to that of the handle. A straight razor is properly balanced when the weight of the blade and handle are equal. Proper balance means greater ease in handling the razor during shaving. The balance may be determined by opening the razor and resting it on the first finger at the pivot. If the razor is not well balanced, the head of the razor will move up or down.

Razor Tempers

Tempering the razor involves a special heat treatment given by the manufacturer. When a razor is properly tempered, it acquires the degree of hardness required for a good cutting edge. Razors can be purchased with a hard, soft, or medium temper. The barber-stylist selects the temper that produces the most satisfactory shaving results.

Hard-tempered razors will hold an edge longer, but are very difficult to sharpen.

Soft-tempered razors are very easy to sharpen, but the sharp edge does not last long.

Razor Grinds

The grind of a razor is the shape of the blade after it has been ground. There are two general types—the concave and the wedge grind. Concave grinds are available in full concave, one-half concave, and one-quarter concave.

The concave grind (often referred to as the hollow ground razor) is generally preferred. The back and edge of the razor looks hollow, being slightly thicker between the hollow part and the extreme edge. The resistance of the beard can more easily be felt with the hollow ground razor, thus warning the stylist to check the sharpness of the cutting edge.

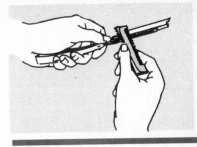

5.38 – Remove the guard. With left hand, hold razor firmly above joint. Catching the blade in the teeth on upper part of guard, push blade out.

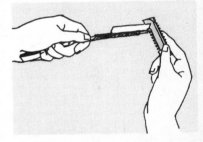

5.39 – Slide blade into groove, pushing the end with your fingers. Place the tooth end of guard into the blade notch and slide the blade in until it clicks into position. (Note: Some razor blade packaging is designed to act as a dispenser. The razor groove is slid over the top of the blade from the side of the dispenser until the blade is in place.)

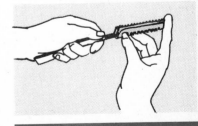

5.40 – Slide the guard over blade, making sure the open end of the guard is over cutting edge of blade.

The one-half and one-quarter concave grinds are less hollow than the full concave. However, there will not be any more thickness between the concave and the extreme edge of the razor.

The wedge grind is neither hollow nor concave. Both sides of the blade form a sharp angle at the extreme edge of the razor. Most older razors were made with a wedge grind. For most barber-stylists learning how to sharpen a wedge grind is quite difficult. Once they become accustomed to using it, however, they usually find that it produces an excellent shave. It is especially preferred for men with coarse, heavy beards. (Fig. 5.41)

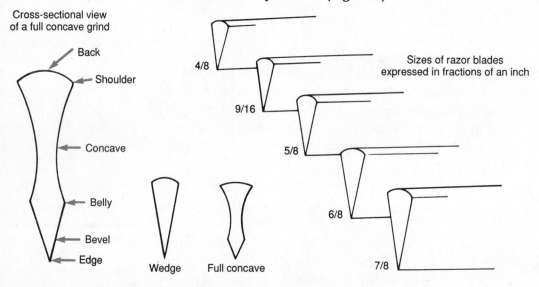

Cross-sectional view of a full concave grind

Back
Shoulder
Concave
Belly
Bevel
Edge

Wedge   Full concave

4/8
9/16
5/8
6/8
7/8

Sizes of razor blades expressed in fractions of an inch

5.41 – Razor grinds

Razor Finish

The finish of a razor is the condition of its surface—plain steel, crocus (polished steel), or metal-plated (nickel or silver). Of these types, the crocus finish is usually the choice of the discriminating barber-stylist. Although the crocus finish is more costly, it lasts longer and does not rust. Metal-plated razors are undesirable because the finish wears off quickly and often hides a poor-quality steel.

Razor Sizes

The size of the razor is measured by the length and width of the blade. The width of the razor is measured either in eighths or sixteenths of an inch, but usually in eighths, such as 4/8, 5/8, 6/8, and 7/8. The 5/8 and 9/16 inch are the two most common sizes, with the 5/8 inch being the more popular.

Razor Styles

The style of a razor indicates its shape and design. Modern razors have such features as a straight, parallel back and edge; a round heel; a square point; a flat or slightly round handle. To prevent scratching the skin, the barber-stylist usually rounds off the square point of the razor slightly by drawing the point of the razor along the edge of the hone.

Razor Care

Razors will maintain their quality if care is taken to prevent corrosion of the extremely fine edge. After use, they should be stropped and a little castor oil applied to the cutting edge. Be careful not to drop the razor—doing so may damage the blade. When closing the razor, be careful that the cutting edge does not strike the handle.

The barber-stylist's tool kit should include several high-grade razors. If one razor is damaged, an immediate replacement should be available.

BARBER-STYLING ACCESSORIES USED IN SHAVING

Hones

Various types of hones are available for the purpose of sharpening razors. A hone is a rectangular block of abrasive material. Since it is harder than steel, the abrasive in the hone cuts or files the edge on the razor.

The final choice of hone is based on personal preference. The question often arises as to which type of hone is best. Generally, any type of hone is satisfactory, provided it is properly used and is capable of producing a sharp cutting edge on the razor.

Students usually practice with a slow-cutting hone, while experienced practitioners generally prefer a faster-cutting hone. In selecting a hone, remember that the finer the abrasive, the slower its action.

Depending on their source, hones are divided into three main groups: natural, synthetic, and combination.

Natural Hones

Natural hones are derived from natural rock deposits. These hones are usually used wet with either water or lather before use.

The water hone is a natural hone cut out of rock formations, usually imported from Germany. Accompanying the water hone is a small piece of slate of the same texture, called the rubber. When the rubber is applied over the hone, which is moistened with water, a proper cutting surface is created. Be careful not to work a bevel into the hone. (Fig. 5.42)

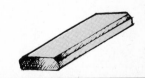

5.42 – Water hone

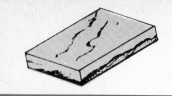

5.43 – Belgian hone

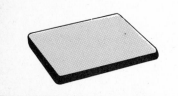

5.44 – Synthetic or manufactured hone

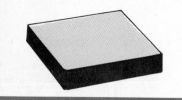

5.45 – Carborundum hone

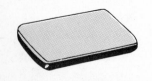

5.46 – Combination hone

The water hone is primarily a slow-cutting hone. When used as directed by the manufacturer, a smooth and lasting edge will result. It is gray or brown in color. Of the two colors, the brown water hone is considered to be slightly superior, and also exerts a slightly faster cutting action.

The Belgian hone is a natural hone cut from rock formations found in Belgium. It is a slow-cutting hone, but a little faster than the water hone, and can create a very sharp edge. Lather is generally applied to the hone to facilitate movement of the razor.

One type of Belgian hone consists of a light yellowish rock top glued on to the back of dark red slate. Its principal advantage is to yield a keen cutting edge on the razor. It can be used either wet or dry. (Fig. 5.43)

Synthetic Hones

Synthetic (sin-**THET**-ick) **hones,** such as the **Swaty hone** and the **carborundum hone,** are manufactured products. These hones can be used dry or a lather can be spread over them before use.

Because they cut faster than the water hone, synthetic hones have the advantage of producing a keen cutting edge in less time. (Fig. 5.44)

Carborundum (kar-bor-**UN**-dum) **hones** are synthetic hones produced in the United States. There are several types, ranging from slow-cutting to fast-cutting. Many practitioners prefer the fast-cutting type because of its quick sharpening action. Carborundum hones should not be used by a beginning student because they may produce a very rough edge if not handled properly. (Fig. 5.45)

Combination Hones

Combination hones consist of both a water and a synthetic hone. The synthetic side is a dark brown and is used first to develop a good cutting edge. To give the razor a finished edge, it is stroked over the side of the water hone. The practitioner can use the synthetic side when the razor is bad, use the water side when the razor needs only a slight touch-up, or use both together, simply by turning it over. (Fig. 5.46)

Most barber-stylists use either carborundum or combination hones. It is advisable, however, to be familiar with the other types of hones and understand the benefits of each.

General Information About Hones

The type of hone used is largely a matter of personal choice. The type of steel in a razor may make some difference as to whether a good edge can be obtained with a particular type of hone. There are a great many other hones available, besides the ones described, which will give very satisfactory results.

Care of Hones

Always clean hones before using. Whenever hones fill with tiny steel particles they must be removed. Use water and a pumice stone to remove them. If a new hone is very rough, the same method can be used to work it into shape.

When wet honing is done, always wipe the hone dry after use. This aids in cleaning and also wipes away the particles of steel that adhere to the cutting surface.

Honing

Honing (HON-ing) is the process of sharpening a razor blade on a hone. The main object is to obtain a perfect cutting edge on the razor.

Prepare hone. Both the razor and the hone should be kept at room temperature. Depending on which type of hone is used, it may be moistened with water or lather, or kept dry. When in use, the hone should be kept perfectly flat. Sufficient space should be provided to permit free arm movements.

Technique of Honing

The razor blade is sharpened by honing the razor with smooth, even strokes of equal number and pressure on both sides of the blade. The angle at which the blade is stroked must be the same for both of its sides. An old, damaged razor may be used for practice.

How to hold the razor. Grasp the razor handle comfortably in the right hand as follows:

1. Rest the index finger on top of the side part of the shank.
2. Rest the ball of the thumb at the joint.
3. Place the second finger at the back of the razor near the edge of the shank.
4. Fold the remaining fingers around the handle to permit easy turning of the razor.

How to hold the hone. Lay the hone firmly and flat in your left hand, using the index finger and little finger. (Fig. 5.47)

CAUTION: Make sure that the fingertips do not project above the hone. If they do, you will cut them.

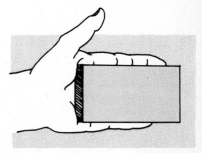

5.47 – Proper way to hold hone

Turning the razor. Place the razor on the hone with the razor's edge facing left. Turn it from one side to the other. The rolling movement across the back of the razor is produced with the fingers, rather than the wrist. Practice the turning action until it is mastered.

First stroke in honing. The razor blade must be stroked diagonally across the hone, drawing the blade toward the cutting edge and heel of the razor. (Fig. 5.48)

Second stroke in honing. After completing the first stroke, the razor is turned on its back with the fingers in the same manner as you would roll a pencil, without turning the wrist. As the razor is rolled over on its back, slide it upward, from left-bottom to left-top of the hone. (Fig. 5.49)

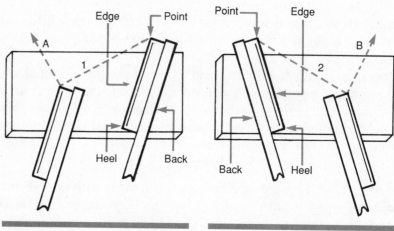

5.48 – First position and stroke in honing   5.49 – Second position and stroke in honing

Completing the second stroke. Draw the razor from the left-top corner to the right-bottom corner of the hone so that the edge faces to the right and the heel leads. Keep equal pressure on the razor at all times. As the razor is rolled over on its back, slide it upward from right-bottom to right-top.

In going from one step to the other, try to maintain four different movements, rather than a sweeping movement. The number of strokes required in honing depends on the condition of the razor's edge.

Testing razor on moistened thumbnail. Depending on the hardness of the hone and the number of strokes taken, the razor edge may be either blunt, keen, coarse, or rough. Different sensations are felt when the razor is passed lightly across the thumbnail, which should be moistened with water or lather. (Fig. 5.50)

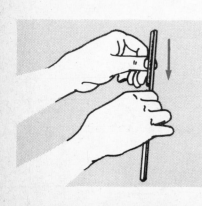

5.50 – Testing razor on moistened thumbnail

Magnified razor edge. While honing, the abrasive material makes small cuts in the sides of the razor blade. The small cuts resemble the teeth of a saw and they point in the same direction as the stroke. (Fig. 5.51)

To test the razor edge, place it lightly on the nail of the thumb and slowly draw the nail from the heel to the point of the razor.

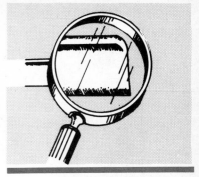

5.51 – Magnified razor edge

1. A perfect or keen edge has fine teeth and tends to dig into the nail with a smooth, steady grip.
2. A blunt or dull razor edge passes over the nail smoothly, without any cutting power.
3. A coarse razor edge digs into the nail with a jerky feeling.
4. A rough (coarse) or over-honed edge has large teeth which stick to the nail and produce a harsh, grating sound.
5. A nick in the razor. A feeling of a slight gap or unevenness in the draw will indicate a nick in the razor.

Correcting an over-honed razor. To correct an over-honed edge, draw the razor backward in a diagonal line across the hone, using the same movement and pressure as in regular honing. One or two strokes each way will usually remove the rough edge. This is called back honing. The razor is then honed again, being careful to prevent over-honing.

Strops

Unlike hones, which are designed to grind the edge of a razor, strops are intended to bring the razor to a smooth, whetted edge.

A good strop is made of durable and flexible material, has the proper thickness and texture, and shows a smooth, finished surface. Some barber-stylists like a thin strop; others prefer a thick, heavy strop. Most strops are made in pairs, one side of leather and the other side of canvas.

Various types of strops are available. Depending upon the material from which they are made, they fall into the following groups: French or German, canvas, cowhide, horsehide, and imitation leather. The finer strops are broken in by the manufacturer. Let us consider these one at a time.

French or German Strop

This is a combination strop with leather on one side and a finishing strop on the other. It is used by many barber-stylists for styling razors. (Fig. 5.52)

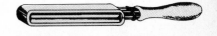

5.52 – French or German strop

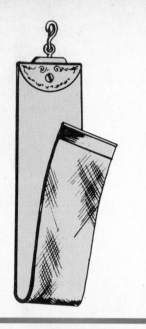

5.53 – Leather and canvas strop

Canvas Strop

The canvas strop is made of high-quality linen or silk, woven into a fine or coarse texture. A fine-textured linen strop is most desirable for putting a lasting edge on a razor. (Fig. 5.53)

To obtain the best results, a new canvas strop should be thoroughly broken in. A daily hand finish will keep its surface smooth and in readiness for stropping.

For a hand finish, the canvas strop is given the following treatment:

1. Attach the swivel end of the strop to a fixed point, such as a nail. (Older barber-styling chairs have a metal loop attached for this purpose.)
2. Hold the other end tightly over a smooth and level surface.
3. Rub a bar of dry soap over the strop, working it well into the grain of the canvas.
4. Rub a smooth glass bottle over the strop several times, each time forcing the soap into the grain and also removing any excess soap.

Cowhide Strop

The cowhide strop was originally imported from Russia. To this day it still bears the name **Russian strop**, even though it may be manufactured in this country. This name usually implies that the strop is made of cowhide and that the Russian method of tanning was employed.

The cowhide or Russian strop is one of the best. When new, it requires a daily hand finish until it is thoroughly broken in. There are several ways to break in a Russian strop. A method frequently used is as follows:

1. Rub dry pumice stone over the strop in order to remove the outer nap and develop a smooth surface.
2. Rub stiff lather into the strop.
3. Rub dry pumice stone over the strop until smooth.
4. Clean off the strop.
5. Rub fresh, stiff lather into the strop.
6. Rub a smooth glass bottle over the strop several times until a smooth surface is developed.

Another method to break in a Russian strop is to omit the pumice stone. Instead, stiff lather is rubbed into the strop with the aid of a smooth glass bottle or with the palm of the hand.

Horsehide Strop

Strops made of horsehide are divided into two main groups: the ordinary horsehide strop and the shell.

1. An ordinary horsehide strop is of medium grade and has a fine grain. It tends to be very smooth. In this condition it does not readily impart the proper edge to a razor. For this reason, it is not recommended for professional use. However, it is suitable for private use.
2. The other type of horsehide strop is called shell or Russian shell. This is a high-quality strop taken from the rump area of a horse. Although it is quite expensive, it makes one of the best strops for the barber-stylist. It always remains smooth and requires very little, if any, breaking in.

Imitation Leather Strop

The imitation leather strop has not proven too satisfactory. Because of the availability of high-quality strops, it is wise to avoid strops made of imitation leather.

Strop Dressing

Strop dressing cleans the leather strop, preserves its finish, and also improves its draw and sharpening qualities. For proper use, apply a very small amount of dressing to the leather strop. Rub it into the pores well and remove any surplus. Always wait at least 24 hours between applications.

Stropping

Stropping a razor is a fine art developed by repeated practice. Its aim is to smooth and shape the razor into a keen cutting implement. After being honed, the razor seldom needs any stropping on the canvas. Instead, the honed razor is stropped directly over the surface of the leather strop. The time to use the canvas strop is when the razor develops a smooth edge from continued use. The effect of the canvas strop is similar to mild honing.

The Technique of Stropping

Hold the end of the strop firmly in the left hand so it cannot sag. Hold it close to the side, and as high as is comfortable. Grasp the razor firmly in the right hand so that the first finger is on the shank, the second finger is on the handle, and the thumb rests lightly on both parts. At the same time, the first finger of the right hand rests at the edge of the strop.

> **NOTE:** The direction of the razor in stropping is the reverse of that used in honing.

Turning the razor. Place the razor on the strop, turning it with fingers and thumb. Practice the turning action until it is mastered.

In stropping the razor, use a long, diagonal stroke with even pressure from the heel to the point.

First stroke. Start the stroke at the top edge of the strop closest to the chair. Draw the razor perfectly flat, with back leading, straight over the surface. (Fig. 5.54) Bear down just heavily enough to feel the razor draw. Do not worry about speed. This will come with practice.

Second stroke. When the first stroke is completed, turn the razor on the back of the blade by rolling it in the fingers without turning the hand. Now draw the razor away from you, toward the hydraulic chair, thus completing the second stroke. (Fig. 5.55)

Make a final test of the razor prior to shaving on the moistened tip of the thumb. Touch the razor's edge lightly, and note the reaction. A dull edge produces no sensation of drawing. A razor with a proper cutting edge tends to stick to the thumb and will not slide along it.

If the razor's edge produces a rough, disagreeable sound upon testing, it indicates that the cutting edge is still coarse. To correct this condition, additional finishing on the leather strop is necessary.

Should the razor's edge yield a smooth feeling upon testing, finish it again on the canvas strop, followed by a few more strokes on the leather strop.

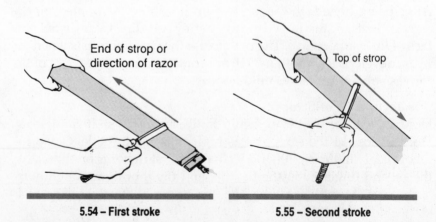

5.54 – First stroke   **5.55 – Second stroke**

Lather Receptacles

Lather receptacles are containers used to hold lather for shaving. (Figs. 5.56–5.58) Those most commonly used are:

1. Electric latherizer
2. Press-button-can latherizer
3. Lather mug with paper lining

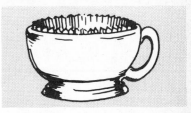

5.56 – Lather mug with paper lining

Lather-making devices such as the electric latherizer are far superior to the lather mug. Not only are these machines cleaner and more sanitary, but they are also more convenient and easier to operate. Clients are favorably impressed by the clean, sanitary, preheated lather coming from these modern machines. For satisfactory performance follow the manufacturer's instructions on their proper use and care.

The electric latherizer is the most widely used lather-making device, to the extent that all other methods are virtually excluded.

Lather mugs are receptacles made out of glass, earthenware, rubber, or metal. When the lather mug is used, shaving soap and warm water are mixed thoroughly with the aid of a lather brush. Since the lather mug is exposed and collects dirt easily, it requires thorough cleansing after each client.

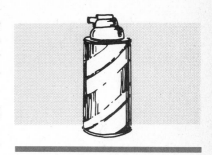

5.57 – Press-button can

To maintain sanitary conditions, a separate paper lining for each client should be used in the lather mug.

Lather mugs or press-button cans are convenient in the absence of electric lather-making devices, or in case the machines malfunction.

> **NOTE:** Lather mugs have a very limited use in the modern styling shop.

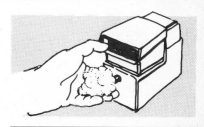

5.58 – Electric latherizer (cream soap type)

Lather Brushes

Lather brushes are used to apply soap lather which softens the beard. Most barber-stylists favor the number three size of lather brush. The vulcanized type is the most durable, since its bristles will not fall apart in hot water.

To guard against contaminated brushes, many states have laws requiring that brushes made from animal hair be free of anthrax germs at the time of purchase. These brushes must contain the imprint **sterilized**. Lather brushes must be sanitized after each use.

> **NOTE:** Like the lather mug, the lather brush has very limited use in modern barber-styling. Check with your state board to determine if the use of lather brushes is permitted.

Shaving Soaps

Shaving soaps can be purchased in various forms and shapes. Hard shaving soaps include those sold in cake, stick, or powdered form, and are similar in composition to toilet soaps. Soft soap is available as shaving cream in a tube, jar, or press-button container. A liquid cream soap is used in the electric latherizer.

Whatever form of shaving soap is used, it usually contains animal and vegetable oils, alkaline substances, and water. The presence of coconut oil improves the lathering qualities of the shaving soap, which helps to keep the hair erect while the alkalinity softens the hair for shaving.

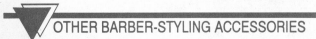

OTHER BARBER-STYLING ACCESSORIES

Styling Brushes

Barber-stylists use a number of different brushes in their work. The choice of bristle texture, spacing, and material will depend on the hairstyle desired. The proper use of brushes can produce waving, added fullness, smoothing, and scalp stimulating effects.

Hair brushes are made out of plastic, wood, or metal and contain either natural or artificial bristles.

> **NOTE:** If made of natural bristles, the brush must bear the marking sterilized.

Some brush styles combine plastic or hard rubber handles with a cushioned rubber base into which either nylon or metal bristles are set. These brushes are very popular with many barber-stylists. (Figs. 5.59–5.62)

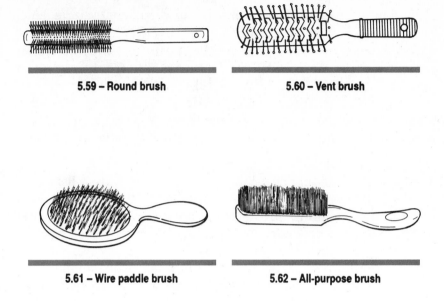

5.59 – Round brush

5.60 – Vent brush

5.61 – Wire paddle brush

5.62 – All-purpose brush

Removing Loose Hair

Since a number of states have forbidden the use of hair dusters, other methods are now used to remove loose hair.

1. A small towel, properly folded, can be used to dust off loose hair.
2. Paper neck strips are popular.
3. Small electric hand vacuums and air hoses are also being employed.

All of these methods are in compliance with state and local health codes.

Electric Hair Vacuum

The electric hair vacuum provides quick clean-up service after a haircut. It can remove all loose hair and some loose dandruff. It is particularly suitable for going over the forehead and around the neck and ears. Make sure to sanitize the nozzle applicator after each use and empty the container as hair accumulates in it.

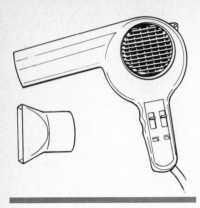

5.63 – Blow-dryer

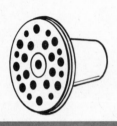

5.64 – A diffuser is an attachment that disperses the air within its conical shape and allows the heat to dry the hair. Diffusers are especially convenient for drying curly or permed hair for a "natural" effect.

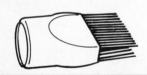

5.65 – Comb attachments, which take the place of the nozzle, are available in several sizes for the purpose of combing through the hair while drying it.

Blow-Dryer

The blow-dryer is designed for drying and styling hair in a single operation. Its parts include a handle, air directional nozzle, small fan, heating element, and controls. (Figs. 5.63–5.65)

The blow-dryer produces a steady stream of temperature-controlled air at various speeds. The controls permit the stylist to make heat and air speed adjustments while operating the dryer. Some blow-dryers offer an automatic cool-down feature. Care should be taken when purchasing a blow-dryer to check the warranty and any service agreements, in addition to the particular features of the unit.

How to Hold the Blow-Dryer

The blow-dryer should be balanced, and fit the barber-stylist's hand comfortably. The dryer is usually held just above the area being dried, nozzle pointing downward at an angle as the hair is dried from the scalp to the ends. Free-style drying is performed by moving the dryer back and forth in a sideways motion, allowing the hair to fall naturally. (See hairstyling chapter for more information.)

Blow-Dryer Safety

To ensure both your safety and that of the client and his or her hair, the following precautions should be observed:

1. Apply a protective setting agent to the hair to shield it from the heat of the blow-dryer.
2. Check the brush bristles for sharp points.
3. Test the temperature controls.
4. Keep the air and the hair moving to prevent burns. Do not concentrate dryer heat too close to the scalp.
5. Follow the brush or comb with the blow-dryer, working in the direction of the desired style, blowing damp hair onto dry hair.
6. Avoid dropping the dryer.
7. Never use the dryer near water.

Thermal Hairstyling Tools

Thermal waving is the process of waving or curling straight or **pressed** hair and requires the use of thermal irons, stoves, or sometimes, brushes. Thermal hairstyling tools are used most often in women's and ethnic hairstyling. The ability to use these tools is an important aspect of the barber-stylist's training.

Thermal Irons

Thermal irons are available in a variety of styles, sizes, and weights, from small to large barrel diameters.

The conventional (Marcel) iron requires the use of a stove to heat it. The electric iron is available with or without a vaporizing action feature and can be purchased with a stationary or rotating handle style. Pressing combs also require the use of the stove and are used for straightening or pressing hair. Electric pressing combs are also available. Both types of combs are constructed in high-quality steel or brass. The electric stove heats both the conventional irons and the metal pressing combs. Stoves become very hot and must be handled carefully. (Figs. 5.66–5.69)

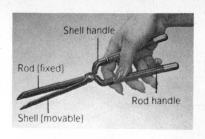

5.66 – Stove-heated curling iron

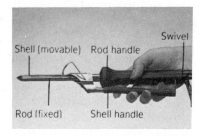

5.67 – Electric curling iron

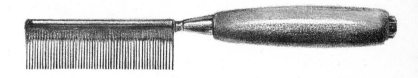

5.68 – Regular pressing comb

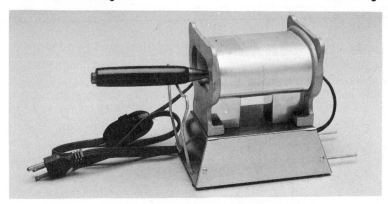

5.69 – Electric stove or heater

Testing Thermal Irons

After heating the irons to the desired temperature, test them on a piece of tissue paper. Clamp the heated irons over the tissue and hold for five seconds. If the paper scorches or turns brown, the irons

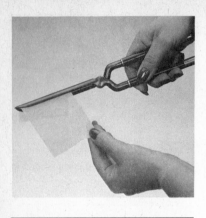

5.70 – Testing the heat of thermal irons

are too hot. Let them cool before using. Remember that fine, lightened, or badly damaged hair withstands less heat than normal hair. (Fig. 5.70)

Care of Thermal Irons

Thermal irons should be kept clean and free from rust and carbon. To remove dirt or grease, wash the irons in a soap solution containing a few drops of ammonia. This cuts the oil and grease that usually adhere to the irons. Fine sandpaper, or steel wool with a little oil, helps to remove rust and carbon. It also polishes the irons. To permit greater facility in movement, oil the joint of the irons.

New thermal irons are **tempered** at the factory in order to hold heat uniformly. If the irons are overheated they usually lose their temper, and, in most cases, are ruined.

Holding Thermal Irons

Hold the irons in a comfortable position that gives you complete control. Grasp the handles of the irons in the right hand, far enough away from the joint to avoid the heat. Place the three middle fingers on the back of the lower handle, the little finger in front of the lower handle, and the thumb in front of the upper handle.

The Galvanic Machine

This is an apparatus with attachments designed to produce galvanic current. The main function of the galvanic machine is to introduce water-soluble products into the skin during a facial. (Fig. 5.71)

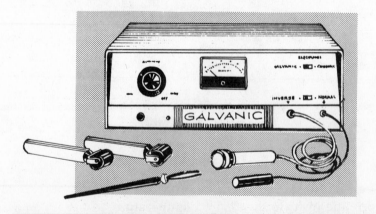

5.71 – Galvanic machine

High-Frequency Machine

This is a machine that produces ultraviolet rays, used for facial and scalp treatments. (Fig. 5.72)

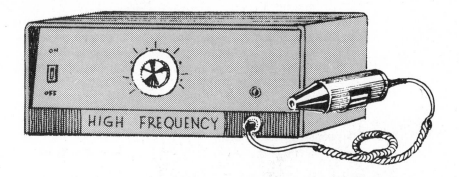

5.72 – High-frequency machine

Facial Cleansing Machine

This is a machine equipped with a magnifying glass-lamp combination used to analyze skin conditions, as well as an apparatus that applies steam to the face at a comfortable temperature during a facial treatment. (Fig. 5.73)

Comedone Extractor

The comedone extractor is a metallic implement having a screwed attachment at each end. A fine needle point is at one end and the opposite end is round, has a hole in the center, and is used to press out blackheads.

Tweezers

The tweezer is a metallic implement having two blunt prongs at one end. The blunt prongs of the tweezer are used to pluck unsightly hair. To remove hair, pull it in the same direction in which it grows. For added comfort, the treated area can be steamed and a little cold cream applied. The tweezer may also be used to pull out ingrown hairs.

The automatic tweezer is a more recent development which is gaining quickly in popularity. The automatic tweezer is set and a spring action quickly and painlessly extracts the hair.

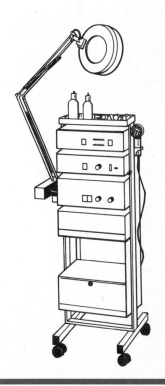

5.73 – Facial cleansing machine

Electric Vibrators

The vibrator is an electric appliance used in facial and scalp massage.

Heating Cap

This is an insulated cap containing interwoven electric wires, which is used for heating the hair and scalp in some corrective treatments. (Fig. 5.74)

Hair-Dryer

A hair-dryer may be necessary for some permanent wave solutions to ensure processing, in addition to drying hair sets and styles. Controls include a timer and heat temperature dial. (Fig. 5.75)

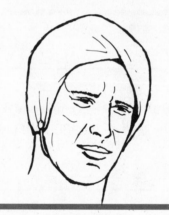

5.74 – Heating cap

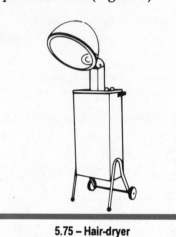

5.75 – Hair-dryer

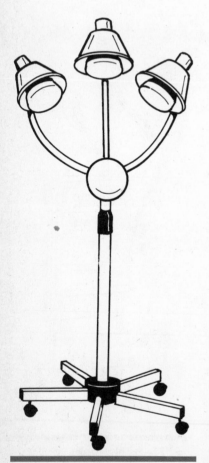

5.76 – Heat lamp

Heat Lamp

This device is used for drying curly or permed hair, and for scalp treatments. (Fig. 5.76)

Hydraulic Chair

A hydraulic chair is an essential fixture for rendering service to clients. It can be easily adjusted both in height and position. Generally, such chairs are spaced about 4 ½ to 5 feet apart from center to center. (Fig. 5.77)

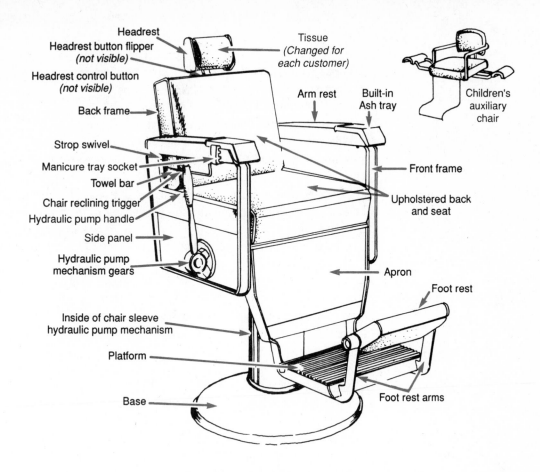

5.77 – Hydraulic chair

To use the chair properly:

1. Lower and lock the chair before a client gets in or out of it.
2. Rotate the chair to the proper position and lock it.
3. Operate the chair's hand pump in a skillful and quiet way.
4. Always lock the chair during any type of service.
5. Press the release when removing or adjusting the headrest.

For effective operation, follow the manufacturer's instructions at all times.

REVIEW QUESTIONS

Implements, Tools, and Equipment

1. Name the principal implements used in barber-styling.
2. For what should the barber-stylist look in the purchase of implements?
3. What determines the correct choice of combs?
4. What style comb is used for general haircutting?
5. Name two ways in which a tapering comb can be used.
6. Which comb is the best to use for flat tops?
7. Name some uses for the tail comb.
8. Name the important parts of haircutting shears.
9. Distinguish between the German and French types of haircutting shears.
10. How are the lengths of shears usually measured? Which sizes are used most often?
11. What are the two main types of shear grinds, and which type is used most frequently?
12. Give the finish of the various plain grinds. Which one is preferred by the barber-stylist?
13. Name one way to determine a comfortable shear length.
14. For what are thinning shears used?
15. Name two types of hair clippers.
16. Name two types of electric clippers.
17. Name the visible parts of an electric clipper.
18. Which type of clipper is recommended for making the outline around the ear?
19. What size clipper blade gives the shortest cut?
20. Name two types of straight razors.
21. Name eight important points about razors.
22. Name the eleven important parts of a razor.
23. What is the proper way to care for razors?
24. What is a hone?
25. Name three types of hones.
26. Name two kinds of natural hones.
27. Which strops can be used by barber-stylists?
28. How are combs and brushes sanitized?
29. How are metal implements sanitized?

Honing and Stropping

1. How does the barber-stylist acquire the right technique of honing and stropping?
2. What is accomplished by proper honing?
3. Describe the manner of stroking a razor on a hone.

4. Describe the first stroke in honing.
5. How is the second stroke performed in honing?
6. What happens to the razor edge as it is honed?
7. Why should a honed razor be tested on a moist thumbnail?
8. What is the sign of a keen edge or a properly honed razor?
9. What is the sign of a blunt razor edge?
10. What is the sign of a coarse razor edge?
11. What is the sign of a rough or over-honed razor edge?
12. What is the proper care of hones?
13. What is the purpose of stropping the razor after honing?
14. How does stropping differ from honing?
15. Which strop is used on a freshly honed razor?
16. What is the proper way to hold the strop?
17. How should the razor be held for stropping?
18. Where should the first stroke be started?
19. Describe the movements used in stropping.
20. Which fingers are used in rolling and turning the razor in the hand?
21. How much pressure should be applied in stropping?
22. How is the razor edge tested after stropping?
23. What is the sign of a smooth, sharp razor edge?
24. What is the sign of a dull razor edge?
25. How can the canvas strop be kept clean and smooth?
26. What is the purpose of stropping the razor before shaving?
27. In what position should the strops be kept?
28. What is used to clean a dirty leather strop?

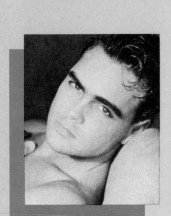

6

Properties and Disorders of the Skin, Scalp, and Hair

Learning Objectives

After completing this chapter, you should be able to:

1. Describe the structure and composition of the skin, scalp, and hair.

2. Define the divisions of skin and hair.

3. List the functions of the skin and hair.

4. Discuss facts relating to hair growth, distribution, and replacement.

5. Identify contagious skin and scalp disorders.

Courtesy of: Hair: Van Michael Salon Artistic Team. Photo: Rick Day.

INTRODUCTION TO THE SKIN AND SCALP

The scientific study of the skin and scalp is of particular importance to the barber-stylist. It forms the basis for an effective program of skin and scalp treatments. **Dermatology** is the study of the skin, its nature, structure, functions, diseases, and treatment. The barber-stylist who has a thorough understanding of the skin will be better able to give clients professional advice on scalp and facial care.

The skin is the largest and one of the most important organs of the body.

Healthy skin is slightly moist, soft, flexible, possesses a slightly acid reaction, and is free of blemishes and other disorders. Its texture should be smooth and soft. The skin is also elastic, resistant, and, under normal and healthy conditions, renews itself.

The skin varies in thickness, being thinnest on the eyelids and thickest on the palms of the hands and soles of the feet. Continued pressure over any part of the skin will cause it to thicken and become calloused.

The skin of the scalp is constructed similarly to the skin elsewhere on the human body. However, larger and deeper hair follicles are present to accommodate the longer hair on the head. (Fig. 6.1)

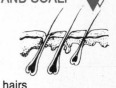

65 hairs

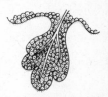

95–100 sebaceous glands

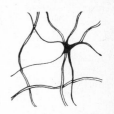

78 yards (70 meters) of nerves

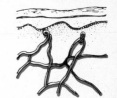

19 yards (17 meters) of blood vessels

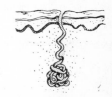

650 sweat glands

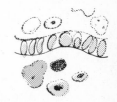

9,500,000 cells

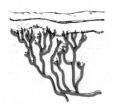

1,300 nerve endings to record pain

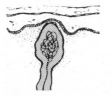

78 sensory apparatuses for heat

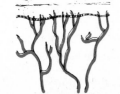

19,500 sensory cells at the ends of nerve fibers

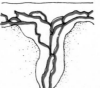

13 sensory apparatuses for cold

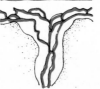

160–165 pressure apparatuses for the perception of tactile stimuli

6.1 – The structure of the skin contained within one square inch (6.452 square centimeters)

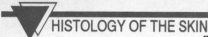

HISTOLOGY OF THE SKIN

The skin is constructed of two clearly defined divisions: the epidermis and the dermis. (Fig. 6.2)

1. The **epidermis** (ep-i-**DUR**-mis) is the outermost, protective

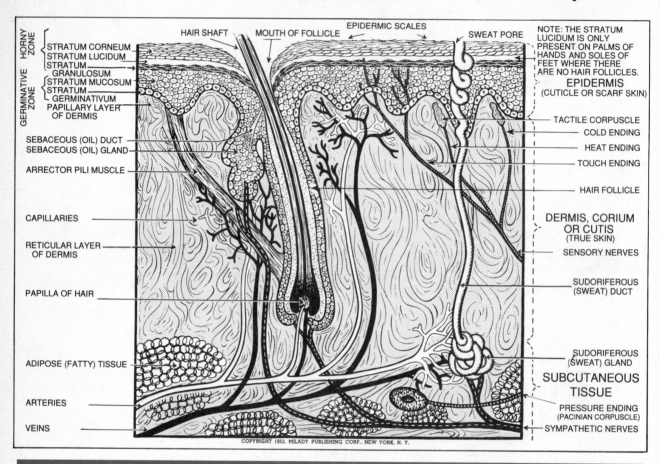

HORNY ZONE
GERMINATIVE ZONE

- STRATUM CORNEUM
- STRATUM LUCIDUM
- STRATUM GRANULOSUM
- STRATUM MUCOSUM
- STRATUM GERMINATIVUM
- PAPILLARY LAYER OF DERMIS

HAIR SHAFT
MOUTH OF FOLLICLE
EPIDERMIC SCALES
SWEAT PORE

NOTE: THE STRATUM LUCIDUM IS ONLY PRESENT ON PALMS OF HANDS AND SOLES OF FEET WHERE THERE ARE NO HAIR FOLLICLES.

EPIDERMIS (CUTICLE OR SCARF SKIN)

SEBACEOUS (OIL) DUCT
SEBACEOUS (OIL) GLAND
ARRECTOR PILI MUSCLE

TACTILE CORPUSCLE
COLD ENDING
HEAT ENDING
TOUCH ENDING

HAIR FOLLICLE

CAPILLARIES

RETICULAR LAYER OF DERMIS

DERMIS, CORIUM OR CUTIS (TRUE SKIN)
SENSORY NERVES

PAPILLA OF HAIR

SUDORIFEROUS (SWEAT) DUCT

ADIPOSE (FATTY) TISSUE

SUDORIFEROUS (SWEAT) GLAND
SUBCUTANEOUS TISSUE

ARTERIES

PRESSURE ENDING (PACINIAN CORPUSCLE)

VEINS

SYMPATHETIC NERVES

COPYRIGHT 1953, MILADY PUBLISHING CORP., NEW YORK, N.Y.

6.2 – Histology of the skin

layer of the skin. It is commonly called **cuticle** or **scarf skin**.

2. The **dermis** (**DUR**-mis) is the underlying, or inner layer of the skin. It is also called **derma, corium, cutis,** or **true skin**

The epidermis contains no blood vessels, but has many small nerve endings, and is made up of the following layers:

1. The horny layer (**stratum corneum—STRAT-um KOHR-nee-um**), consists of tightly packed, scale-like cells that are shed and replaced continually. As these cells develop layers

beneath, they form **keratin** (**KER**-a-tin), a chemical substance that acts as a waterproof covering.

2. The clear layer (**stratum lucidum**—**LOO**-si-dum) consists of small, transparent cells through which light can pass. It is not present where there are hair follicles.

3. The granular layer (**stratum granulosum**—gran-yoo-**LOH**-sum) consists of cells that look like distinct granules. These cells are almost dead and change into a horny substance.

4. The reproductive layer (**stratum germinativum**—jur-mi-nah-**TIV**-um) is composed of several layers of differently shaped cells. The deepest layer is responsible for the growth of the epidermis. It also contains a dark pigment called **melanin** (**MEL**-a-nin), which protects the sensitive cells below from the destructive effects of ultraviolet rays.

The **dermis** is called the true skin. It is a highly sensitive and vascular layer of connective tissue. It contains numerous blood vessels; nerves; lymph, sweat, and oil glands; hair follicles; arrector pili muscles (described later in this chapter); and papillae. The dermis consists of two layers: the papillary, or superficial layer; and the reticular, or deeper layer.

1. The **papillary** (pa-**PIL**-ah-ry) **layer** lies directly beneath the epidermis. It contains small, cone-shaped projections of elastic tissue that point upward into the epidermis. These projections are called **papillae** (pa-**PILL**-ee). Some of these papillae contain looped capillaries, or small blood vessels. Others contain many nerve fiber endings. This layer also contains some melanin skin pigment.

2. The **reticular** (re-**TIK**-u-lar) **layer**, within its network, contains the following structures.

   a. fat cells   e. sweat glands
   b. blood vessels   f. hair follicles
   c. lymph glands   g. arrector pili muscles
   d. oil glands

Subcutaneous (sub-kyoo-**TAY**-nee-us) **tissue** is a layer of fatty tissue found below the dermis. This fatty tissue varies in thickness according to age, sex, and general health. It gives smoothness and contour to the body, contains fats for use as energy, and also acts as a protective cushion for the outer skin. Circulation is maintained by a network of arteries and lymphatics.

> **NOTE:** Some histologists regard the subcutaneous tissue as a continuation of the dermis.

How the Skin is Nourished

Blood and lymph supply nourishment to the skin. From one-half to two-thirds of the body's blood supply is distributed to the skin. The blood and lymph, as they circulate through the skin, contribute essential materials for growth, nourishment, and repair of the skin, hair, and nails. In the subcutaneous tissue are found networks of arteries and lymphatics which send their smaller branches to hair papillae, hair follicles, and skin glands. Capillaries in the skin are quite numerous.

Nerves of the Skin

The skin contains the surface endings of many nerve fibers classified as:

1. Motor nerve fibers, which are distributed to the arrector pili muscles of the hair follicles.
2. Sensory nerve fibers which react to heat, cold, touch, pressure, and pain. (Fig. 6.3)
3. Secretory nerve fibers which are distributed to the sweat and oil glands of the skin.

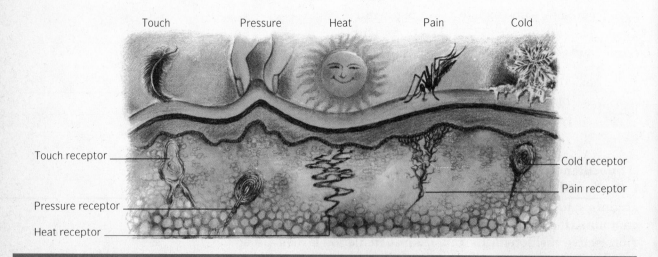

6.3 – Sensory nerves of the skin

Sense of touch. The papillary layer of the dermis provides the body with the sense of touch. Nerves supplying the skin register basic sensations, such as touch, pain, heat, cold, pressure, or deep touch. Nerve endings are most abundant in the fingertips. Complex sensations, such as sense of vibration, seem to depend on a combination of these nerve endings.

Skin Elasticity

Pliability of the skin depends upon the elasticity of the dermis fibers. For example, when healthy skin expands, it regains its former shape almost immediately.

Aging skin. The aging process of the skin is a subject of vital importance to everyone. Perhaps the most outstanding characteristic of the aged skin is its loss of elasticity.

Skin Color

The color of the skin, whether fair or dark, depends partly upon the blood supply, but primarily upon the melanin, or coloring matter, which is deposited in the reproductive layer and the papillary layer of the dermis. The pigment varies in different people. In various races and nationalities, the distinctive color of the skin is a hereditary trait.

Melanocytes

Special cells called **melanocytes** (MEL-uh-no-sights) produce pigment granules that are scattered throughout the basal layer (germinativum) of the epidermis. The basal layer is the layer of cells at the base of the epidermis closest to the dermis. Melanocytes are derived from nerve tissue and produce the pigment granules that are passed on to **keratinocytes** (ke-RAT-i-no-sights) (epidermal cells that synthesize keratin) to give the skin most of its color. These granules are called **melanosomes** (MEL-uh-no-sohms) and produce a complex protein called melanin, a brown-black pigment that serves as the skin's protective screen.

People of different races have approximately the same number of melanocytes but they are more active in dark-skinned people. The lighter the skin, the fewer the melanocyte pigment cells. The darker the skin, the more protection the melanin provides from the ultraviolet rays of the sun and from premature aging.

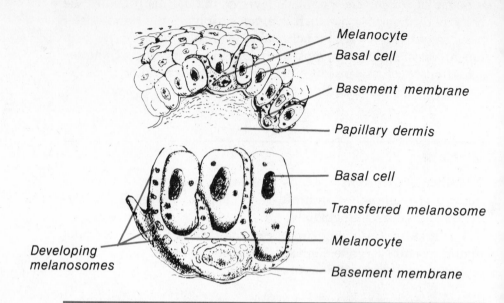

6.4 – Melanocytes transfer pigment to the keratinocytes, the epidermal cells that synthesize keratin, to give the skin most of its color.

Dark-skinned people also have fewer incidences of skin cancer. (Fig. 6.4)

The Glands of the Skin

The skin contains two types of duct glands that extract materials from the blood to form new substances.

1. The **sweat glands (sudoriferous**—sue-dur-**IF**-ur-us) excrete sweat.
2. The **oil glands (sebaceous**—si-**BAY**-shus) secrete sebum.

The sweat glands (tubular type) consist of a coiled base and a tube-like duct that terminates at the skin surface to form the **sweat pore**. Practically all parts of the body are supplied with sweat glands. They are more numerous on the palms, soles, forehead, and armpits. The sweat glands regulate body temperature and help to eliminate waste products from the body. Their activity is greatly increased by heat, exercise, emotion, and certain drugs. The excretion of sweat is under the control of the nervous system. Normally,

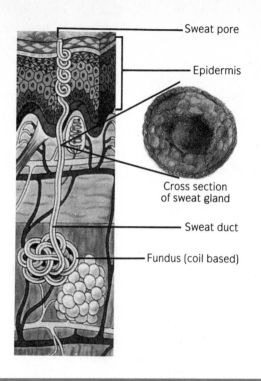

6.5 – Sweat gland

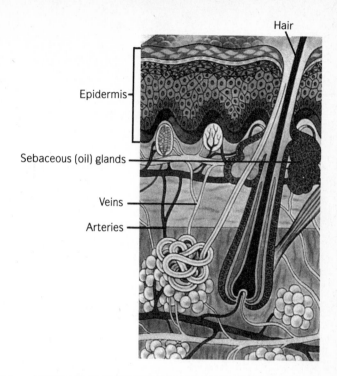

6.6 – Scalp hair, follicle, and oil glands

one to two pints of liquid, containing salts, are eliminated daily through the sweat pores in the skin. (Fig. 6.5)

The oil glands consist of little sacs with ducts that open into the hair follicle. They secrete **sebum** (**SEE**-bum), that lubricates the skin and preserves the softness of the hair. With the exception of the palms and soles, these glands are found in all parts of the body, particularly the face. (Fig. 6.6)

Sebum is a semi-fluid, oily substance produced by the oil glands. Ordinarily it flows through the oil ducts leading to the mouths of the hair follicles. However, when the sebum becomes hardened and the duct becomes blocked, a blackhead is formed. Cleanliness is of prime importance in keeping the skin free of blemishes.

Absorption of the Skin

Although the skin is an intact outer layer of the body, it is, in fact, indented by hair follicles with their sebaceous (oil) glands and by the pores of the sudoriferous (sweat) glands. These pockets, although normally resistant to bacterial attack (except in certain cases where they show as pimples, boils, blackheads, or acne), will allow the entry of special drugs and chemicals into the body. These chemicals may be absorbed in order to combat infections of the skin (e.g., antiseptic creams and ointments), or they may be used as skin conditioners to help overcome dryness or damage (e.g., vitamin and hormone creams).

Functions of the Skin

The principal functions of the skin are: protection, sensation, heat regulation, excretion, secretion, and absorption.

1. **Protection.** The skin protects the body from injury and bacterial invasion. The outermost layer of the epidermis is covered with a thin layer of sebum, thus rendering it waterproof. It is resistant to ranges of temperature, minor injuries, chemical substances, and many microbes. If they do invade, the skin becomes inflamed and gets rid of them.

2. **Sensation.** Through its sensory nerve endings, the skin responds to heat, cold, touch, pressure, pain, and location. Stimulation of a sensory nerve ending produces pain. A minor burn is very painful, but a deep burn that destroys the nerves may be painless. Sensory endings responsive to touch and pressure lie in close relation to hair follicles.

3. **Heat regulation.** The healthy body maintains a constant internal temperature of about 98.6 degrees fahrenheit. As changes occur in the outside temperature, the blood and sweat glands of the skin make necessary adjustments. Heat regulation is a function of the skin, the organ that protects the body from the environment. Heat is lost by the evaporation of sweat.

4. **Excretion.** Perspiration is excreted from the skin. Water lost by perspiration carries salt and other chemicals with it.

5. **Secretion.** Sebum is secreted by the sebaceous glands. Excessive flow of oil from the oil glands may produce **seborrhea** (seb-o-REE-ah). Emotional stress may increase the flow of sebum.

6. **Absorption** is limited, but it does occur. Fatty materials, such as lanolin creams, are absorbed largely through the hair follicles and sebaceous gland openings.

The skin has an immune response to many things that touch it or are absorbed by it.

The appendages of the skin are hair, nails, sweat glands, and oil glands.

INTRODUCTION TO HAIR

As a barber-stylist, a technical understanding of hair is vitally important in order to provide knowledgeable and professional service. To keep hair in a healthy condition, proper attention must be given to its care and treatment. Abusing the hair by harmful cosmetic applications or faulty hair treatments can cause the hair structure to become weakened or damaged. Knowledge and analysis of the client's hair, tactful suggestions for its improvement, and a sincere interest in maintaining its health and appearance should be the concern of every barber-stylist.

THE STUDY OF HAIR

The study of hair is called **trichology** (treye-**KOL**-o-jee). In addition to being used as an adornment, hair protects the head from heat, cold, and injury. It is an appendage of the skin in the form of a slender, thread-like outgrowth of the skin and scalp.

Composition of Hair

Hair is composed chiefly of a **protein** (**PRO**-teen) called **keratin** (**KER**-a-tin), which is present in all horny growths such as nails, claws, and hoofs. The chemical composition of average hair is: carbon, 50.65 percent; hydrogen, 6.36 percent; nitrogen, 17.14 percent; sulphur, 5.0 percent; and oxygen, 20.85 percent. The chemical composition varies with color. Light hair contains less carbon and hydrogen, and more oxygen and sulphur. Conversely, dark hair has more carbon and less oxygen and sulphur.

Division of Hair

Full-grown human hair is divided into two principal parts: the hair root and hair shaft.

1. The **hair root** is that portion of the hair found beneath the skin surface. This is the portion of the hair enclosed within the follicle.
2. The **hair shaft** is that portion of the hair extending above the skin surface.

Structures Associated with the Hair Root

Structures closely associated with the hair root are the hair follicle, hair bulb, and hair papilla. (Fig. 6.7)

The **hair follicle** (FOL-i-kel) is a tube-like depression or pocket in the skin or scalp encasing the **hair root**. The bottom of this pocket contains a finger-like projection called the **papilla** (pa-PIL-ah), from which the new hair develops. One or more oil glands are attached to each hair follicle. Follicles vary in depth, depending upon the thickness and location of the skin. There is a follicle for every hair. The funnel-shaped mouths of hair follicles are favorite breeding places for germs, sebum, and dirt.

The follicle does not run straight down into the skin or scalp. It is set at an angle so that the hair above the surface has a natural flow to one side. This natural flow is sometimes called the **hair stream**. Since the angles run according to set areas, hair emerges from the scalp slanting naturally in a particular given direction.

The **hair bulb** is a thickened, club-shaped structure forming the lower part of the hair root. The lower part of the hair bulb is hollow. It fits over and covers the hair papilla.

The **hair papilla** is a small, cone-shaped elevation at the bottom of the hair follicle that fits into the hair bulb. Within the hair papilla is a rich blood and nerve supply, which contributes to the growth and regeneration of the hair. It is through the papilla that nourishment reaches the hair bulb. As long as the papilla is healthy and well nourished, it produces hair cells that enable new hair to grow.

Structures Connected to Hair Follicles

The **arrector pili** (a-REK-tohr PIGH-ligh) is a small involuntary muscle attached to the underside of a hair follicle. Fear or cold contracts it, causing the hair to stand up straight, and giving the skin the appearance of *goose flesh*. Eyelash and eyebrow hairs lack arrector pili muscles.

Sebaceous (si-BAY-shus) or oil glands consist of little sack-like structures located in the dermis. Their ducts are connected to hair follicles. They secrete an oily substance, **sebum** (SEE-bum), which gives luster and pliability to the hair and keeps the skin surface soft and supple. However, the sebaceous glands frequently become troublemakers. By over-producing sebum, they bring on a common form of oily dandruff and can be a contributing cause of hair loss or baldness.

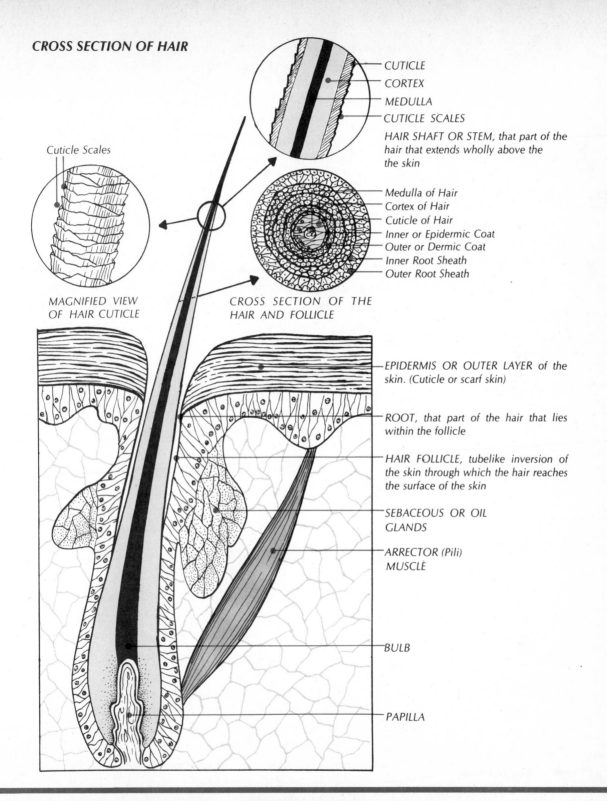

CROSS SECTION OF HAIR

CUTICLE
CORTEX
MEDULLA
CUTICLE SCALES

HAIR SHAFT OR STEM; that part of the hair that extends wholly above the the skin

Medulla of Hair
Cortex of Hair
Cuticle of Hair
Inner or Epidermic Coat
Outer or Dermic Coat
Inner Root Sheath
Outer Root Sheath

Cuticle Scales

MAGNIFIED VIEW
OF HAIR CUTICLE

CROSS SECTION OF THE
HAIR AND FOLLICLE

EPIDERMIS OR OUTER LAYER of the skin. (Cuticle or scarf skin)

ROOT, that part of the hair that lies within the follicle

HAIR FOLLICLE, tubelike inversion of the skin through which the hair reaches the surface of the skin

SEBACEOUS OR OIL
GLANDS

ARRECTOR (Pili)
MUSCLE

BULB

PAPILLA

6.7 – Cross section of hair

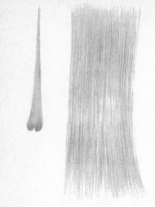

Straight hair

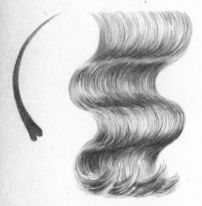

Wavy hair

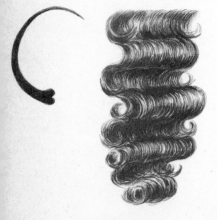

Curly hair

6.8 – Three general hair shapes

The production of sebum is influenced by five factors, some of which are subject to personal control:

1. diet
2. blood circulation
3. emotional disturbance
4. stimulation of endocrine glands
5. drugs

Diet influences the general health of the hair. Overindulgence in sweet, starchy, and fatty foods may cause the sebaceous glands to become overactive and secrete too much sebum.

The hair derives its nourishment from the blood supply, which in turn depends upon the foods eaten for certain elements. In the absence of necessary food elements, the health of the hair declines.

Emotional disturbances are linked with health of the hair through the nervous system. The hair's condition is affected by stress. Healthy hair is an indication of a healthy body.

Endocrine (EN-do-krin) **glands** are ductless glands. Their secretions go directly into the bloodstream, which in turn influences the welfare of the entire body. The condition of the endocrine glands influences their secretion. During adolescence, they become very active. Their activity usually decreases after middle age. Endocrine gland disturbances influence the hair, as well as other aspects of health.

Drugs such as the hormones may adversely affect the hair.

Hair Shapes

As a rule, hair has one of three general shapes. The hair as it grows out assumes the shape, size, and direction of the follicle. (Fig. 6.8) A cross-sectional view of the hair under the microscope reveals that usually:

1. Straight hair is round.
2. Wavy hair is oval.
3. Curly or kinky hair is almost flat.

There is no strict rule regarding cross-sectional shapes of hair. Wavy, straight, or curly hair has been found in all shapes.

Layers of the Hair

The structure of the hair is composed of cells, arranged in three layers:

1. **Cuticle (KYOO**-ti-kel), the **outside horny layer,** is composed of transparent, overlapping, protective, scale-like cells which point away from the scalp, toward the hair ends. Chemical solutions raise these scales so that solutions can be absorbed by the hair shaft.
2. **Cortex (KOR**-teks), the **middle** or **inner layer,** provides strength and elasticity. It is made up of a fibrous substance formed by elongated cells. This layer contains the pigment that gives the hair its color.
3. **Medulla** (mi-**DUL**-ah), the **innermost layer,** is referred to as the pith or marrow of the hair shaft, and is composed of round cells. The medulla may be absent in fine and very fine hair.

Hair Distribution

Hair is found all over the body except on the palms, soles, lips, and eyelids. It forms a cushion for the head.

There are three types of hair on the body:

1. Long hair grows from the scalp, protects it against the sun and injury, adorns the head, and frames the face. Soft, long hair also grows in the armpits of both sexes, and on men's faces.
2. Short or bristly hair, such as the eyebrows and eyelashes, enhances the appearance of the face. Eyebrows divert sweat from the eyes. The eyelashes help protect the eyes from foreign bodies and light.
3. **Lanugo** (lah-**NOO**-goh) **hair** is the fine, soft, downy hair found on cheeks, forehead, and nearly all areas of the body. It helps in the efficient evaporation of perspiration.

Hair Growth

If hair is normal and healthy, each individual strand goes through a cycle of events: **growth, fall,** and **replacement.**

The formation and growth of hair cells depend upon proper nourishment and oxygen which only the bloodstream can supply. Therefore, the function of blood is indispensable to the health and life of hair.

When the body is healthy, hair flourishes. If the body is ill, hair papilla weaken. When the bloodstream provides hair with food, it grows long and strong. If inadequately nourished, it becomes weak, and eventually hair loss occurs.

The average growth of healthy hair on the scalp is about one-half inch per month. The rate of growth will differ on specific parts of the body, between sexes, among races, and with age. Scalp hair will also differ among individuals in strength, elasticity, and waviness.

The growth of scalp hair occurs more rapidly between the ages of 15 and 30, and declines sharply between 50 and 60. Scalp hair grows faster in women than in men. Hair growth is also influenced by such factors as the seasons of the year, nutrition, and hormonal changes.

Climatic conditions will affect the hair in the following ways:

1. Moisture in the air will deepen the natural wave.
2. Cold air will cause the hair to contract.
3. Heat will cause the hair to swell or expand, and absorb moisture.

Hair growth is not increased by any of the following:

1. Close clipping, shaving, trimming, cutting, or singeing.
2. The application of ointments or oils. They act as lubricants to the hair shaft, but do not feed the hair.
3. Hair does not grow after death. The flesh and skin contract, thus giving the appearance of some growth.

Normal Hair Shedding

A certain amount of hair is shed daily, thus making room for new hair, at an average rate of 50 to 80 hairs per day. Hair loss beyond this estimated average indicates some problem.

Eyebrow hairs and eyelashes are replaced every four to five months.

Definitions of Directional Hair Growth

Hair stream. Hair that slopes in the same direction is known as a hair stream. It is caused by the follicles being arranged in a uniform manner. When two such streams slope in opposite directions, they form a natural part.

Whorl. Hair that forms a swirl, as at the crown, is called a whorl.

Cowlick. Tufts of hair standing up are known as cowlicks. They are noticeable most often at the front hairline. However, they may be located in other areas. Cowlicks must be considered when choosing styles, to minimize their effects.

Replacement of Hair

Material necessary for hair growth comes from the papilla. As long as the papilla is not destroyed, the hair will grow. If the hair is pulled out at the root, it will grow again. Should the papilla be destroyed, however, the hair will not be replaced.

In human beings, new hair replaces old hair in the following ways:

1. The bulb loosens and separates from the papilla.
2. The bulb moves upward in the follicle.
3. The hair moves slowly to the surface, where it is shed.
4. The new hair is formed by cell division from a growing point at the root around the papilla. (Figs. 6.9 and 6.10)

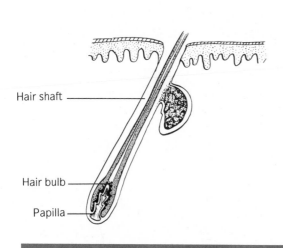

Hair shaft

Hair bulb

Papilla

6.9 – At an early stage of shedding, the hair shows its separation from the papilla.

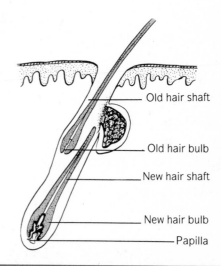

Old hair shaft

Old hair bulb

New hair shaft

New hair bulb

Papilla

6.10 – At a later stage of the hair shedding, you will note a new hair growing from the same papilla.

Life and Density of Hair

The exact life span of hair is not known, but it seems to average from two to four years. Some authorities estimate its life span as up to seven years. Factors such as sex, age, type of hair, heredity, and health have a bearing on the duration of hair life.

The average area of the head is about 120 square inches. There are an average of 1,000 hairs to a square inch.

The number of hairs on the head varies with the color of the hair: blond, 140,000; brown, 110,000; black, 108,000; red, 90,000.

Hair Color

The natural color of hair, its strength and texture, depend mainly on hereditary factors. The color, an inherited characteristic, is one that is easy to observe and classify. To be successful in coloring hair, the barber-stylist should understand the color and distribution of hair pigmentation, as well as hair texture, porosity, and elasticity.

The cortex of the hair contains coloring matter, minute grains of melanin, or pigment. Although there is some disagreement, the derivation of pigment is probably from color-forming substances in the blood. The color of the hair, light or dark, depends upon the color and amount of the grains of pigment it contains.

An **albino** (al-**BEYE**-no) is a person born with white hair, the result of an absence of pigment in the hair shaft, accompanied by no marked pigmentation in the skin or iris of the eyes.

Graying of Hair

Canities (ka-**NISH**-ee-eez), or gray hair, is due mainly to the absence of hair pigment in the cortical layer. Gray hair is really mottled hair—spots of white or whitish-yellow scattered about in the hair shafts. Normally, gray hair grows out in this condition from the hair bulb. Graying does not take place after the hair has grown.

In most cases, gray hair is a result of the natural aging process. It is not related to the hair's texture or growth. Graying can also occur as a result of serious illness or emotional shock.

Premature grayness is usually due to a defect in pigment formation occurring at birth. Often it will be found that several members of the same family are affected with premature grayness.

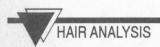

HAIR ANALYSIS

Because barber-styling services include coloring and styling hair, it is essential to be able to recognize the client's hair texture, hair porosity, and hair elasticity. It is of utmost importance to be able to recognize and distinguish the various types and conditions of hair.

Condition of the Hair

Knowledge and skill in determining hair condition can be acquired by observation and practice, using the senses of sight, touch, hearing, and smell.

1. **Sight.** Observation will impart some knowledge immediately. However, sight alone cannot allow accurate judgment of hair quality. The sense of sight comprises approximately 15 percent of the process of hair analysis.
2. **Touch.** This is the final determining factor in analyzing hair condition. Without developing this sense to its fullest capacity, the barber-stylist cannot provide truly professional services.
3. **Hearing.** Some clients like to talk about their hair, health problems, their hair's reaction to applied lotions, and its reaction to certain medications. Since all of these factors are important when deciding how to treat the hair, it is advisable to listen carefully.
4. **Smell.** Uncleanliness and certain scalp disorders will create an odor. If the client is in good health generally, and the scalp is clean, the hair will be odor-free.

Qualities of the Hair

Qualities by which hair is analyzed are texture, porosity, and elasticity.

Texture

Hair texture refers to the degree of coarseness or fineness of hair, which varies on different parts of the head. Variations in hair texture are due to:

1. **Diameter of the hair**, whether coarse, medium, fine, or very fine. Coarse hair has the widest diameter and very fine hair has the narrowest.
2. **Feel of the hair**—harsh, soft, or wiry.

Coarse hair contains three layers: the medulla, cortex, and cuticle. Usually the scales on the outside layer are closely overlapped and raised away from the hair shaft, which is the reason that coarse hair readily absorbs water.

Medium textured hair is the most common type. The medulla, cortex, and cuticle layers are present to a lesser degree than in coarse hair. This type of hair does not present any unusual problem.

Fine or very fine hair requires special care. A microscopic study of its structure reveals that only two layers, the cortex and cuticle, are present.

Wiry hair, whether coarse, medium, or fine, has a hard, glassy finish because the cuticle scales lie flat against the hair shaft. It takes longer to give this type of hair a coloring treatment.

Porosity

Hair porosity (po-**ROS**-i-tee) is the ability of hair of any texture to absorb moisture. In hair with **good porosity**, the cuticle layer is raised from the hair shaft. Hair of this type is fairly absorbent.

Hair with **moderate porosity** (normal hair) is less porous than hair with good porosity. Usually hair with good or moderate porosity presents no special problems for the barber-stylist.

In hair with **poor porosity** (resistant hair) the cuticle layer lies close to the hair shaft. This type of hair absorbs the least amount of moisture. Hair with poor porosity requires thorough analysis and strand tests before the application of any chemical.

Hair that is in **poor condition** or **extremely porous** often has been damaged by continuous or faulty treatments. This hair absorbs liquids very easily and quickly, and requires special care.

Elasticity

Hair elasticity (e-las-**TIS**-i-tee) is the ability of the hair to stretch and return to its original form without breaking. Hair with normal elasticity is springy and has a live and lustrous appearance. Normal hair is capable of being stretched about one-fifth its length and will spring back when released. However, wet hair can be stretched 40 to 50 percent of its length. Porous hair will stretch more than hair with poor porosity. Hair is classified as having good, normal, or poor elasticity.

DISORDERS OF THE SKIN, SCALP, AND HAIR

The following section has been compiled to familiarize the barber-stylist with certain common skin, scalp, and hair disorders. The barber-stylist must be able to recognize certain skin conditions and should know how to deal with them properly. Some skin and scalp disorders may be treated in cooperation with, and under the supervision of a physician. Treatments for scalp, skin, or hair disorders requiring a prescription may be applied only as prescribed, and with the permission of a physician. Any condition that the practitioner does not recognize with assurance as positively one that can be treated properly and safely in the barber-styling shop should be referred tactfully, but firmly, to a physician.

Most important, no person with an infectious or contagious skin disorder should be served in the barber-styling shop. The barber-stylist should be able to recognize such conditions and suggest that the affected person seek appropriate medical treatment. By doing so, the barber-stylist safeguards personal and public health.

Definitions Pertaining to Disease

Before describing the specific diseases of the skin and scalp so they will be recognized by the barber-stylist, it is important to understand what is meant by disease.

A **disease** is any departure from a normal state of health. An **acute disease** is one with symptoms of a more or less violent character and of short duration. A **chronic (KRON-ick) disease** may be mild, but is long-lasting or recurring.

An **infectious (in-FEK-shus) disease** is caused by a pathogenic microorganism or virus (see chapter 3, Bacteriology) which can be spread by contact with a lesion or contaminated object. A **contagious (kon-TAY-jus) disease** is one that is readily spread to other persons by contact.

> **NOTE:** The terms infectious disease, **communicable** (kuh-MEW-ni-kuh-bul) disease, and contagious disease are often used interchangeably.

A **skin disease** is usually characterized by skin lesions that may take the form of scales, pimples, or pustules.

A **congenital (kun-JEN-i-tul) disease** is one that is present at birth.

A **seasonal disease** is one that is influenced by the weather or seasonal changes.

An **occupational disease** is caused by exposure to substances used in certain types of employment.

A **parasitic (par-uh-SIT-ick) disease** is caused by vegetable or animal parasites such as for lice, scabies, or ringworm.

A **pathogenic (path-uh-JEN-ick) disease** is produced by bacteria.

A **systemic (sis-TEM-ick) disease** is one that affects the entire body. It can be caused by viruses or bacteria, or a number of other agents.

A **venereal** (ve-**NEER**-ee-ul) **disease**, such as syphilis or gonorrhea, is a contagious disease commonly acquired by contact with an infected person during sexual intercourse.

An **epidemic** (ep-i-**DEM**-ick) is the occurrence of a particular disease simultaneously attacking a large number of persons living in a particular locality.

An **allergy** (**AL**-ur-jee) is a sensitivity to normally harmless substances. Skin allergies are quite common. Contact with certain types of cosmetics, medicines, and tints, or eating certain foods may cause an allergic reaction—often an itching eruption, accompanied by redness, swelling, blisters, oozing, or scaling.

An **inflammation** (in-fluh-**MAY**-shun) is characterized by redness, pain, swelling, and heat.

> CAUTION: To avoid the transmission of disease in the barber-styling shop, be sure to practice sanitation and sanitization at all times.

Pigmentations of the Skin

In abnormal conditions, **pigment** (**PIG**-munt) may come from inside or outside the body. Abnormal colors are seen in every skin disease and in many systemic disorders. Pigmentation due to foreign substances is observed when certain drugs are being taken internally.

Tan is caused by excessive exposure to the sun.

Freckles (**lentigines**—len-ti-**JEE**-neez), (singular, **lentigo**) are small, light brown spots appearing on those parts of the body exposed to sunlight, principally the face, hands, and arms.

Stains are abnormal brown skin patches having a generally circular, somewhat irregular shape. Their color is due to the presence of blood pigment. They occur during aging, after certain diseases, and after the disappearance of moles, freckles, and liver spots. The cause of these stains is unknown.

Liver spots (**chloasma**—kloh-**AZ**-mah) are caused by increased deposits of pigment in the skin. They are found mainly on the forehead, nose, and cheeks.

Birthmarks (**naevus**—**NEE**-vus) are malformations of the skin due to pigmentation or dilated capillaries. They vary widely in size and appearance.

Leucoderma (loo-ko-DUR-mah) refers to abnormal white patches due to congenital pigmentation defects. They are classified as follows:

1. **Vitiligo** (vit-i-LEYE-goh) is an acquired condition affecting skin or hair. There is no treatment except the application of a matching cosmetic color.
2. **Albinism** (AL-bi-niz-em) is a congenital absence of melanin pigments in the body, including the skin, hair, and eyes. This condition may be partial or complete. The hair is silky and white, or pale yellow. The skin is pinkish-white, and will not tan.

Lesions of the Skin

A lesion is a structural change in the tissues caused by injury or disease. There are three types: primary, secondary, and tertiary. The barber-stylist is concerned only with primary and secondary lesions. (Fig. 6.11)

Symptoms (SIMP-tums) are signs of disease. Symptoms of skin disorders generally are divided into two groups. **Subjective** (sub-JECK-tiv) symptoms can be felt by the patient, such as in itching,

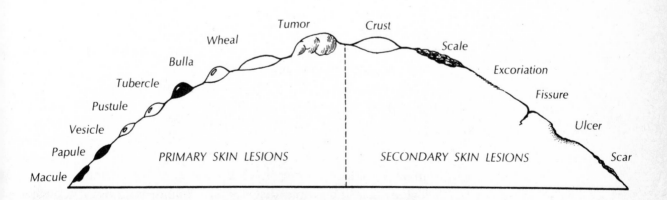

6.11 – Primary and secondary skin lesions.

burning, or hurting. **Objective** (ub-JECK-tiv) symptoms can be observed—for instance, pimples or boils.

Primary Lesions

A **macule** (**MAK**-ul) is a small, discolored spot or patch on the surface of the skin. It is neither raised nor sunken.

A **papule** (**PAP**-yool) is a small, elevated pimple containing no fluid, but which may develop pus.

A **wheal** (**WHEEL**) is an itchy, swollen lesion that lasts only a few hours. Hives and insect bites are examples of wheals.

A **tubercle** (**TOO**-ber-kel) is a solid lump larger than a papule. It projects above the surface or lies within or under the skin. It varies in size from a pea to a hickory nut. An example of a tubercle is a thick scar, usually caused by a healed injury or previous infection.

A **tumor** (**TOO**-mohr) is an abnormal cell mass varying in size, shape, and color. **Nodules** are also referred to as tumors, but they are smaller.

A **vesicle** (**VES**-i-kel) is a blister with clear fluid in it. Vesicles lie within or just beneath the epidermis. Poison ivy produces small vesicles.

A **bulla** (**BYOO**-lah) is a blister containing a watery fluid, similar to a vesicle, but larger.

A **pustule** (**PUS**-chool) is an elevation of the skin having an inflamed base and containing pus, such as the common pimple.

Secondary Lesions

Secondary lesions are those that develop in the later stages of disease.

A **scale** (**SKAIL**) is an accumulation of dry or greasy flakes, such as abnormal or excessive dandruff.

A **crust** or **scab** is a dried accumulation of sebum and pus.

An **abrasion** (uh-**BRAY**-zhun) is a skin sore produced by scratching or scraping. The skin's surface becomes raw due to the loss of superficial skin after an injury.

A **fissure** (**FISH**-ur) is a crack in the skin penetrating into the derma, such as chapped hands or lips.

An **ulcer** (**UL**-cer) is an open lesion on the skin or mucous membrane of the body, accompanied by pus and loss of skin depth.

A **scar** or **cicatrix** (**SIK**-a-triks) is likely to form after the healing of an injury or skin condition that has penetrated the derma.

A **stain** is an abnormal discoloration remaining after the disappearance of moles, freckles, or liver spots. Sometimes stains are a result of previous diseases.

Hypertrophies (New Growths)

A **callous** (**keratoma**—ker-a-**TAH**-ma) is a superficial, thickened patch of skin occurring, for the most part, in regions subject to friction such as the hands and feet.

A **mole** is a small, brownish spot or blemish on the skin. Some moles are believed to be inherited. They range in color from pale tan to brown, or bluish black. Some are small and flat, resembling freckles, while others are more deeply seated and darker in color. Large, dark hairs often grow in moles. If a mole grows in size, gets darker, or becomes sore or scaly, medical attention is needed.

> CAUTION: Do not treat or remove hair from moles.

Verruca (ve-**ROO**-kah) is the technical term for a **wart**. It is caused by a virus and is infectious. It can spread from one location to another, particularly along a scratch in the skin.

Inflammations

Dermatitis (dur-mah-**TEYE**-tis) is a general term for an inflammation of the skin. The lesions may appear in various forms, such as vesicles or papules.

Eczema (**EK**-se-mah) is an inflammation of the skin of acute or chronic nature, presenting many forms of dry or moist lesions. It is frequently accompanied by itching or burning. All cases of eczema should be referred to a physician for treatment. Its cause is unknown.

Psoriasis (so-**REYE**-a-sis) is a chronic, inflammatory skin disease, the cause of which is unknown. It is usually found on the scalp, elbows, knees, chest, and lower back, rarely on the face. The lesions are round, dry patches covered with coarse, silvery scales. If irritated, bleeding points occur. It is not contagious.

Fever blisters (**herpes simplex**—**HUR**-peez **SIM**-pleks) are caused by a viral infection. They appear as vesicles with red, swollen bases. The blisters usually appear on the lips, nostrils,

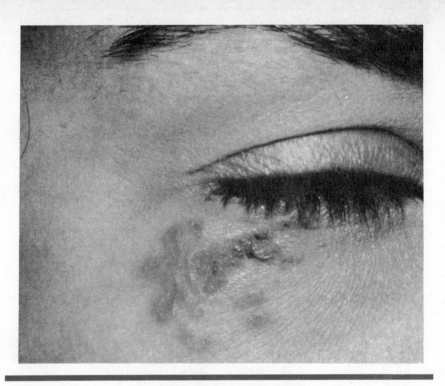

6.12 – Herpes simplex, or fever blisters

or other part of the face, and rarely last more than a week. (Fig. 6.12)

Anthrax (**AN**-thraks) is an inflammatory skin disorder. It can be spread, among other ways, by the use of an infected shaving brush. It is characterized by the presence of a small, red papule, followed by the formation of a pustule, vesicle, and hard swelling. It is accompanied by itching and burning at the point of infection. It is contagious.

Ivy dermatitis is a skin inflammation caused by exposure to the poison ivy, poison oak, or poison sumac leaves. Blisters and itching develop soon after contact occurs. The condition can be spread to other parts of the body by contact with contaminated hands, clothing, objects, and anything that was exposed to the plant itself. It also can be spread from one person to another by direct contact. Serious cases should be referred to a physician.

Occupational disorders in barber-styling refer to abnormal conditions resulting from contact with chemicals or tints. Certain ingredients in cosmetics, antiseptics, and aniline derivative tints may cause eruptive skin infections known as **dermatitis venenata** (**VEN-**e-na-tah). It is important that barber-stylists use rubber gloves or protective creams, whenever possible.

Alopecia

Alopecia (al-oh-**PEE**-shee-ah) is the technical term for any abnormal hair loss. The natural loss of hair should not be confused with alopecia. When hair has grown to its full length, it comes out and is replaced by a new hair. This natural shedding occurs most frequently in spring and fall. On the other hand, the hair lost in alopecia does not come back unless special treatments are given to encourage hair growth.

Alopecia senilis (se-**NIL**-is) is baldness occurring in old age. The loss of hair is permanent.

Alopecia prematura (pre-mah-**CHUR**-ah) is baldness beginning any time before middle age. It occurs by a slow, thinning process, and is due to hairs that fall out being replaced by weaker ones.

Alopecia areata (air-ee-**AH**-tah) is the loss of hair in round patches, or bald spots. It can be caused by anemia, scarlet fever, typhoid fever, or syphilis. Affected areas are slightly depressed, smooth, and very pale due to the decreased blood supply. Patches may be round or irregular, and vary in size from one-half inch to two or three inches in diameter. In most cases of alopecia areata, there has been injury to the nervous system. Since the flow of blood is influenced by the nervous system, the affected area is usually poorly nourished as well.

Alopecia may appear in different forms, resulting from a variety of abnormal conditions. Sometimes alopecia can be treated successfully by proper scalp treatments. (Fig. 6.13)

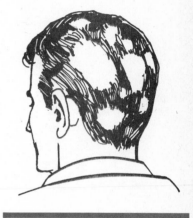

6.13 – Alopecia areata

Disorders of the Sebaceous (Oil) Glands

There are several common diseases of the sebaceous glands that the barber-stylist should be able to identify and understand.

Comedones (**KOM**-e-donz), or **blackheads**, are a mass of hardened sebum appearing most frequently on the face, forehead, and nose.

Blackheads accompanied by pimples often occur in youths between the ages of 13 and 20. During adolescence the activity of the sebaceous glands is stimulated, thereby contributing to the formation of blackheads and pimples. When the hair follicle is filled with excess oil from the sebaceous gland, a blackhead forms and creates a blockage at the mouth of the follicle. (Fig. 6.14) This causes irritation and may result

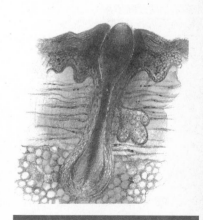

6.14 – Blackhead (plug of sebaceous matter and dirt) forming around the mouth of hair follicle

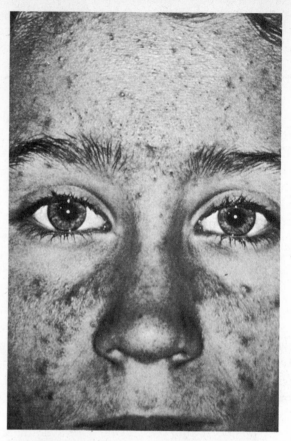

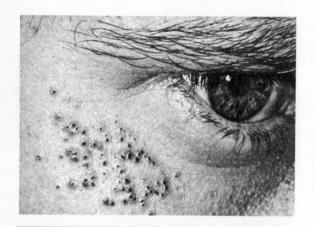

6.15 – A cluster of comedones in the eye area (Reprinted from *Acne Morphogenesis and Treatment* by Gerd Plewig, MD and Albert M. Klingman, MD, Ph.D; permission of Publishers, Springer-Verlag, New York, U.S.A., Heidelberg, Berlin, Germany.)

6.16 – Acne in the young (Reprinted from *Acne Morphogenesis and Treatment* by Gerd Plewig, MD and Albert M. Klingman, MD, Ph.D; permission of Publishers, Springer-Verlag, New York, U.S.A., Heidelberg, Berlin, Germany.)

in an inflamed pimple filled with pus. Such a lesion is known as acne. (Figs. 6.15, 6.16)

The treatment for blackheads is to reduce the skin's oiliness by local applications of cleansers, and the removal of blackheads under sterile conditions. Thorough skin cleansing each night is very important. Cleansing creams and lotions often achieve better results than common soap and water. Should this condition become severe, medical attention is necessary.

Milia (MIL-ee-uh), or **whiteheads**, is a disorder of the sebaceous glands caused by the accumulation of sebaceous matter beneath the

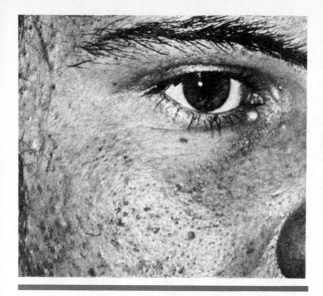

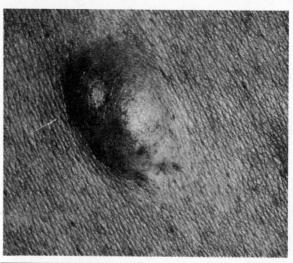

6.17 – Combination of milia and comedones (Reprinted from *Acne Morphogenesis and Treatment* **by Gerd Plewig, MD and Albert M. Klingman, MD, Ph.D; permission of Publishers, Springer-Verlag, New York, U.S.A., Heidelberg, Berlin, Germany.)**

6.18 – A cyst (Reprinted from *Acne Morphogenesis and Treatment* **by Gerd Plewig, MD and Albert M. Klingman, MD, Ph.D; permission of Publishers, Springer-Verlag, New York, U.S.A., Heidelberg, Berlin, Germany.)**

skin. This may occur on any part of the face and neck, and occasionally on the chest and shoulders. Whiteheads are often associated with dry skin types. (Fig. 6.17)

Steatoma (stee-ah-**TOH**-mah), or **sebaceous cyst**, is a subcutaneous tumor of the sebaceous glands, the contents consisting of **sebum** (**SEE**-bum). The tumors range in size from that of a pea to that of an orange, and usually occur on the scalp, neck, and back. A steatoma is sometimes called a **wen**. (Fig. 6.18)

Asteatosis (as-tee-ah-**TOH**-sis) is a condition of dry, scaly skin, characterized by absolute or partial deficiency of sebum, due either to senile (**SEE**-nile) (old age) changes or some bodily disorders. It may also be caused by exposure to alkalies, such as are found in soaps and washing powders.

Seborrhea (seb-o-**REE**-ah) is a skin condition due to over-activity and excessive secretion of the sebaceous glands. An itching or burning sensation may accompany it. An oily or shiny nose, forehead, or scalp indicates the presence of seborrhea. On the scalp, it is readily detected by the presence of an unusual amount of oil on the hair.

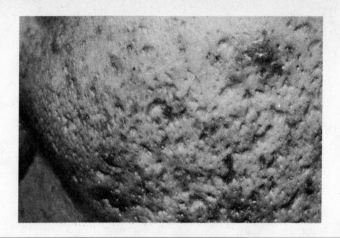

6.19 – Crater-like depressions and pits are characteristic of facial scarring in severe acne (Reprinted from *Acne Morphogenesis and Treatment* by Gerd Plewig, MD and Albert M. Klingman, MD, Ph.D; permission of Publishers, Springer-Verlag, New York, U.S.A., Heidelberg, Berlin, Germany.)

Acne (**AK**-nee) is a chronic inflammatory disease of the sebaceous glands, occurring most frequently on the face, back, and chest. The cause of acne is generally held to be **microbic** (migh-**KRO**-bick), but predisposing factors are adolescence and disturbances of the digestive tract.

Acne appears in a variety of types, ranging from the simple (non-contagious) pimple to serious, deep-seated skin conditions. It is always advisable to seek diagnosis and treatment by a competent physician before any facial service is given in the barber-styling shop. (Fig. 6.19)

Acne rosacea (ro-**ZA**-se-a) is a chronic, inflammatory congestion of the cheeks and nose. It is characterized by redness, dilation of the blood vessels, and the formation of papules and pustules. (Figs. 6.20, 6.21) The cause of rosacea is unknown. Certain things are known to aggravate rosacea in some individuals. These include consumption of hot liquids, spicy foods, or alcohol; being exposed to extremes of heat and cold; exposure to sunlight; and stress.

The first stage starts with a slight pinkness all over the face, varying with the temperature and the temperament of the individual.

The second stage affects the **capillaries**. Often they become so dilated that they are apparent to the naked eye. At this stage the sebaceous glands are affected. Large pores, oiliness, and comedones invariably result.

The third stage is very disfiguring. The entire face becomes congested, and the condition may remain chronic, although dormant for years.

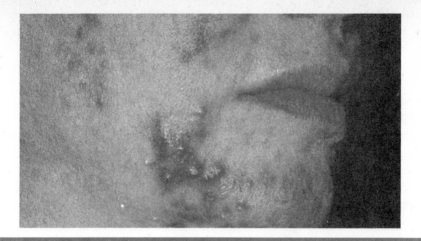

6.20 – Acne rosacea

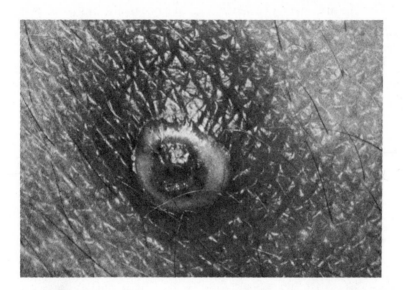

6.21 – A pustule (Reprinted from *Acne Morphogenesis and Treatment* by Gerd Plewig, MD and Albert M. Klingman, MD, Ph.D; permission of Publishers, Springer-Verlag, New York, U.S.A., Heidelberg, Berlin, Germany.)

Disorders of the Sudoriferous (Sweat) Glands

Bromidrosis (broh-mi-**DROH**-sis), or **osmidrosis** (ah-smi-**DROH**-sis), refers to foul-smelling perspiration, usually noticeable in the armpits or on the feet.

Anidrosis (an-i-**DROH**-sis), or lack of perspiration, is often a result of fever, or certain skin diseases. It requires medical attention.

Hyperidrosis (heye-per-heye-**DROH**-sis), or excessive perspiration, is caused by excessive heat or general body weakness. The parts of the body most commonly affected are the armpits, joints, and feet. It requires medical treatment.

Miliaria rubra (mil-ee-**AY**-ree-ah **ROOB**-rah), (prickly heat), is an acute inflammatory disorder of the sweat glands characterized by the eruption of small, red vesicles, accompanied by burning and itching of the skin. It is caused by exposure to excessive heat and obesity.

Dandruff

Dandruff (**DAN**-druf) is the presence of small, white scales, usually on the scalp and hair. Dandruff is also known by the medical term of **pityriasis** (pit-i-**REYE**-ah-sis). Just as the skin is being shed and replaced continually, the uppermost layer of the scalp is being cast off. Ordinarily, these horny scales are loose, and fall off freely. Their natural shedding should not be mistaken for dandruff. Long-neglected dandruff frequently leads to baldness. (Fig. 6.22)

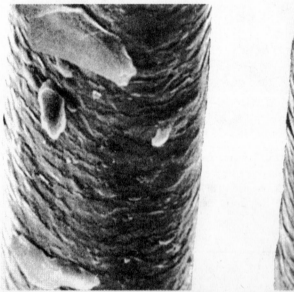
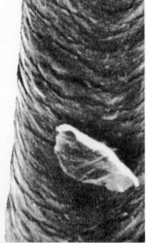

6.22 – Normal hair with dandruff flakes adhering to hair fibers (Courtesy: Gillette Company Research Institute)

Dandruff is caused by:

1. the excessive shedding of the **epithelial** (ep-i-**THEEL**-ee-ul) scales—instead of growing to the surface and falling off, the horny scales accumulate on the scalp; or,
2. a sluggish condition of the scalp caused by poor circulation, infection, injury, lack of nerve stimulation, improper diet, or uncleanliness. Contributing causes are the use of strong shampoos and rinsing the hair incompletely after a shampoo.

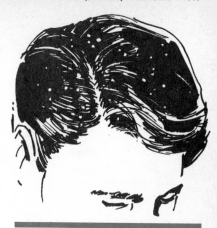

6.23 – Dry dandruff

The two principal types of dandruff are:

1. **Dry dandruff** (pityriasis capitis—**KAP**-i-tis)
2. **Greasy (waxy) dandruff** (pityriasis steatoides—ste-a-**TOY**-dez)

Dry dandruff is characterized by an itchy scalp and small, white scales, usually attached in masses to the scalp or scattered loosely in the hair. Occasionally, they are so profuse that they fall to the shoulders. (Fig. 6.23)

Treatment for dry dandruff includes frequent scalp treatments and mild shampoos, regular scalp massage, daily use of antiseptic scalp lotions, applications of scalp ointment, and electrical treatments.

Greasy (waxy) dandruff is scaliness of the epidermis, mixed with sebum which causes it to stick to the scalp in patches. The associated itchiness causes the person to scratch the scalp. If the greasy scales are torn off, bleeding or oozing of sebum may follow. Medical treatment is advisable. (Fig. 6.24)

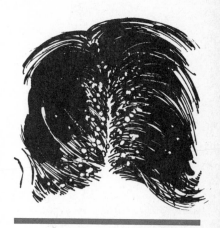

6.24 – Greasy (waxy) dandruff

CAUTION: The nature of dandruff is not clearly defined by medical authorities. It is generally believed to be of infectious origin. Some authorities hold that it is due to a specific microbe. However, a barber-stylist should consider both forms of dandruff to be contagious and transmittable by use of common brushes, combs, and other articles. Therefore, the barber-stylist must take extreme care to sanitize everything that comes into contact with the client.

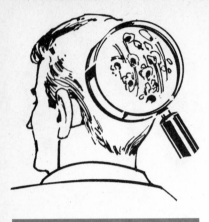

6.25 – Tinea capitis

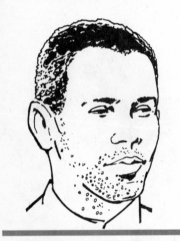

6.26 – Tinea sycosis (barber's itch)

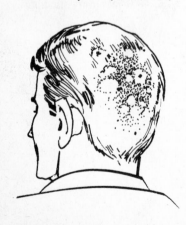

6.27 – Tinea favosa

Contagious Disorders

Common contagious disorders with which a barber-stylist may have to deal include:

1. **Ringworm**, due to **fungi** (plant or vegetable parasites)
2. **Scabies** and **head lice**, due to animal parasites
3. **Boil**, **carbuncle**, and **inflammations**, traceable to bacterial infections

Vegetable Parasitic Infections

Tinea (TIN-ee-ah) is the medical term for **ringworm**. Ringworm is caused by **vegetable parasites**. All forms are contagious. Tinea can be transmitted from one person to another. The disease is commonly passed by scales or hair containing fungi. Public showers, swimming pools, and unsanitized articles are also sources of transmission. Any case of ringworm should be referred to a physician.

Ringworm starts with a small, reddened patch of little blisters. They spread outward and heal in the middle, with scaling. Several such patches may be present.

Tinea capitis (ringworm of the scalp) is a contagious, vegetable parasitic disease characterized by red papules or spots at the opening of the hair follicles. The patches spread, the hair becomes brittle and lifeless, and breaks off leaving a stump, or falls from the enlarged, open follicles. (Fig. 6.25)

Tinea sycosis (sigh-KO-sis) (barber's itch) is a fungus infection occurring chiefly over the bearded area of the face. Beginning as small, round, slightly scaly, inflamed patches, the areas enlarge, clearing up somewhat at the center with elevation at the borders. As the parasites invade the hairs and follicles, hard, lumpy swellings develop. In severe cases, pustules form around the hair follicles and rupture, forming crusts. In the later stage, the hairs become dry, break off, and fall out, or are readily extracted. Being highly contagious, medical treatment is required. (Fig. 6.26)

Tinea favosa (fa-VO-shah) also **favus** (FA-vus) or **honeycomb ringworm** is an infectious growth caused by a vegetable parasite. It is characterized by dry, sulphur-yellow, cup-like crusts on the scalp, having a peculiar, musty odor. Scars from favus are bald patches, pink or white, and shiny. It is very contagious and should be referred to a physician. (Fig. 6.27)

Tinea unguium (UN-gwee-um) (ringworm of the nails) is a localized infectious disease. As the disease spreads, the nails thicken, become brittle, and lose their natural shape. It is very contagious. (Fig. 6.28)

Ringworm (tinea) of the foot or **athlete's foot** is a localized infectious disease. The inflamed areas of the sole of the foot and between the toes show signs of redness, blisters, and cracking of the skin. Itching and excessive sweating are also present. It is very contagious. (Fig. 6.29)

Ringworm of the feet may spread and infect other parts of the body. Anyone with this infection must take special precautions to prevent its spread.

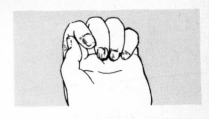

6.28 – Tinea unguium

Animal Parasitic Infections

Scabies (SKAY-beez) is a highly contagious, animal parasitic skin disease caused by the itch mite. Vesicles and pustules may form from irritation caused by the parasites, or from scratching the affected areas. Any person suffering from scabies needs medical treatment.

Pediculosis (pe-dik-yoo-LOH-sis) **capitis** is a contagious condition caused by the infestation by the head louse (animal parasite) of the hair and scalp. the parasites feed on the scalp and cause severe itching. The head louse is transmitted from one person to another by contact with personal articles of a person suffering from the condition. There are several preparations sold over the counter for treatment of head lice. However, it is best to seek the advice of a physician. Head lice are tenacious creatures that can live off of the human body for up to 48 hours. It is important, therefore, to disinfect clothing, bedclothes, furniture, etc., in order to avoid becoming reinfected. (Fig. 6.30)

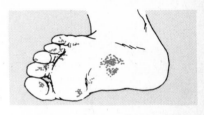

6.29 – Ringworm of the foot

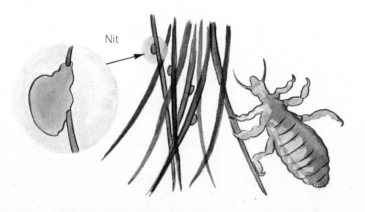

Nit

6.30 – Head louse

Bacterial Infections

Sycosis vulgaris (vul-GA-ris) is a chronic bacterial infection involving the hair follicles of the beard and mustache areas. It is transmitted by the use of unsanitized towels or implements, and can be worsened by irritation, such as shaving or a continual nasal discharge. The main lesions are papules and pustules pierced by hairs. The surrounding skin is tender, reddened, swollen at times, and tends to itch. Medical care is required. (This infection must not be confused with tinea sycosis, which is due to ringworm fungus.)

A **furuncle** (FEW-rung-kul), or **boil**, is an acute bacterial infection of a hair follicle, producing constant pain. A furuncle is the result of an active inflammatory process limited to a definite area and subsequently producing a pustule perforated by a hair. (Fig. 6.31)

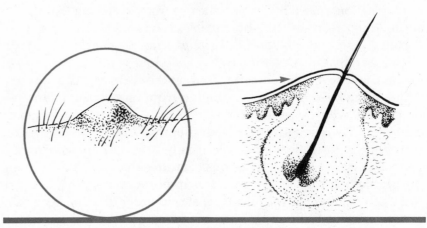

6.31 – Furuncle (boil)

A **carbuncle** (KARH-bunk-ul) is the result of an acute, deep-seated bacterial infection and is larger than a furuncle, or boil. It should be referred to a physician.

Venereal Diseases

Syphilis (SIF-i-lis) is a dangerous infectious disease. The disease germs enter the body through the skin or mucous membranes of the body by way of sexual intercourse with a person having the disease.

If there is the slightest suspicion of syphilis, it is imperative that a person seek medical treatment. Delay reduces the chances of a cure.

Only a physician is qualified to diagnose and prescribe treatment for this condition. If in doubt as to who is qualified to treat syphilis, consult your local health department.

The symptoms or signs of syphilis appear in three stages.

First stage. Several weeks after the germs enter the body, a sore usually appears at the spot where they entered. Little discomfort is experienced in early syphilis. After a few weeks, the sore heals and leaves a scar. In the meantime, the disease spreads throughout the body.

Second stage. This stage of syphilis develops about three to six weeks after the sore has appeared. As the disease progresses, the following symptoms may occur, ranging from mild to severe:

1. Skin rash
2. Sores in mouth and throat
3. Swollen glands
4. Loss of hair
5. Fever and headache

Third stage. If syphilis has not been treated and cured by the time the disease enters the third stage, damage may occur to the vital organs.

Syphilis is most infectious in the primary and secondary stages, especially when the lesions (sores and mucous patches) are located on an exposed part of the body or in the mouth.

Gonorrhea (gon-uh-**REE**-uh) is a contagious disease that generally attacks the mucous membranes covering the mouth, eyes, sex organs, and other internal body structures. Gonorrhea, like syphilis, is usually spread by sexual contact.

The first symptoms of gonorrhea usually appear from two to five days after exposure. At first, itching and burning are experienced. Shortly afterward, a discharge of pus is noticeable from the inflamed area. At this stage, gonorrhea is highly contagious.

The best assistance the barber-stylist can give is to recommend medical treatment as soon as possible. Failure to treat gonorrhea in its early stages may cause the disease to spread. Occasionally, in the later stages, gonorrhea attacks the lining of the heart, the joints, and the lining around the liver.

CAUTION: A barber-stylist infected with gonorrhea or syphilis must not work during this period because of the possibility of spreading it to other persons.

The Control of Venereal Disease

Penicillin and sulfa drugs are being used for the treatment of **venereal** (ve-**NEER**-ee-ul) diseases. Patients may now be treated in hospitals and rendered non-infectious within a short period of time. Health departments give free treatment to those who cannot afford a private doctor.

Syphilis and gonorrhea can be treated as soon as the first sign of infection is detected. If treatment is either neglected or delayed, however, the treatment may take a long time and permanent damage may occur. Only a reliable physician can safely decide which treatment is best.

The barber-stylist can make contributions to public health by:

1. Eliminating the sources of infection in the barber-styling shop.
2. Encouraging early medical treatment as needed.
3. Urging the infected person to follow the doctor's instructions.
4. Cooperating with health officials to try to control venereal diseases.

Non-Contagious Hair Disorders

Six non-contagious disorders of the hair are:

- **Grayness—canities** (ka-**NISH**-ee-eez)
- **Split hair ends—trichoptilosos** (tri-ko-ti-**LOH**-sis)
- **Superfluous hair—hypertrichosis** (hi-per-tri-**KOH**-sis)
- **Knotted hair—trichorrhexis nodosa** (**TRIK**-o-rek-sis no-**DO**-sa)
- **Brittle hair—fragilitas crinium** (frah-**JIL**-i-tas **KRI**-nee-um)
- **Beaded hair—monilethrix** (moh-**NIL**-e-thriks)

Grayness of the hair is caused by the loss of natural pigment in the hair. It may be either of two types:

1. **Congenital**—grayness exists at or before birth. It occurs in albinos and occasionally in persons with perfectly normal hair. The patchy type of congenital canities may develop slowly or rapidly, according to the cause of the condition.
2. **Acquired**—grayness may be due to the natural aging process or it may be premature. Several causes of acquired grayness are worry, anxiety, nervous strain, prolonged illness, and heredity.

Ringed hair is alternate bands of gray and dark hair.

Superfluous hair, also called **hirsuties** (hur-**SUE**-shee-eez), is an abnormal development of hair on areas of the body normally bearing only downy hair. Treatments include:

1. Dark hairs—tweeze or remove by depilatories.
2. Severe cases—remove by electrolysis, shaving, or epilation.

> CAUTION: Do not treat or remove hair from small, pigmented areas.

For split ends, treatment involves oiling the hair well to soften and lubricate it, since split ends are a result of excessive dryness. The split hair may also be removed by cutting. (Fig. 6.32)

Knotted hair is a dry, brittle condition with formation of nodular swellings along the hair shaft. The hair breaks easily and the fibers of the broken hair spread out and become brush-like. Softening hair with ointments may be beneficial. (Fig. 6.33)

Beaded hair breaks between the beads or nodes. Scalp and hair treatments may be beneficial. (Fig. 6.34)

Brittle hair may split at any part of the hair shaft. Scalp and hair treatments may be given.

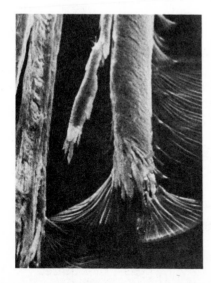
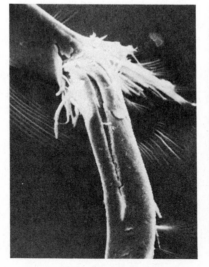
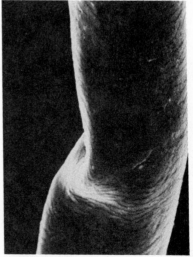

6.32 – Split hair ends   6.33 – Knotted hair   6.34 – Beaded hair

REVIEW QUESTIONS

The Skin and Scalp

1. Briefly describe healthy skin.
2. What is the appearance of a good complexion?
3. Name the two main divisions of the skin.
4. Locate the epidermis and give its main function.
5. Name the four layers of the epidermis.
6. Which epidermal layer is continually being shed and replaced?
7. Where is the coloring matter of the skin found?
8. Describe the structure of the dermis.
9. Name the two layers of the dermis.
10. What renders the skin flexible?
11. Name the four appendages of the skin.
12. How is the skin nourished?
13. Name three types of nerve fibers found in the skin.
14. Which part of the body is abundantly supplied with nerve endings?
15. To what structures in the skin are the motor nerve fibers distributed?
16. To what five things will the sensory nerves of the skin react?
17. What are the functions of the nerve fibers distributed to sweat and oil glands?
18. What regulates the temperature of the body?
19. Give an example of a complex sensation.
20. Upon what do complex sensations depend?
21. What is meant by pliability of the skin?
22. What is the characteristic of aged skin?
23. What determines the color of the skin?
24. Name one cosmetic that the skin can absorb in small amounts.
25. What are the six important functions of the skin?

Sweat and Oil Glands

1. What is a gland? Name two types of glands found in the skin.
2. Describe the structure of the sweat glands.
3. Where are the sweat glands found?
4. What is the function of the sweat glands?
5. What four things will increase the activity of the sweat glands?
6. Describe the structure of the oil glands.
7. Which substance is secreted by the oil glands?
8. What is the chief function of sebum?
9. On what parts of the body are oil glands found?

The Hair

1. Why is the study of hair important to the barber-stylist?
2. What is the technical term for the study of hair?
3. Define hair.

4. What is melanin?
5. Give the name of the protein found in the hair.
6. How is each layer of hair held together?
7. What kind of treatment may cause the hair structure to become weakened?
8. How do strongly alkaline solutions harm the hair shaft?
9. Name the two parts into which the length of the hair is divided.
10. What is the hair shaft?
11. What is the hair root?
12. What is the hair follicle?
13. What muscle and gland are attached to the hair follicle?
14. What is the hair bulb?
15. What is the hair papilla?
16. How does the hair receive its nourishment?
17. What is the function of the papilla?
18. What is meant by a hair stream?
19. What is a: a) cowlick; b) whorl?
20. The mouths of hair follicles are favorite breeding places for _____ and dirt.
21. What causes *goose pimples*?
22. What function is performed by the oil glands on the scalp?
23. List five factors that influence the production of sebum.
24. What determines the size and shape of the hair?
25. Name three general shapes of hair.
26. Name three layers found in hair.
27. Which layer is sometimes missing in hair?
28. Which hair layer contains coloring matter?
29. Which hair layer serves to protect its inner structure?
30. Which parts of the body do not contain any hair?
31. Briefly describe the appearance of lanugo hair. Where is it usually found?
32. What is the function of lanugo hair?
33. Briefly explain the hair replacement process.
34. What is meant by *hair cycle*?
35. What is the average rate of growth of hair on the head?
36. About how many square inches does an average scalp area contain?
37. List three ways in which climatic conditions will affect the hair.
38. What is the average number of hairs shed daily?
39. What is the average life span of scalp hair?
40. What causes the hair to turn gray?
41. What is an albino?
42. Name the four senses used when analyzing the hair.
43. Name the four important qualities by which hair is judged.
44. Which two senses are used to judge these qualities?

45. Define hair texture.
46. About how many hairs are there on a head of: a) blond hair; b) black hair; c) brown hair?
47. Define hair porosity.
48. Define hair elasticity.
49. To what extent can normal dry hair be stretched; wet hair be stretched?
50. Which layer of the hair gives strength and elasticity?

Disorders of the Skin, Scalp, and Hair

1. Why should the barber-stylist be able to recognize the common skin, scalp, and hair disorders?
2. Why should the barber-stylist refuse to treat a client with an infectious or contagious disease?
3. What is the purpose of studying infectious diseases of the skin, scalp, and hair?
4. Define disease.
5. What is a lesion?
6. Name eight primary lesions of the skin.
7. What is the difference between objective and subjective symptoms? Give one example of each.
8. Name seven secondary lesions of the skin.
9. a) What are scales? b) In that scalp disorder are scales present?
10. Which of the following terms apply to diseases of the sebaceous (oil) glands? Milia, acne, hypertrophies, leucoderma, comedones, seborrhea, and hyperidrosis.
11. Define acne.
12. What are the common terms for a) comedones; b) milia?
13. Briefly describe bromidrosis, anidrosis, and hyperidrosis.
14. What causes the formation of comedones?
15. Name and briefly describe the two principal types of dandruff.
16. List six conditions that may be the cause of dandruff.
17. Define dermatitis.
18. What is the characteristic appearance of psoriasis?
19. On which five parts of the body is psoriasis usually found?
20. Define alopecia.
21. What is the common term for tinea?
22. What is the cause of tinea?
23. Briefly describe ringworm.
24. What is meant by canities?
25. Briefly describe two types of canities.
26. Briefly describe trichoptilosis.
27. By what two terms is superfluous hair known?
28. By what other two terms is acne, the common pimple, known?

29. What is the medical term for a boil?
30. Name the types of bacteria that cause a boil.
31. What is the common term for pediculosis capitis?
32. Describe vitiligo.
33. Define albinism.
34. What is the common name for naevus?
35. What is the technical term for a wart?
36. What is a mole?

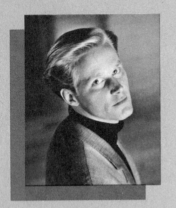

Treatment of Hair and Scalp

Learning Objectives

After completing this chapter, you should be able to:

1. *Demonstrate proper draping procedures for hair services.*
2. *Discuss the pH factor.*
3. *Discuss shampoo chemistry.*
4. *Identify the different types of shampoos, rinses, and conditioners.*
5. *Demonstrate the shampoo service.*
6. *Demonstrate scalp massage and treatments.*
7. *Discuss treatments for alopecia.*

Courtesy of: Hair: Xenon, Attractions International Creative Director. Photo: Gina Uhlmann. Makeup: James of che Seguro. Fashion styling: Donna Forst.

The comfort and protection of the client must always be considered during barber-styling services. Protection of the skin and clothing assures clients that the barber-stylist is concerned about their comfort and safety.

The method of draping chosen depends on the service being provided. Several procedures are presented in this text, although those taught by your instructor are also acceptable. Consideration for the client should be one of your highest priorities.

The following instructions are important before draping a client for any type of service:

1. Prepare materials and supplies for the service.
2. Sanitize your hands.
3. Ask the client to remove all neck and hair jewelry, and store it in a safe place.
4. Remove objects, if any, from the client's hair.
5. Turn the client's collar to the inside.
6. Proceed with the appropriate draping method.

In the following procedures the purpose of the towel or neck strip is sanitary, to prevent the cape having contact with the client's skin.

Draping for Wet Hair Services

Shampooing and Scalp and Hair Care

1. Place a towel lengthwise across the client's shoulders, crossing the ends beneath the chin. (Fig. 7.1)
2. Place a plastic cape over the towel and fasten it in the back so that the cape does not touch the client's skin. A plastic cape should be used to protect the client's skin and clothing from water or other liquids.
3. Place another towel over the cape and secure it in front.

Haircutting

For haircutting, the towel should be removed after shampooing and replaced with a neck strip. This allows the hair to fall naturally, without obstruction. Replace the plastic cape with a nylon or cotton

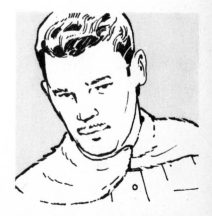

7.1 – Placing towel across client's shoulder

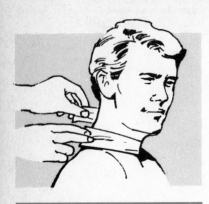

7.2 – Placing neck strip around neck; folding ends over and tucking in

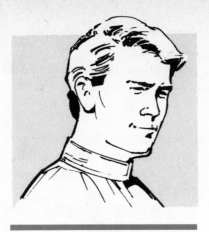

7.3 – Tieing, pinning, or attaching cape over neck strip

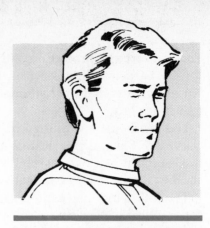

7.4 – Folding neck strip down over cape neck band. Cape should not touch the client's skin.

chair cloth, since wet hair will not adhere as easily to these fabrics. (Figs. 7.2–7.4)

Draping for Chemical Services

Hair Color, Perms, and Relaxers

1. Slide a towel down from back of client's head and place it lengthwise across the client's shoulders. (Fig. 7.5)
2. Cross the ends of the towel beneath the chin and place the cape over the towel. Fasten it in the back and adjust the towel over the cape. (Fig. 7.6)

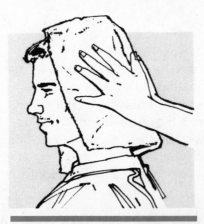

7.5 – Sliding towel down around client's neck

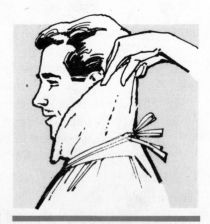

7.6 – Adjusting towel over cape

3. Fold the towel over the top of the cape and secure in front. (Fig. 7.7)
4. It is advisable to apply a protective cream around the hairline immediately prior to the application of chemicals to the hair. This helps to prevent possible skin irritation.

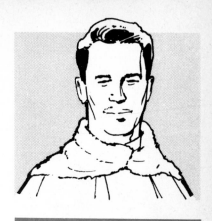

7.7 – Folding towel over cape

SHAMPOO

The primary purpose of shampooing is to clean the scalp and hair. To be effective, a shampoo must remove all dirt, oil, perspiration, and skin debris, without adversely affecting either the scalp or the hair.

The hair collects dust particles, natural oils from the sebaceous glands, perspiration, and dead skin cells which accumulate on the scalp. This accumulation creates a breeding place for disease-producing bacteria which, in turn, can lead to scalp disorders. The hair and scalp should be thoroughly shampooed as frequently as is necessary to keep them clean, healthy, and free from bacteria.

Four Requirements of a Shampoo

1. It should cleanse the hair of oils, debris, and dirt.
2. It should work efficiently in hard as well as soft water.
3. It should not irritate the eyes or skin.
4. It should leave the hair and scalp in their natural condition.

It is important that the barber-stylist knows how the shampoo cleanses the hair. However, no discussion of the action of shampoos and how they function can be meaningful unless the structure of a shampoo molecule is understood.

Shampoo Molecules

Shampoo molecules are large molecules that have been specially treated. They are composed of a head and tail, each with its own special function.

The tail of the shampoo molecule attracts dirt, grease, debris, and oil, but repels water. The head of the shampoo molecule attracts water, but repels dirt. Working together both parts of the molecule effectively cleanse the hair. (Figs. 7.8–7.11)

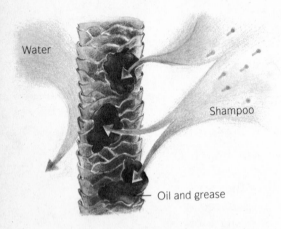

7.8 – Tail of shampoo molecules is attracted to hair, grease, and dirt.

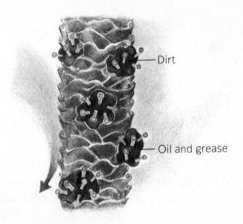

7.9 – Shampoo causes grease and oils to roll up into small globules.

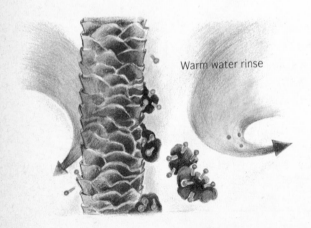

7.10 – While rinsing, shampoo heads attach to water molecules and cause debris to roll off.

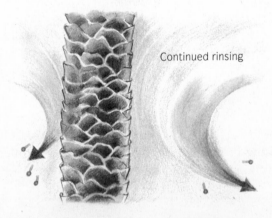

7.11 – Thorough rinsing ensures that debris and excess shampoo are washed away.

Water

For efficiency in shampooing, it is important that the barber-stylist know what type of water is available and whether the water is hard or soft.

Soft water is rain water or water that has been chemically softened, containing very small amounts of minerals. It therefore lathers freely. For this reason, it is preferred for soap shampooing.

Hard water contains certain minerals, and as a result soap shampoo does not readily lather in it. Depending on the kind of hard water available in your community, it usually can be softened by a chemical process and made suitable for shampooing.

Chemistry of Water

Water (H_2O) is the most abundant and important element on earth. It is essential to the life process. The human body is made of approximately 70 percent water, and water covers almost 75 percent of the earth's surface. Water is a solvent, meaning that it has the ability to dissolve another substance.

Water Purification

Fresh water from lakes and streams is purified by sedimentation (a treatment that causes mass to sink to the bottom) and filtration (passing through a porous substance, such as a filter paper or charcoal) to remove suspended clay, sand, and organic material. Small amounts of chlorine are then added to kill bacteria. Boiling water at a temperature of 212° fahrenheit (100° celsius) will also destroy most microbic life.

Water can be treated further by distillation, which is a process of heating water so that it becomes a vapor, then condensing the vapor so that it collects as a liquid. This process is often used in the manufacture of cosmetics.

Why is water so important in the hair care industry? Although the answer is obvious—water is used for shampooing, mixing solutions, and other functions—it is interesting to learn more about its make-up. How does water help chemical or other solutions that are used in the shop or salon? Water is made of protons and electrons (also neutrons, but here we are only concerned with protons and electrons), which are electrically charged. Protons are positive charges; electrons are negative charges. If a solid particle is added to water—for example, salt—the positive and negative charges work together to pull apart, or dissolve, the salt. The same process occurs when other solids or liquids are combined with water. Only oil and wax cannot be dissolved with water.

pH Factor

To a barber-stylist, pH is a value used to indicate the acidity or alkalinity of water-based solutions. This pH value can be measured through the use of meters and indicators. The acidity or alkalinity of cosmetic products is important because it influences how that product will affect various layers of the hair and skin. Acidic solutions (below pH 7.0) will shrink, constrict, and harden. An alkaline solution (above pH 7.0) will soften, swell, and expand.

The pH scale ranges from 0.0 to 14.0. Each increase of one indicates a tenfold increase of alkalinity and a tenfold decrease of acidity.

Acidity. Anything below pH 7.0 is acidic. The lower the pH, the greater the degree of acidity.

Alkalinity. Anything above pH 7.0 is alkaline. The higher the pH, the greater the degree of alkalinity.

Along with cosmetic ingredients, pH can be considered a means for achieving the desired results. (Fig. 7.12)

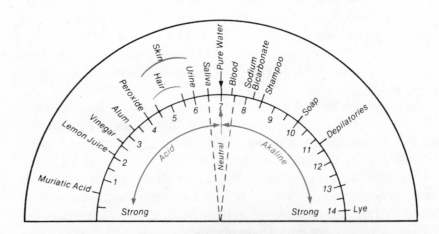

7.12 – The pH scale. The symbol is used to express the hydrogen-ion concentration of a solution, which determines the relative degree of its acidity or alkalinity. The pH scale ranges from 0 to 14. A pH of 7 represents neutrality; numbers less than 7, down to 0, represent increasing acidity, and numbers greater than 7, up to 14, represent increasing alkalinity.

Chemistry of Shampoos

To determine which shampoo will leave hair in the best condition for the intended service an understanding of the chemical ingredients of shampoos is necessary. Most shampoos have many common ingredients. It is often the small differences in formulation that make one shampoo better than another for a particular hair texture or condition.

The ingredient that most shampoos have in common (and it usually is number one on the list to show that there is more of it than any other ingredient) is water. Generally, it is not just plain water, but purified or de-ionized water. From there, ingredients are listed in descending order according to the percentage of each ingredient in the shampoo.

Classifications of Shampoos

The second ingredient that most shampoos have in common is the **base surfactant** (sir-**FAK**-tant) or **base detergent**. These two terms, surfactant and detergent, mean the same thing, cleansing or surface active agent. The term surfactant describes organic compounds brought together by chemical synthesis to create wetting, dispersing, emulsifying, solubilizing, foaming, or washing agents (detergents).

The base surfactant or combination of surfactants determines into which class a shampoo will fall. The base surfactants used in shampoos fall into four broad classifications: **anionic** (an-i-**ON**-ik), **cationic** (**KAT**-i-on-ik), **nonionic** (non-i-**ON**-ik), and **ampholytic** (**AM**-fo-li-tik).

Most manufacturers use detergents from more than one classification. It is customary to use a secondary surfactant to complement, or offset, the negative qualities of the base surfactant. For example, an **amphoteric** (**AM**-fo-ter-ik) that is nonirritating to the eyes can be added to a harsh anionic to create a product that is more comfortable to use.

Anionics. Sodium lauryl sulfate (**SO**-dee-um **LAW**-ril **SUL**-fate) and **sodium laureth sulfate** (**SO**-dee-um **LAW**-reth **SUL**-fate), which fall into the first classification known as **anionic surfactants**, are the most commonly used detergents. Sodium lauryl sulfate is a relatively harsh cleanser that produces a rich foam. It is suitable for use in hard or soft water because it rinses easily from the hair. Sodium laureth sulfate is also a strong, rich, foaming detergent. However, because it is less alkaline than the lauryl sulfates, it is often used in shampoos that are designed to be milder or less drying to the hair shaft.

Cationics. The second classification of detergents or surfactants, cationics, is made up almost entirely of quarternary ammonium compounds or quats. Practically all the quarternary compounds have some antibacterial action; therefore they are sometimes included in the chemical composition of dandruff shampoos.

Nonionics. The third classification, nonionics, are valued as surfactants for their versatility, stability, and ability to resist shrinkage, particularly in cold temperatures. They have a mild cleansing action and low incidence of irritation to human tissues. **Cocamide** (DEA, MEA) is one of the most widely used nonionics in the industry, not only in shampoos but also in lipstick and permanent waving lotions.

Ampholytes. The fourth type of cleanser, the ampholyte, is important commercially because it can behave as an anionic or a cationic substance, depending on the pH of the solution. The ampholytes have a slight tendency to cling to hair and skin, and thus are conducive to hair manageability. They possess germicidal properties that vary between derivatives. Amphoteric surfactants are used in several baby shampoos because they do not sting the eyes. Many amphoterics are identified on the ingredient list by Amphoteric 1–20.

A familiarity with these four classifications of detergents or surfactants and their use in shampoo products will enable the barber-stylist to make a professional decision when selecting the appropriate product to use on a client.

Categories of Shampoos

Cleansing the scalp and hair may be accomplished by either a wet or dry shampoo. Wet shampoos are watery solutions comprised of soap and various other cleansing agents. Dry shampoos do not use water, but contain either powdery substances or cosmetic products in dry form.

Wet shampoos, depending on their composition, are of three basic types:

1. Soap shampoos
2. Soapless shampoos (foaming or foamless)
3. Cream shampoos

Soap shampoos are available in various forms—cake, powder, jelly, or liquid. The active cleansing agent is a soap made from olive oil, coconut oil, or other oils. Liquid soap shampoos contain more than 50 percent water. When used on the hair, a soap shampoo will produce an alkaline reaction. With soft water, soap shampoos lather readily. When used with hard water, soap shampoos will not lather and tend to produce an insoluble soap residue on the hair.

Soapless shampoos come in the form of a powder, jelly, cream, or liquid. They are effective cleansing agents. Their main ingredient is a sulfonated oil. Both lathering and non-lathering types of soapless shampoos are available.

Soapless shampoos are equally effective in soft, hard, cold, or hot water. They should be used with discretion, since frequent applications not only dry the scalp and hair, but also render the hair more absorbent than usual.

The cleansing action of cream or paste shampoo is created by soap, a synthetic detergent, or a combination of both. They may also contain a reconditioning agent for the hair. Cream shampoos or pastes without soap are usually acid in reaction.

Choice of Shampoo

The shampoo service should be individualized for each client. The barber-stylist should examine the client's hair and scalp, and understand the various types of shampoos well enough to determine which would do the most effective job. The selection of a shampoo for a client is an important matter of judgment. Conditions that must be considered in the selection of a shampoo are:

1. Excessively dry hair—Use an oil shampoo or one with a neutral base.
2. Oily condition—Green soap shampoo or plain shampoo.
3. Tender scalp—Cream or egg shampoo.
4. Sensitive scalp—Egg, oil, or mild shampoo.
5. Normal scalp—Plain shampoo.

Types of Shampoos

Plain Shampoos

Plain shampoos are usually clear and may be an amber shade or a greenish yellow. They may contain a plain liquid soap or a detergent-based product. These shampoos seldom have lanolin or other special agents used to leave a gloss on the hair. A plain shampoo may be used on hair that is in good condition. It should never be used on colored hair because it will strip or fade the color.

Liquid Cream Shampoos

Liquid cream shampoos are usually fairly thick white liquids. Generally, they contain either soap or soap jelly. **Magnesium stearate** is also used as a whitening agent. They often contain oily compounds, to make the hair feel silky and softer. Use this type of shampoo as directed by your instructor or manufacturer.

Liquid Dry Shampoos

Liquid dry shampoos are cosmetic products used for cleansing the scalp and hair when the client is prevented by illness from having a regular shampoo.

> CAUTION: Be sure the shop is well ventilated when using liquid dry shampoo.

Procedure for Liquid Dry Shampoo

1. Brush the hair thoroughly and comb it lightly.
2. Part the hair into small sections.
3. Saturate a piece of cotton with the liquid, squeeze it out lightly, then rub it over the scalp briskly, along each part. Follow by rubbing the scalp with a towel swiftly along the part. Repeat this procedure over the entire head. Next, apply liquid with a cotton pledget down the length of the hair strands.
4. Rub the hair strands with a towel to remove the soil.
5. Re-moisten the hair lightly with liquid, and comb it into the desired style.

Such a dry shampoo will freshen the hair and tone the scalp without endangering the client. (When using any type of shampoo, carefully read and follow the manufacturer's directions.)

Powder Dry Shampoo

A powder dry shampoo is usually given when the client's health will not permit a wet shampoo. A commercial powder dry shampoo containing **orris root powder** is freely sprinkled into the hair and worked in, one section at a time. This powder, which soaks up the oil in the hair, is then brushed out of the hair with a long-bristled brush. Brush the hair, strand by strand, until every trace of powder has been removed. Between strokes, the brush should be wiped on a clean towel to remove the dust and dirt.

Other Shampoos

For dry or damaged hair, use one of the following:

1. **Egg shampoo.** Apply a mixture of one or two whole eggs to the hair and scalp in the same manner as for a regular shampoo. Use only tepid water, as hot water will congeal the egg on the hair.
2. A commercial shampoo containing a small amount of egg. Apply as directed by the manufacturer.
3. Any other commercial shampoo that contains ingredients helpful to dry scalp and hair.

Castile and olive oil shampoos contain a coconut oil soap solution, dissolved flakes of castile soap, and a small amount of olive oil to prevent the excessive drying produced by the high alkali content of the soap. They are neutral and mild in action, provided they contain a high-grade castile soap. Be guided by your instructor.

Medicated shampoos. These shampoos are usually in the form of a liquid or jelly. They contain a medicinal agent such as sulphur, tar, cresol, a small percentage of phenol, or another antiseptic agent.

Therapeutic medicated shampoos contain special chemicals or drugs that are very effective in reducing excessive dandruff. They must be used only by prescription and instructions should be followed carefully.

Hot oil shampoos are used very seldom today. They are being replaced by improved shampoos capable of cleansing and correcting dry scalp and hair.

Acid-balanced (non-strip) shampoos are formulated to prevent the stripping of hair color from the hair. They are mild, contain conditioners, and are low in alkaline content. They are recommended also for brittle, dry, or damaged hair. Follow the manufacturer's directions.

Special Shampoos

There are a number of shampoos available for professional use. At times, the barber-stylist may be uncertain as to which shampoo to use. To avoid making mistakes, carefully read the label and literature accompanying the shampoo. Such information will reveal the principal ingredients and the advantages claimed for the product.

One way to test a shampoo is to give it a fair trial. Make sure to follow the manufacturer's instructions. Keeping a written record of the shampoo used and the results obtained will eliminate guesswork as to its effectiveness.

HAIR RINSES

The barber-stylist is engaged in the business of selling services. The more services the stylist has to offer, the more satisfied clients will be. Hair rinses are a profitable service that can be easily learned and applied.

A hair rinse is an agent that can cleanse and condition the hair and scalp, bring out the luster of the hair, or add highlights and color.

Water Rinse

A tepid, soft water rinse is generally used after a shampoo. The object is to remove any residue present on the hair.

Acid Rinses

Acid rinses are used to restore the pH balance to the hair and to remove soap scum. The fatty acids found in soap combine with the minerals in water to form a soap scum that cannot be completely removed from the hair with plain water. Therefore, the hair tends to become coated, dull, and difficult to comb. Because soap is not currently used in the manufacture of professional shampoos, you will not find acid rinses in many shops or salons.

The types of acids used in prepared acid hair rinses are:

Citric acid from the juice of a lime, orange, or lemon.
Tartaric acid, which is obtained from residues in wine making.
Acetic acid, which is present in vinegar.
Lactic acid, which is lactose or sugar of milk.

Vinegar (Acid) Rinse

A vinegar (acetic) rinse is used to separate the hair, dissolve soap curds, give hair brightness, and make hair soft and pliable. A vinegar rinse may also be used to counteract the alkalinity of hair after a bleach (lightening), tint, or cold wave.

Formula: Two tablespoons of white vinegar to one pint of tepid water.

Use as a last rinse after a shampoo. After using the vinegar rinse, run water quickly over the hair to remove the odor.

Lemon (Acid) Rinse

A lemon rinse has a slight lightening quality, is effective on bleached (lightened) and blond hair, and separates the hair strands.

Formula: Use the strained juice of one or two lemons or a few drops of concentrated lemon extract in one quart of warm water.

Rinse the hair with the lemon mixture several times. Finally, rinse the hair with clear warm water to remove all the lemon juice.

Citric Acid Rinse

A citric acid rinse is often used in place of a lemon rinse.

Formula: Place one tablespoonful of citric acid crystals into a pint container, and pour four ounces of boiling water over them. Fill the rest of the container with warm water, stirring while you add the water. Apply as for lemon rinse.

Bluing Rinse

A prepared rinse, containing a blue base color, is used to give yellowed hair a silvery gray or white tone. The porosity of the hair must be taken into consideration to avoid a two-toned effect on the porous ends. Follow the manufacturer's directions when mixing to achieve the desired silver or slate tone.

Color Rinses

Color rinses are prepared rinses used to highlight or add temporary color to the hair. These rinses remain on the hair until the next shampoo.

Medicated Rinses

These are formulated to control minor dandruff. A **dandruff rinse** is a commercial product applied following a shampoo. It removes and controls dandruff. Many such rinses, of good quality, are on the market. Some rinses are used in a prepared form while others are diluted with water. Always follow the manufacturer's directions.

Cream Rinse

A cream rinse is a commercial product having a creamy appearance and is used as a last rinse. It tends to soften the hair, adds luster, and makes tangled hair easier to comb.

Cream rinses depend for their effectiveness on one or more chemicals having one property in common—that of being substantive to hair. Some substances will adhere to the hair shaft and will not wash off in the course of ordinary rinsing. This is specifically so in the materials used in a cream rinse. The result is that the hair has a nice, soft feel and is much easier to comb and handle.

A cream rinse does not have the same function as an acid rinse. While cream rinses are slightly acid in reaction, this is due to the nature of the ingredients used. Moreover, the acidity is so low that, in the dilutions used, it would have no effect as a soap film remover.

Rinses in Connection with Hair Coloring

An **acid-balanced (non-strip) rinse** is formulated to prevent the stripping of a hair coloring treatment. Most manufacturers formulate this type of rinse for use in connection with their particular tint product.

A **reconditioning rinse** may be used following a hair coloring treatment. Follow the manufacturer's directions.

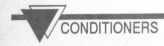

CONDITIONERS

The professional hair treatment requires the use of many chemicals. Certain chemicals remove natural oils as well as protein from the hair, causing it to become dry, brittle, and damaged. Hair conditioners help to restore some of these natural oils and proteins and moisturize the hair, preparing it to receive other hair services. Clients with naturally dry, brittle hair will benefit also from regular conditioning treatments.

Conditioners are designed to deposit protein or moisturizers in damaged areas, giving the hair body and sheen while making it easier to comb. They are available in both cream and liquid forms. The formulations of the products vary. They may contain lanolin, moisturizers, fatty acids, quats, vegetable oils, proteins, herbs, or various combinations of these. For the best results, it is important that each product be applied as indicated by the manufacturer. Most conditioners are applied to hair that has been shampooed or towel dried.

There are four general groups of hair conditioners available: instant, protein, neutralizing, and moisturizing. The selection of the type to use depends on the texture and condition of the hair and the results desired.

Instant Conditioners

These conditioners are applied to hair, allowed to stay on for one to five minutes, then rinsed out. They usually have an acid pH. They do not penetrate into the hair shaft but add natural oils, moisture, and sometimes protein to the hair.

Conditioners Combined with Styling Lotions

Protein or resin-based conditioners are contained in some styling lotions and applied as part of the hair styling process. A little water, added during the styling procedure, helps to facilitate styling by keeping the hair soft and manageable. These conditioners are designed to increase hair diameter slightly by a coating action, and to give it body. They are available in several strengths to accommodate various textures, conditions, and hair qualities.

Protein Penetrating Conditioners

These conditioners utilize hydrolized protein (very small fragments), moisturizers, and oils. They pass through the cuticle, penetrate the cortex, and replace the keratin that has been lost from the hair. They improve texture, equalize porosity, and increase elasticity. Any excess conditioner must be rinsed well from the hair before setting.

> **NOTE:** Care should be taken not to overuse protein penetrating conditioners as the hair may become brittle or "over-proteinized." The use of a moisturizing conditioner combined with the protein conditioner has proved effective for the prevention of adverse conditions.

Neutralizing Conditioners (pH Balancers)

These conditioners neutralize alkalinity created by strong alkaline hair products. They have an acid pH and are designed to prevent damage to the hair and alleviate scalp irritation. Neutralizing conditioners are allowed to remain on the hair from one to five minutes and then are rinsed out.

Moisturizing Conditioners

These conditioners draw moisture into the hair with **humectants** (hew-**MECK**-tunts), chemical compounds that absorb and hold moisture from the hair, or seal moisture inside damp hair by coating the cuticle. Natural moisturizing ingredients may include oils, essential fatty acids, sodium PCA, and sometimes herbs. Coating moisturizers usually contain wax or glycerin in addition to other ingredients.

Other Conditioners

In addition to the above, there are a number of other vegetable, protein, and synthetic polymer conditioners available. These are usually highly specialized conditioners.

Synthetic polymer conditioners are designed for use on badly damaged hair. A polymer is a compound consisting of many (poly) repeating units that form a chain. When the hair, a natural polymer, is so severely damaged that it cannot be conditioned by normal protein conditioners, a synthetic polymer may be necessary to prevent breakage and correct excessive porosity.

Chelators are used as a pre-treatment, before certain chemical services. They are designed to neutralize metallic elements in or on the hair that could interfere with the chemicals to be applied. Chelators can be either a separate conditioner or an ingredient in a pretreatment product. Be guided by your instructor's information and the manufacturer's directions.

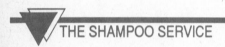

THE SHAMPOO SERVICE

Physical Presentation While Shampooing

Most barber-styling shops are equipped with shampoo bowls, either within a working booth area or in a separate section of the shop. The stylist stands beside the client while performing a shampoo.

To prevent muscle aches, back strain, fatigue, and other problems, it is extremely important to maintain good posture.

1. Stand as close as possible to the back of the client's head.
2. The knees should be flexed slightly, positioned directly over the feet to maintain good balance.
3. The head should be raised, with the chin at a level with the floor. The chest should be up, the abdomen flat, and the shoulders relaxed.
4. Do not bend or twist sideways from the waist or lean forward too far.

Superior Shampoo Service

Excellence in shampoo services requires the barber-stylist to give individual attention to each client's needs. In addition to selecting

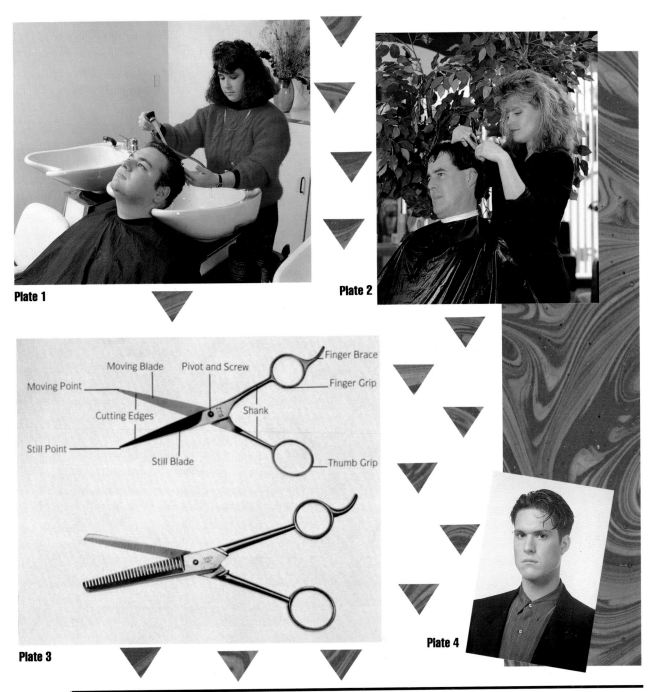

Plate 3 — Haircutting scissors (top); thinning shears, one blade notched (bottom).

Within the scissors diagram:
Moving Point · Moving Blade · Cutting Edges · Pivot and Screw · Finger Brace · Finger Grip · Shank · Thumb Grip · Still Point · Still Blade

Plate 1 · **Plate 2** · **Plate 3** · **Plate 4**

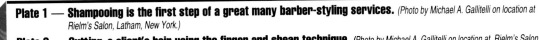

Plate 1 — Shampooing is the first step of a great many barber-styling services. *(Photo by Michael A. Gallitelli on location at Rielm's Salon, Latham, New York.)*

Plate 2 — Cutting a client's hair using the finger and shear technique. *(Photo by Michael A. Gallitelli on location at Rielm's Salon, Latham, New York.)*

Plate 3 — Haircutting scissors (top); thinning shears, one blade notched (bottom). *(Photo by Michael A. Gallitelli .)*

Plate 4 — Finished hairstyle. *(Hair: Julie Biafore, Photo: Timm Eubanks. Courtesy John Paul Mitchell Systems.)*

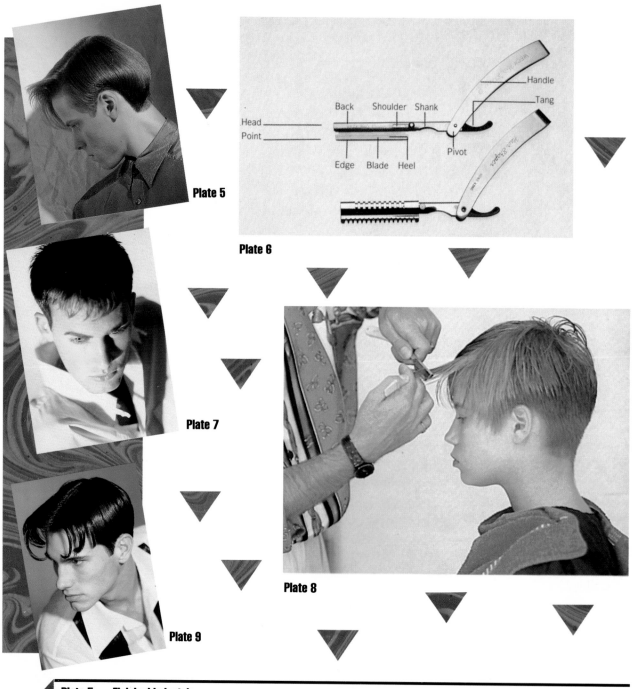

Plate 5

Plate 6

Head
Point
Back Shoulder Shank Handle
Tang
Edge Blade Heel Pivot

Plate 7

Plate 8

Plate 9

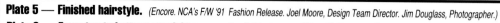

Plate 5 — **Finished hairstyle.** *(Encore. NCA's F/W '91 Fashion Release. Joel Moore, Design Team Director. Jim Douglass, Photographer.)*

Plate 6 — **From top to bottom: straight razor; straight razor with safety guard.** *(Photo by Michael A. Gallitelli.)*

Plate 7 — **Finished hairstyle.** *(Hair: Doyle Wilson Salon, Los Angeles, for Joico International. Photo: Albert Sanchez.)*

Plate 8 — **Razor haircutting.** *(Photo by Steven Landis, with direction from Vincent and Alfred Nardi of Nardi Salon.)*

Plate 9 — **Finished hairstyle.** *(Hair: Doyle Wilson Salon, Los Angeles, for Joico International. Photo: Albert Sanchez.)*

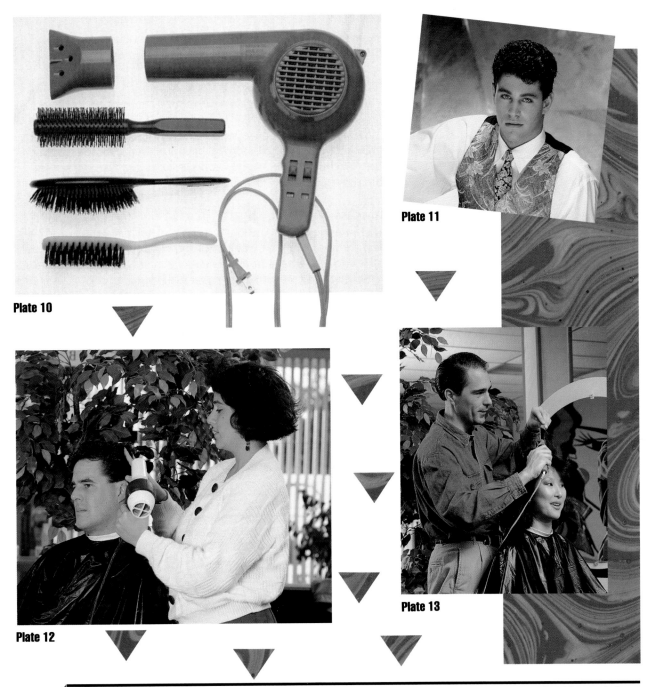

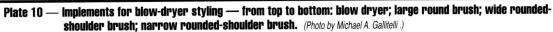

Plate 10 — **Implements for blow-dryer styling — from top to bottom: blow dryer; large round brush; wide rounded-shoulder brush; narrow rounded-shoulder brush.** *(Photo by Michael A. Gallitelli .)*

Plate 11 — **Finished hairstyle.** *(Courtesy of Matrix Essentials, Inc.)*

Plate 12 — **For successful blow-dry styling, the air should be directed from the scalp area to the hair ends.** *(Photo by Michael A. Gallitelli on location at Rielm's Salon, Latham, New York.)*

Plate 13— **Styling the hair with an electric curling iron.** *((Photo by Michael A. Gallitelli on location at Rielm's Salon, Latham, New York.)*

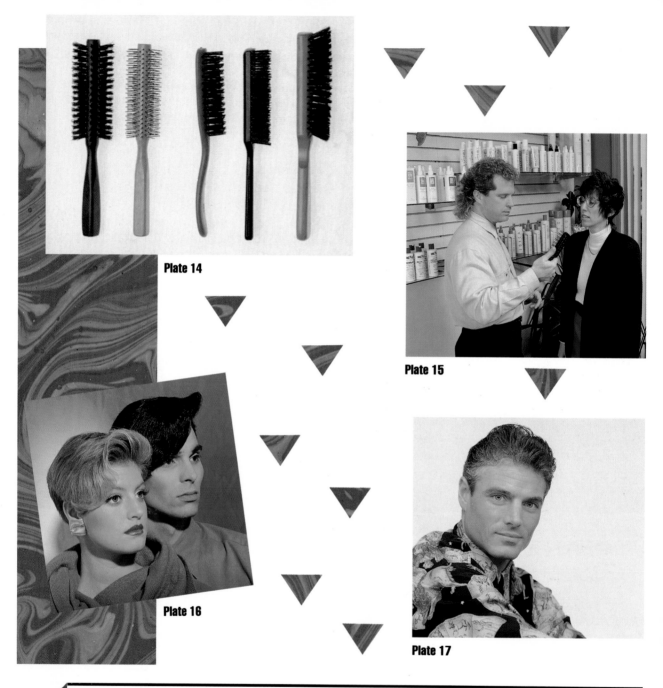

Plate 14

Plate 15

Plate 16

Plate 17

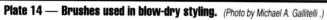

Plate 14 — **Brushes used in blow-dry styling.** *(Photo by Michael A. Gallitelli .)*

Plate 15 — **Barber-stylists use a number of different brushes in their work. The texture of such brushes vary with the type of service they are expected to perform and their quality.**
(Photo by Michael A. Gallitelli on location at Rielm's Salon, Latham, New York.)

Plate 16 — **Finished hairstyles.** *(Encore. NCA's F/W '91 Fashion Release. Joel Moore, Design Team Director. Jim Douglass, Photographer.)*

Plate 17 — **Finished hairstyle.** *(Courtesy of Matrix Essentials, Inc.)*

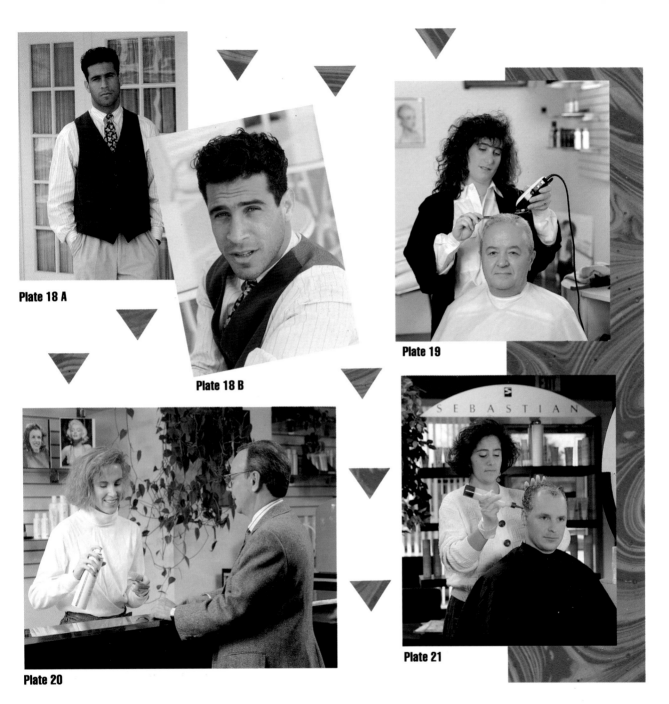

Plate 18 A

Plate 18 B

Plate 19

Plate 20

Plate 21

Plates 18 A & B — **Finished hairstyle.** *(Hair: Pamela Perettie. Photo: Gary Lyons. Courtesy John Paul Mitchell Systems.)*

Plate 19 — **Cutting the hair using the clipper-over-comb technique.** *(Photo by Michael A. Gallitelli on location at Rielm's Salon, Latham, New York.)*

Plate 20 — **Selling in the barber-styling shop.** *(Photo by Michael A. Gallitelli on location at Rielm's Salon, Latham, New York.)*

Plate 21 — **Applying hair coloring tint to client's hair.** *(Photo by Michael A. Gallitelli on location at Rielm's Salon, Latham, New York.)*

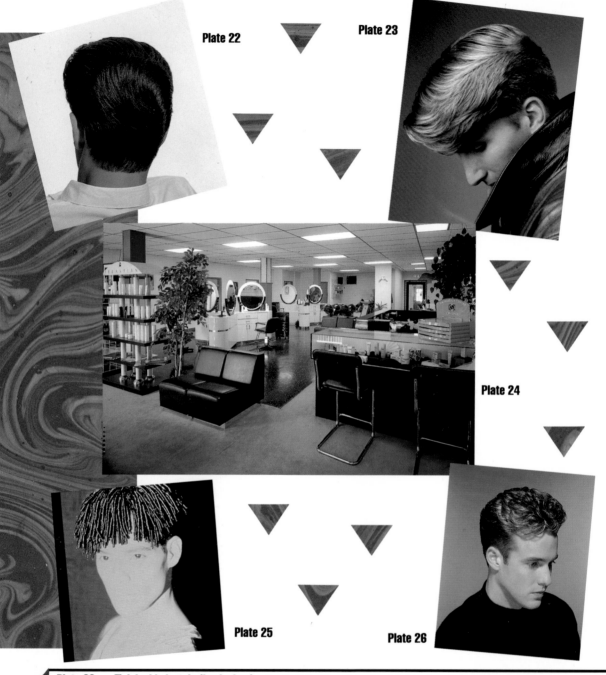

Plate 22

Plate 23

Plate 24

Plate 25

Plate 26

Plate 22 — Finished hairstyle (back view). *(From the National Cosmetology Association's Ice Cream Collection. Danny Ewert, Design Team Director. Jim Douglass, Photographer.)*

Plate 23 — Finished hairstyle (side view). *(Photo Courtesy of Clairol.)*

Plate 24 — Barber-styling shop interior. *(Photo by Michael A. Gallitelli on location at Rielm's Salon, Latham, New York.)*

Plate 25 — Finished hairstyle. *(Hair: Tony Lacey and Marian Crowell, North American Hairdresser Award winners in the Ethnic Category.)*

Plate 26 — Finished hairstyle. *(Courtesy of Matrix Essentials, Inc.)*

Men's Makeover Winners

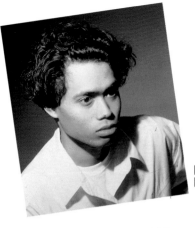

**Plate 27
Before**

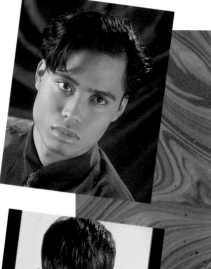

**Plate 28
After**

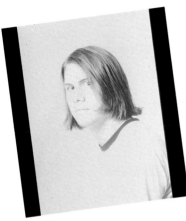

**Plate 29
Before**

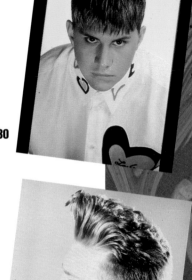

**Plate 30
After**

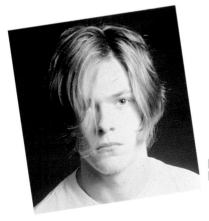

**Plate 31
Before**

**Plate 32
After**

Plate 27

Plate 28 — *(Hair: Sabrina Hill, North American Hairdresser Award winner in the Men's Makeover Category.)*

Plate 29

Plate 30 — *(Hair: Tony Lacey , North American Hairdresser Award winner in the Men's Makeover Category.)*

Plate 31

Plate 32 — *(Hair: Tony Lacey , North American Hairdresser Award winner in the Men's Makeover Category.)*

Men's Makeover Winners

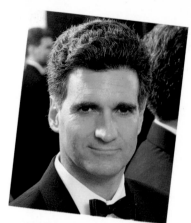

Plate 33
Before

Plate 34
After

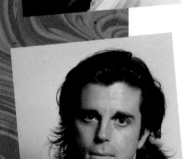

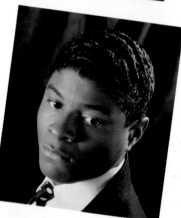

Plate 35
Before

Plate 36
After

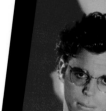

Plate 37
Before

Plate 38
After

Plate 33

Plate 34 —— *(Hair: Frederic Fekkai. Color: Mark Wofford both for Keralogie L'Oreal Technique Professionnelle. Photo: Keith Trumbo.)*

Plate 35

Plate 36 —— *(Hair: Sabrina Hill, North American Hairdresser Award winner in the Men's Makeover Category.)*

Plate 37

Plate 38 —— *(Hair: Tony Lacey , North American Hairdresser Award winner in the Men's Makeover Category.)*

the shampoo best suited to the condition of the scalp, the effectiveness of the shampoo will depend on:

1. The way the shampoo is applied.
2. The way the scalp is massaged.
3. The way the shampoo is rinsed from the hair.

A good shampoo not only removes dirt and dandruff from the scalp and hair, but also helps to keep them healthy.

Preparation

Adequate preparation is the first step in giving a good shampoo. Before starting, the barber-stylist should assemble all necessary supplies. Following a definite procedure saves time and increases efficiency.

The essential supplies needed for a shampoo are:

1. The shampoo, conditioner, and/or other products selected.
2. Soft, warm water capable of producing an abundance of lather with the shampoo. (Remember, hard water will not produce lather unless softened by boiling or chemical treatment.)
3. Shampoo bowl or tray, chair cloth, and towels.

How to Prepare the Client for Shampoo

1. Seat the client in a comfortable and relaxed position.
2. Drape the client according to textbook or your instructor's procedures.
3. Consult with the client concerning any problems or questions he or she may have, what type of shampoo he or she uses, etc.
4. Examine the condition of the client's hair and scalp. Briefly massage the scalp. This procedure loosens the epidermal scales, debris, and scalp tissues.
5. Determine the type of shampoo and other products to be used.

Water Temperature

The water should be comfortably warm for the client. Cold water, in addition to causing discomfort, tends to reduce lathering. Hot water can cause the scalp to flake or become dry. Warm water is not only comfortable and relaxing for the client; it also reacts favorably in the foaming process.

Shampooing at the Chair

The shampoo may be applied while the client is sitting upright in the hydraulic chair or is seated at the shampoo bowl. The method used is usually that preferred by the barber-stylist or required by the facilities available.

Application of Shampoo

The shampoo is applied by spreading sections of the hair apart with the thumb and fingers of the left hand and applying the shampoo directly onto the scalp. Make sure that the entire scalp is covered. The shampoo should be massaged completely into the scalp. Warm water is added gradually to work up a rich, creamy lather.

As a lather is created and the scalp manipulated, be careful that the shampoo lather does not run onto the client's forehead or into the eyes or ears.

All shampoo movements must be executed with the cushion tips of the fingers. The scalp manipulations are repeated several times, until the lather is completely worked into the hair and scalp. The excess lather is then removed by a sweep with the palm, from the front to the back of the head and rinsed from the practitioner's hand. Rinse hair thoroughly with a strong spray.

Two Methods of Shampooing and Rinsing

There are two methods used for shampooing and rinsing at the shampoo bowl. These are the **inclined method** and the **reclined method**.

The Inclined Method

While shampooing or rinsing, the client's head is bent forward over the shampoo bowl. The following procedures are necessary for the inclined position.

1. Place a clean towel over the edge of the shampoo bowl.
2. Have the client sit on a stool close to the shampoo bowl.
3. Massage the scalp to loosen dandruff and to increase the blood circulation.
4. Follow steps 1 through 8 for a plain shampoo.

The Reclined Method

The reclined method requires that the entire shampoo and rinse procedure be performed at the bowl. The hydraulic chair is reclined, with the client's head lying on the headrest or in the neckrest of the bowl. This method is favored because it is more comfortable for the client and it permits greater speed and efficiency. (Fig. 7.13)

The following procedures are intended for use of the reclined position.

1. Remove the headrest.
2. Massage the scalp to loosen dandruff and to increase the blood circulation.
3. Turn the chair around, with its back facing the shampoo bowl.
4. Place a folded towel in the groove of the shampoo bowl to support the client's neck, or attach a shampoo tray to the bowl.
5. Recline the chair until the client's head rests comfortably in the groove of the shampoo bowl or on the tray.
6. Follow steps 1 through 8 for a plain shampoo, described in next section.

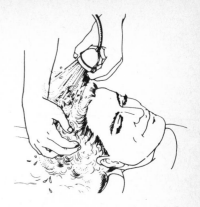

7.13 – Reclined position

Procedure for a Plain Shampoo

1. Wet the hair.
2. Apply shampoo to all parts of the scalp.
3. Massage the scalp for several minutes as described in next section.
4. Rinse the hair thoroughly with warm water and repeat the lathering if necessary. (Figs. 7.14–7.16) (Suggest a hair rinse or hair conditioner at this time.)

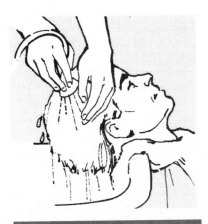

7.14 – Protecting the face

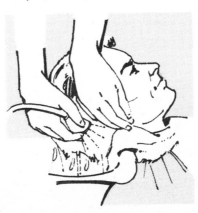

7.15 – Protecting the ears

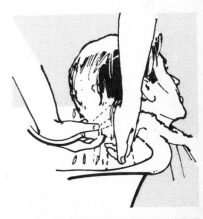

7.16 – Protecting the neck

5. Rinse the hair with cool water.
6. Wipe the face and ears thoroughly.
7. Towel dry the hair.
8. Comb the hair.

Massage Manipulations During Shampoo

The proper way to massage the scalp during a shampoo is as follows:

1. After lathering the scalp and hair, stand behind, or to the side of the client.
2. Place the fingertips at the back of the head just below the ears.
3. Use rotary movements from the ears to the temples, up to the forehead, then over the top of the head down to the neck. (Figs. 7.17–7.19)
4. Repeat these movements for several minutes.

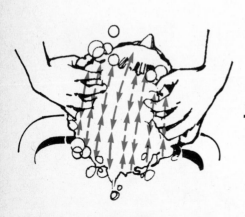

7.17 – Manipulate the scalp from hairline at ears to the top of the head.

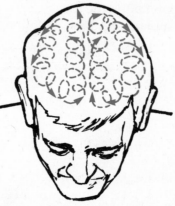

7.18 – Use a rotary type movement

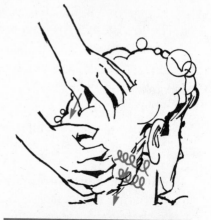

7.19 – Lift the client's head to shampoo and massage the nape area. Stylist's hand should be placed at the base of the occipital area while shampooing the nape with the other hand. Reverse hands for shampooing the occipital area.

Common Faults in Shampooing

Good barber-stylists make every effort to please their clients. A dissatisfied client may find fault with a shampoo for any of the following reasons:

1. Improper shampoo selection
2. Insufficient scalp massage

3. Insufficient rinsing
4. Water too cold or too hot
5. Allowing shampoo or water to run down the client's forehead, or into the eyes or ears
6. Wetting or soiling the client's clothing
7. Scraping or scratching the client's scalp with fingernails
8. Improper hair drying
9. Not getting the scalp and hair clean

SCALP TREATMENTS

The purpose of scalp and hair treatments is to preserve the health and appearance of the hair and scalp. These treatments also help to prevent and combat scalp disorders such as dandruff, hair loss, dryness, or oiliness.

Cleanliness Essential

A basic requirement for a healthy scalp is cleanliness. The scalp and hair should be kept clean by frequent shampooing. A clean, healthy scalp will resist a wide variety of disorders. Because the scalp and hair are vitally related, many scalp disorders need correction in order to keep the hair healthy. A healthy scalp will usually produce healthy hair. Even a healthy person should have scalp treatments to preserve the natural health of the hair. While shampooing will keep the hair clean, it will not prevent the hair from becoming dry and brittle.

A scalp and/or hair treatment may be given separately, or in connection with other services. Depending on the client's needs, the treatment may include:

1. Cleansing with a suitable shampoo
2. Massage with the hands or electrical appliance
3. Use of electrical appliances, such as an electric steamer, infrared lamp, ultraviolet lamp, high-frequency current, or dermal lamp
4. The application of cosmetic preparations, such as hair tonics, astringents, antiseptics, etc.

CAUTION: Do not suggest a scalp treatment if there are scalp abrasions or a scalp disease present. Advise clients with serious or contagious scalp ailments to consult a physician.

Conditions caused by neglect, such as tight scalp, overactive or underactive oil glands, and tense nerves, can be corrected by proper scalp treatments.

Scalp Massage (Manipulations)

Since scalp manipulations are the same for all scalp treatments, the barber-stylist should become skillful at performing them with a continuous, even motion. Scalp massage should be performed as a series of treatments—once a week for a normal scalp, and more frequently for scalp disorders under the direction of a dermatologist.

A thorough scalp massage is beneficial in the following ways:

1. The blood and lymph (LIMF) flow are increased.
2. Nerves are rested and soothed.
3. Scalp muscles are stimulated.
4. The scalp is made more flexible.
5. Hair growth is promoted and the hair is made lustrous.

Knowing the muscles and location of blood vessels and nerves in the scalp and neck will help guide the barber-stylist to those areas in which massage movements should be directed. As for other treatments, the barber-stylist should gather all the equipment needed before beginning a scalp treatment.

Prepare the client as for a shampoo.

Procedure for a Scalp Massage

In scalp massage apply firm pressure on upward strokes. Firm rotary movements loosen the scalp tissues. These movements improve the health of hair and scalp by increasing the blood's circulation to the scalp and hair papillae. When giving a scalp massage, care should be taken to give the manipulations slowly without pulling the hair in any way. With each movement, the hands are placed under the hair. Thus, the length of the fingers, the balls of the fingertips, and the cushions of the palms stimulate the muscles, nerves, and blood vessels in the scalp area.

NOTE: The following is one method of scalp massage. However, your instructor may have developed a different routine that is equally correct.

1. Place the fingertips of each hand at the hairline on each side of the client's head, hands pointing upward. Slide the fingers firmly upward, spreading the fingertips. Continue until the fingers meet at the center or top of the scalp. Repeat three or four times. (Fig. 7.20)

2. Place the fingers of each hand on the sides of the head, behind the ears. Use the thumbs to massage from behind the ears toward the crown. Repeat four or five times. Move the fingers until both thumbs meet at the hairline at the back of neck. Rotate the thumbs upward toward the crown. (Fig. 7.21)

3. Move to the right of the client. Place the left hand at the back of the head. Place the thumb and fingers of the right hand against and over the forehead, just above the eyebrows. With the cushion tips of the thumb and fingers of the right hand, massage slowly and firmly in an upward direction toward the crown while keeping the left hand in a fixed position at the back of the head. Repeat four or five times. (Fig. 7.22)

4. Move behind the client. Place the hands on each side of the head, at the front hairline. Rotate the fingertips three times. On the fourth rotation, apply a quick, upward twist, firm enough to move the scalp. Continue this movement on the sides and top of the scalp. Repeat three or four times. (Fig. 7.23)

5. Place the fingers of each hand below the back of each ear. Rotate the fingers upward from behind the ears to the crown. Repeat three or four times. Move the fingers toward the back of the head and repeat the movement with both hands. Apply rotary movements in an upward direction toward the crown. (Fig. 7.24)

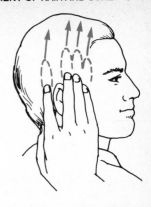

7.20 – Sliding movement

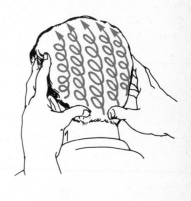

7.21 – Sliding and rotating movement

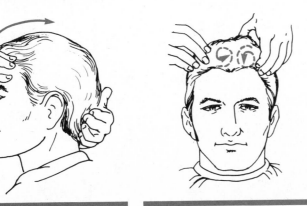

7.22 – Forehead movement

7.23 – Hairline movement

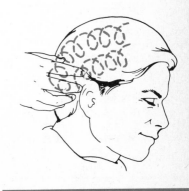

7.24 – Rotary movement of the scalp

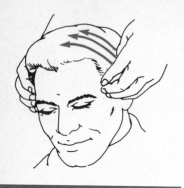

7.25 – Ear-to-ear movement

6. Place one hand at either side of the head. Keep the fingers close together and hold the index finger at the hairline, above the ears. Firmly move the hands directly upward to the top of the head. Repeat four times. Move the hands to above the ears and repeat the movement. Move the hands again to back of ears and repeat the movement. (Fig. 7.25)

When to Recommend Scalp Treatments

Scalp treatments may be advised for any of the following reasons:

1. to keep the scalp clean and healthy;
2. to promote hair growth;
3. to try to prevent excessive hair loss.

> **CAUTION:** No barber-stylist should treat scalp diseases caused by parasitic or staphylococcus infections. If the client has an abnormal scalp condition, it is safest to suggest medical treatment.

MASSAGE AND ITS INFLUENCE ON THE SCALP

Massage Movements	Muscles	Nerves	Arteries
Sliding Movement (Fig. 7.20)	Auricularis superior	Posterior auricular	Frontal Parietal
Sliding and Rotating Movement (Fig. 7.21)	Auricularis posterior Occipitalis	Greater occipital	Occipital
Forehead Movement (Fig. 7.22)	Frontalis	Supra-orbital	Frontal
Hairline Movement (Fig. 7.23)	Frontalis	Supra-orbital	Frontal Parietal
Rotary Movement of the Scalp (Fig. 7.24)	Auricularis posterior Occipitalis	Greater occipital	Posterior auricular Parietal
Ear-to-Ear Movement (Fig. 7.25)	Auricularis anterior and superior	Temporal auricular	Frontal Parietal

Treatment for Normal Scalp and Hair

The purpose of a general scalp treatment is to keep the scalp and hair clean and healthy. Regular scalp treatments also help to prevent baldness.

Procedure after a Shampoo

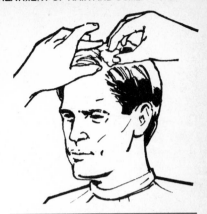

1. Dry the hair and scalp thoroughly.
2. Part the hair and apply a scalp ointment directly to the scalp. (Fig. 7.26)
3. Place both thumbs about three-quarters of an inch apart, on each side of the parted hair.
4. Rotate the thumbs in a circular manner, pressing firmly against the scalp.
5. Make another hair part about one inch away from the first one. Apply ointment and massage.
6. Repeat steps 2 through 5 and continue until the entire scalp has been treated.
7. Adjust the infrared lamp.
8. Expose the scalp to red dermal light or an infrared lamp for three to five minutes, parting the hair to permit maximum exposure. (Fig. 7.27)
9. Stimulate the scalp with high-frequency current for two to three minutes.
10. Apply a suitable hair tonic and work it well into the scalp.
11. Comb the hair.

7.26 – Applying scalp ointment with a swab

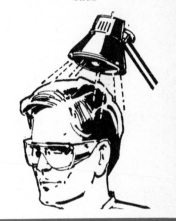

7.27 – Applying heat with infrared lamp

Scalp Treatment with Vibrator

A **vibrator** (VYE-bray-tur) is an effective tool in giving a stimulating scalp massage. Before using, adjust the vibrator on the back of the hand, leaving the thumb and fingers free. Then turn on the current. The vibrations are transmitted through the cushions of the fingertips. The same movements are followed as for a regular hand scalp massage.

When using the vibrator on the scalp, be careful to regulate the intensity and duration of the vibrations, as well as the pressure applied.

Oily Scalp Treatment

The main cause of an oily scalp is an excess of fatty foods in the diet and the resultant overactivity of the oil glands.

Procedure

1. Gently massage the scalp.
2. Shampoo the scalp and hair with a shampoo suitable for an oily scalp.
3. Towel dry the hair, leaving it damp.
4. Part the hair and apply medicated lotion or ointment to the scalp only.
5. Steam the scalp with hot towels or a scalp steamer.
6. Dry excess moisture from the hair with a towel.
7. Expose the scalp to an infrared lamp for about five minutes.
8. Apply an astringent or alcoholic scalp lotion.
9. Dress the hair in the desired style.

CAUTION: Creams or ointments can be applied before using high-frequency current. Hair tonics or lotions with alcoholic content may be applied only after the application of high-frequency current.

Dandruff Treatment

The principal signs of dandruff are the appearance of white scales on the hair and scalp and accompanying itching. Dandruff may be associated with either a dry or an oily condition. The more common causes of dandruff are poor blood circulation to the scalp, improper diet, neglect of cleanliness, and infection.

CAUTION: To prevent the spread of dandruff in the shop, the barber-stylist must sanitize all implements and avoid the common use of combs, brushes, and scalp applicators.

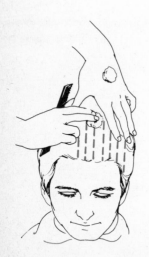

7.28 – Applying scalp lotion with cotton pledget

Procedure

1. Shampoo according to the condition of the scalp (dry or oily dandruff).
2. Dry the hair thoroughly.
3. Apply dandruff or antiseptic lotion to the scalp with a cotton pledget. (Fig. 7.28)
4. Apply four or five steam towels or use a scalp steamer over the scalp.

5. Dry the hair thoroughly.
6. Both the barber-stylist and the client should put on tinted safety goggles.
7. Expose the scalp to ultraviolet rays for five to eight minutes, parting the hair every half inch. (Fig. 7.29)
8. Massage the scalp for five minutes.
9. Apply dandruff ointment to the scalp and retain it until the next shampoo.
10. Expose the scalp to red dermal light or an infrared lamp for five minutes. **Alternate Step.** In place of Step 10, high-frequency current may be applied for three to five minutes.
11. Comb hair in desired style.

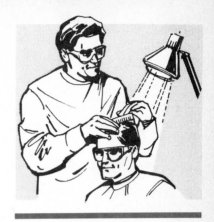

7.29 – Applying ultraviolet rays

Dry Scalp and Hair Treatment

Inactivity of the oil glands or excessive removal of natural oil produce a dry condition of the hair and scalp. Causes contributing to dry hair and scalp are leading an indoor life, frequent washing with strong soaps or alcoholic shampoos, and the continued use of drying tonics or lotions.

Select scalp preparations containing moisturizing and emollient materials. Avoid the use of strong soaps, preparations containing a mineral oil or sulfonated oil base, or greasy preparations and lotions with a high alcoholic content.

Procedure

1. Massage and stimulate the scalp for three to five minutes.
2. Apply a scalp preparation for this condition. If olive oil is used, work it gently but thoroughly into the scalp.
3. Steam the scalp with hot towels or scalp steamer for seven to ten minutes.
4. Wash the hair, using a shampoo suitable for dry scalp.
5. Towel dry the hair, making sure the scalp is thoroughly dried.
6. Apply scalp cream sparingly with a rotary, frictional motion.
7. Apply a red dermal or infrared lamp over the scalp for three to five minutes.
8. Stimulate the scalp with direct, high-frequency current, using a glass rake electrode, for about five minutes. (Fig. 7.30)
9. Comb the hair into the desired style.

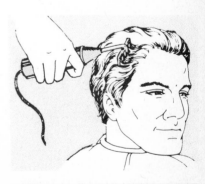

7.30 – Applying high-frequency current

Corrective Hair Treatment

A corrective hair treatment deals with the hair shaft, rather than the scalp. Dry and damaged hair can be greatly improved by reconditioning (corrective) treatments. Hair treatments are especially beneficial to make the hair soft and pliable. Dry hair may be softened quickly with a reconditioning preparation applied directly on the outside of the hair shaft. The product used for this purpose is usually an emulsion containing cholesterol and related compounds.

Procedure

1. Prepare the client as for a normal scalp treatment.
2. Massage and stimulate the scalp for three to five minutes.
3. Apply a mild shampoo.
4. Blot the hair with a towel.
5. Apply a reconditioning agent according to the manufacturer's directions.
6. Dry the hair with a hand dryer.
7. Comb the hair into the desired style.

Treatment for Alopecia

Alopecia is premature baldness or excessive hair loss. The chief causes of alopecia are heredity, poor circulation, lack of proper stimulation, improper nourishment, certain infectious skin diseases such as ringworm, or constitutional disorders. Alopecia is treated by stimulating the blood supply and reviving the hair papillae involved in hair growth. (Figs. 7.31–7.34)

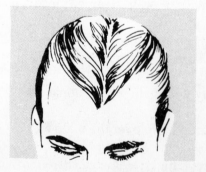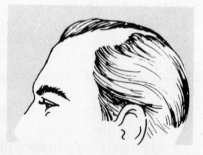

7.31 – Beginning baldness in men age 30 to 40. Scalp treatments are most beneficial at this stage.

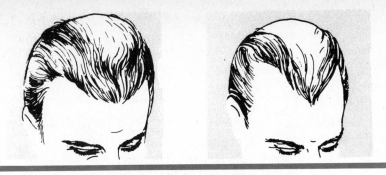

7.32 – Partial baldness in men age 40 to 50. Scalp treatments are worth trying at this stage.

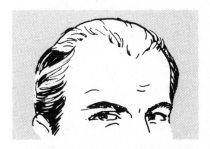
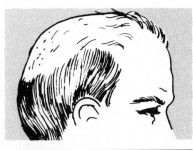

7.33 – Extensive baldness in men from age 50 to 60. Too late for scalp treatments.

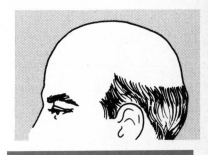

7.34 – Extensive baldness in men from age 61 and over. Too late for scalp treatments.

Procedure

1. Apply regular scalp manipulations.
2. Shampoo the hair and scalp as required (dry or oily).
3. Dry the scalp thoroughly.
4. Protect client's and barber-stylist's eyes with goggles.
5. Expose the scalp to ultraviolet rays for about five minutes.
6. Apply a medicated scalp ointment as directed by a physician.
7. Apply indirect high-frequency current for about five minutes.
8. Comb the hair into the desired style.

Hair Tonics

The term *hair tonic* indicates almost any type of cosmetic solution that stimulates the scalp, helps to correct a scalp condition, or is used in grooming. Since numerous hair tonics are available, an understanding is needed of the ingredients and actions of the various types, and the specific use of each. The barber-stylist should be prepared to advise clients concerning the use of tonics and the specific purpose of each.

While hair tonics are essentially cosmetic solutions that are used primarily on the hair, the scalp also benefits in a number of ways from their use.

In order for maximum benefit to be gained from a tonic application the scalp should be prepared by scalp manipulation, applied with the cushion tips of the fingers. The fingers should be worked through the hair to the surface of the scalp and then manipulated to move the skin with firm, upward pressure.

Purposes of Hair Tonics

Hair tonics are applied for various reasons. Different types of tonics may serve to:

1. Groom the hair.
2. Help correct an oily dandruff condition.
3. Help correct a dry dandruff condition.
4. Stimulate the scalp.
5. Offset an itchy scalp.
6. Maintain a normal, healthy scalp.

Types of Hair Tonics

1. **Non-alcoholic.** This type is usually an antiseptic solution, with hair grooming ingredients added.
2. **Alcoholic.** This type usually contains an antiseptic and alcohol, which acts as a mild astringent.
3. **Cream.** This type is an emulsion containing lanolin and mineral oils.
4. **Oil mixture.** This type contains considerable amounts of alcohol with a small portion of oil floating on the top. It is used as a grooming agent.

Along with a hair tonic, the barber-stylist may use:

1. Steam applications (scalp steamer or steaming towels).
2. An electric vibrator.
3. Scalp manipulations.

Scalp Steam

Steam relaxes the pores, softens the scalp and hair, and increases blood circulation. The **scalp steamer** assures a constant and controlled source of steam. To use, fill the container with water, fit the hood over the client's head, and turn on the current. Many hoods have openings on the side so that hands can be inserted in order to give a scalp massage together with the scalp steam.

Steaming towels are used in the absence of a scalp steamer. They are prepared, one at a time, by soaking the towel in steaming water. The excess water is wrung out and the steaming towel is wrapped around the client's head. As the towel cools, another one is applied in its place. (Figs. 7.35–7.37)

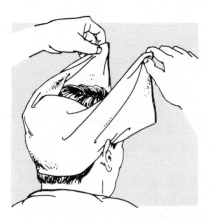

7.35 – Placing the center of towel on the back part of the client's head

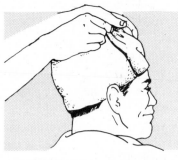

7.36 – Bring both ends of the towel to overlap over the forehead

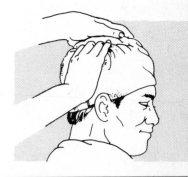

7.37 – Placing the center of towel along the left side of head and wrapping it so the ends will overlap on the right side of head

Procedure for a Scalp Steam

1. Use regular scalp manipulations to increase circulation.
2. Steam the scalp with two hot towels or a scalp steamer.
3. Apply hair tonic carefully and massage it well into the scalp.
4. Comb the hair into the desired style.

Procedure for Hair Tonic Treatment

1. Wash hands.
2. Arrange linen and supplies.
3. Massage the scalp with the hands or a vibrator.
4. Apply steam towels twice, or use a scalp steamer.
5. Apply a suitable tonic directly to the scalp.
6. Massage the scalp with hands or a vibrator.
7. Comb the hair into the desired style.

REVIEW QUESTIONS

Draping

1. What is the purpose of draping a client?
2. Name one of the most important responsibilities of the barber-stylist.
3. What is the purpose of the towel/neck strip?
4. List five instructions a barber-stylist should follow before draping a client.
5. What type of cape should be used for wet hair services?
6. What type of cape should be used for haircutting services? Why?

Shampoo Chemistry

1. What are the two parts of the shampoo molecule?
2. What purpose is served by each of these two parts?
3. Describe the action of the two parts of the shampoo molecule in cleansing the hair.
4. What is the chemical composition of shampoo?
5. What are the three types of shampoos?
6. Describe a base surfactant or base detergent.
7. What determines the class into which a shampoo will be classified?
8. Name four classifications of base surfactants.
9. Identify the surfactants most commonly used in shampoos.
10. What are the characteristics of anionic surfactants? cationic? nonionic? ampholyte?

Water

1. What is water? What ability does it have?
2. Name two substances that cannot be dissolved in water.

pH

1. What is pH? What does the symbol pH express?
2. How is pH value measured?
3. Why is the acidity or alkalinity of products important to the barber-stylist?
4. What effect do acidic solutions have on hair and skin? alkaline solutions?
5. What is the acidic range on the pH scale? the alkaline range?

6. What is the pH value of the following: water; hair/skin; shampoo; conditioners; lemon juice?

1. What is the purpose of a plain shampoo?
2. How often should the hair be shampooed?
3. What kind of soap should be used in a shampoo?
4. Outline the important steps in giving a shampoo.
5. Briefly outline the massage manipulations applied to the scalp during a shampoo.

1. What value does a rinse have on the hair?
2. Name four types of hair rinses.
3. Which hair rinse is best for hard water areas?
4. What benefits are received from a bluing rinse?

1. What type of hair requires reconditioning treatments?
2. What is the function of hair conditioners?
3. What do conditioners deposit on the hair?
4. Name two forms in which conditioners are available.
5. List seven ingredients conditioners may contain.
6. Most conditioners are applied to hair that has been _____ or _____.
7. Name the four general groups of hair conditioners.
8. Identify the two important aspects of hair condition to be considered when choosing a hair conditioner.
9. How long should instant hair conditioners be left on the hair?
10. How do conditioning styling lotions affect the hair?
11. What ingredients do protein penetrating conditioners utilize? How do these conditioners restore keratin to the hair? What conditions of the hair can they improve?
12. What are neutralizing conditioners? What type of pH do these conditioners have? How long is a neutralizing conditioner allowed to remain on the hair?
13. What is the function of moisturizing conditioners?
14. Synthetic polymers should be used for what hair type?
15. What are chelators?

1. What is the purpose of scalp massage?
2. In what ways does scalp massage benefit the blood and nerves?
3. What is the purpose of general scalp treatments?
4. What is accomplished by using a scalp steam?
5. When is a dry scalp treatment recommended?

6. What are some of the common causes of a dry scalp?
7. What is the main cause of an oily scalp?
8. What are the principal signs of dandruff?
9. What are the common causes of dandruff?
10. What are the chief causes of alopecia?
11. What is the aim in treating alopecia?

Hair Tonics

1. What are hair tonics?
2. What is a scalp steam?

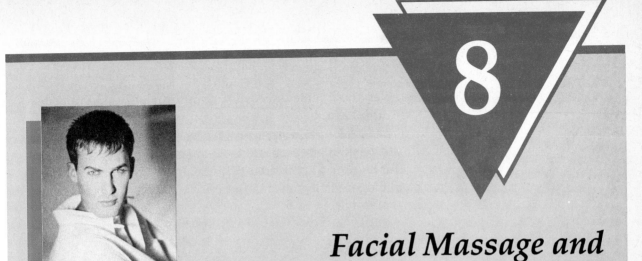

8

Facial Massage and Treatments

Learning Objectives

After completing this chapter, you should be able to:

1. *Describe the purpose of facial massage.*

2. *Identify the basic anatomy of the head, face, and neck.*

3. *List the muscles and nerves that are affected by massage.*

4. *Describe the forms and types of muscle and nerve stimulation.*

5. *Define massage.*

6. *Discuss and analyze when a massage should or should not be given.*

7. *Identify the location of the motor points of the face.*

8. *Identify and demonstrate massage manipulations and procedures.*

9. *Demonstrate a complete facial.*

10. *Identify facial treatment equipment.*

11. *Describe the various types of facial treatments.*

12. *List the physiological effects of massage.*

Courtesy of: Hair: Doyle Wilson Salon, Los Angeles, CA, for Joico International. Photo: Albert Sanchez.

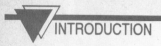

INTRODUCTION

A facial massage is probably the most relaxing and restful service offered in the barber-styling shop. When received regularly, facials result in very noticeable improvement in the client's skin tone, texture, and appearance.

To give a facial with competence, the barber-stylist should be able to analyze the skin condition and recommend the most effective treatment. This requires a knowledge of the anatomy of the head, face, and neck and the correlating muscles, nerves, and arteries that are affected by facial massage.

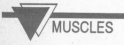

MUSCLES

Muscles are fibrous tissues that have the ability to stretch, contract, and produce all body movements.

There are three parts to a muscle: the origin, the insertion, and the belly. The **origin** does not move. It is attached to the skeleton, and is usually part of a skeletal muscle. The **insertion** moves, and the **belly** is the middle of the muscle. Pressure in massage is usually directed from the insertion to the origin.

Stimulation of Muscles

Muscular tissue can be stimulated by any of the following:

- **Massage** (hand massage and electric vibrator)
- **Electric current** (high-frequency and faradic current)
- **Light rays** (infrared rays and ultraviolet rays)
- **Heat rays** (heating lamps and heating caps)
- **Moist heat** (steamers or moderately warm steam towels)
- **Nerve impulses** (through the nervous system)
- **Chemicals** (certain acids and salts)

Muscles Affected by Massage

The barber-stylist is concerned with the voluntary muscles of the head, face, and neck. It is essential to know the location of these muscles, and what they control.

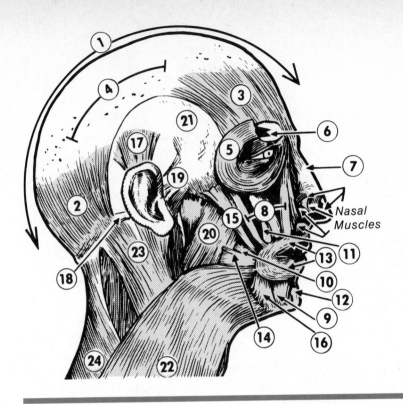

8.1 – Diagram of the muscles of the head, face, and neck

Muscles of the Scalp

The muscles are numbered to correspond with the muscles shown on Fig. 8.1.

1. The **epicranius** (ep-i-**KRAY**-ne-us), or **occipito-frontalis** (ok-**SIP**-i-toh fron-**TAY**-lis), is a broad muscle that covers the top of the skull. It consists of two parts:
2. The **occipitalis** (ok-**SIP**-i-ta-lis), or back part.
3. The **frontalis** (fron-**TAY**-lis), or front part.

The frontalis raises the eyebrows, draws the scalp forward, and causes wrinkles across the forehead. Both the occipitalis and the frontalis are connected by a tendon called

4. The **aponeurosis** (ap-o-noo-**ROH**-sis)

Muscles of the Eyebrows

5. The **orbicularis oculi** (or-bik-yoo-**LAY**-ris **OK**-yoo-leye) completely surrounds the margin of the eye socket and closes the eyelid.

6. The **corrugator** (KOR-oo-gay-tohr) muscle is beneath the frontalis and orbicularis oculi and draws the eyebrows down and in. It produces vertical lines and causes frowning.

Muscles of the Nose

7. The **procerus** (proh-SEE-rus) covers the top of the nose, depresses the eyebrow, and causes wrinkles across the bridge of the nose.

The other nasal muscles are small muscles around the nasal openings, which contract and expand the opening of the nostrils.

Muscles of the Mouth

8. The **quadratus labii superioris** (kwah-DRAY-tus LAY-bee-eye suu-PEER-ee-or-ihs) consists of three parts. It surrounds the upper part of the lip, raises and draws back the upper lip, and elevates the nostrils.
9. The **quadratus labii inferioris** (in-FEER-ee-or-ihs) surrounds the lower part of the lip. It depresses the lower lip and draws it a little to one side.
10. The **buccinator** (BUK-si-nay-tor) is the muscle between the upper and lower jaws. It compresses the cheeks and expels air between the lips.
11. The **caninus** (kay-NIGH-nus) lies under the quadratus labii superioris. It raises the angle of the mouth.
12. The **mentalis** (men-TAL-is) is situated at the tip of the chin. It raises and pushes up the lower lip, causing wrinkling of the chin.
13. The **orbicularis oris** (or-bik-yoo-LAY-ris OH-ris) forms a flat band around the upper and lower lips. It compresses, contracts, puckers, and wrinkles the lips.
14. The **risorius** (ri-ZOHR-ee-us) extends from the masseter muscle to the angle of the mouth. It draws the corner of the mouth out and back.
15. The **zygomaticus** (zeye-goh-MAT-i-kus) extends from the zygomatic bone to the angle of the mouth. It elevates the lip.
16. The **triangularis** (treye-an-gyoo-LAY-ris) extends along the side of the chin. It draws down the corner of the mouth.

Muscles of the Ear
The three muscles of the ear are as follows:

17. The **auricularis** (aw-rik-yoo-LAHR-is) **superior** is above the ear.
18. The **auricularis posterior** is behind the ear.

19. The **auricularis anterior** is in front of the ear.

Muscles of Mastication

20. The **masseter** (ma-**SEE**-tur) and
21. The **temporalis** (tem-po-**RAY**-lis) are muscles that coordinate in opening and closing the mouth, and are referred to as chewing muscles.

Muscles of the Neck

22. The **platysma** (pla-**TIZ**-mah) is a broad muscle that extends from the chest and shoulder muscles to the side of the chin. It depresses the lower jaw and lip.
23. The **sterno-cleido-mastoid** (**STUR**-noh-**KLE**-i-doh-**MAS**-toid) extends from the collar and chest bones to the temporal bone in back of the ear. It rotates and bends the head.
24. The **trapezius** (tra-**PEE**-zee-us) allows movement of the shoulders and covers the back of the neck.

NERVES

Nerves are long, white fibrous cords that originate in the brain and spinal column, distributing nerve branches to all parts of the body. Nerves act as message carriers to and from all parts of the body.

Nerve Stimulation

Stimulation to the nerves causes muscles to contract and expand.
Heat on the skin causes relaxation; cold causes contraction.
Nerve stimulation may be accomplished by any of the following:

- Chemicals (certain acids or salts)
- Massage (hand massage or electric vibrator)
- Electrical current (high-frequency)
- Light rays (infrared)
- Heat rays (heating lamps, and heating caps)
- Moist heat (steamers or moderately warm steam towels)

Cranial Nerves

There are 12 pairs of cranial nerves. All are connected to a part of the brain surface. They emerge through openings on the sides and base of the cranium and reach various parts of the head, face, and neck. They are classified as motor, sensory, and mixed nerves, and contain both motor and sensory fibers.

The cranial nerves are numbered according to the order in which they emerge from the brain, and are named by description of their nature or function.

First: Olfactory (ol-**FACK**-tur-ee)—A sensory nerve that controls the sense of smell.

Second: Optic (**OP**-tick)—A sensory nerve that controls the sense of sight.

Third: Oculomotor (ock-yoo-lo-**MO**-tur)—A motor nerve that controls the motion of the eye.

Fourth: Trochlear (**TROCK**-lee-ur)—A motor nerve that controls the motion of the eye.

Fifth: Trigeminal (trye-**JEM**-i-nul) or **trifacial** (trye-**FAY**-shul)—A sensory-motor nerve that controls the sensations of the face, tongue, and teeth.

Sixth: Abducent (ab-**DEW**-sunt)—A motor nerve that controls the motion of the eye.

Seventh: Facial (**FAY**-shul)—A sensory-motor nerve that controls the motion of the face, scalp, neck, ear, and sections of the palate and tongue.

Eighth: Acoustic (uh-**KOOS**-tick) or **auditory** (**AW**-di-tor-ee)—A sensory nerve that controls the sense of hearing.

Ninth: Glossopharyngeal (glos-o-fa-**RIN**-jee-ul)—A sensory-motor nerve that controls the sense of taste.

Tenth: Vagus (**VAY**-gus) or **pneumogastric** (new-mo-**GAS**-trick)—A sensory-motor nerve that controls motion and sensations of the ear, pharynx, larynx, heart, lungs, and esophagus.

Eleventh: Accessory (ack-**SES**-uh-ree)—A motor nerve that controls the motion of the neck muscles.

Twelfth: Hypoglossal (high-po-**GLOS**-ul)—A motor nerve that controls the motion of the tongue.

The three cranial nerves most important in the massaging of the head, face, and neck are the fifth cranial (trifacial), seventh cranial (facial), and the eleventh cranial (accessory). The **spinal (cervical)** (**SUR**-vi-kal) nerve, which originates in the spinal cord, is also involved in scalp and neck massage.

Fifth Cranial Nerve

The **fifth cranial (trifacial or trigeminal) nerve** is the largest of the cranial nerves. It is the chief sensory nerve of the face, and the motor nerve of the muscles that control chewing. It consists of three branches: ophthalmic, mandibular, and maxillary.

The following important branches of the fifth cranial nerve are affected by massage. They are numbered according to their appearance on Fig. 8.2.

1. The **supra-orbital** (soo-proh-**OHR**-bi-tahl) **nerve** affects the skin of the forehead, scalp, eyebrows, and upper eyelids.
2. The **supra-trochlear** (soo-prah-**TROK**-lee-ahr) **nerve** affects the skin between the eyes and upper sides of the nose.
3. The **infra-trochlear** (in-frah-**TROK**-lee-ar) **nerve** affects the membrane and skin of the nose.
4. The **nasal** (**NAY**-zal) **nerve** affects the point and lower sides of the nose.
5. The **zygomatic** (zeye-goh-**MAT**-ik) **nerve** affects the skin of the temples, sides of the forehead, and upper part of the cheeks.
6. The **infra-orbital** (in-frah-**OR**-bi-tal) **nerve** affects the skin of the lower eyelids, sides of the nose, upper lip, and mouth.

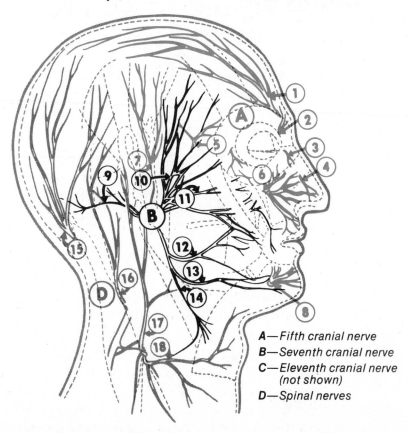

A—Fifth cranial nerve
B—Seventh cranial nerve
C—Eleventh cranial nerve (not shown)
D—Spinal nerves

8.2 – Nerves of the head, face, and neck

7. The **auriculo-temporal** (o-**RIK**-yoo-loh **TEM**-po-rahl) **nerve** affects the external ear and the skin from above the temples to the top of the skull.
8. The **mental** (**MEN**-tahl) **nerve** affects the skin of the lower lip and chin.

Seventh Cranial Nerve

The **seventh cranial (facial) nerve** is the chief motor nerve of the face. It emerges near the lower part of the ear. Its divisions and their branches control all the muscles used for facial expression and extend to the muscles of the neck. Of all the branches of the facial nerve, the following are the most important:

9. The **posterior auricular nerve** affects the muscles behind the ears at the base of the skull.
10. The **temporal nerve** affects the muscles of the temples, sides of the forehead, eyebrows, eyelids, and upper part of the cheeks.
11. The **zygomatic nerve (upper and lower)** affects the muscles of the upper part of the cheeks.
12. The **buccal nerve** affects the muscles of the mouth.
13. The **mandibular nerve** affects the muscles of the chin and lower lip.
14. The **cervical nerve** affects the sides of the neck.

Eleventh Cranial Nerve

The **eleventh cranial (accessory) nerve**—spinal branch—affects the muscles of the neck and back. The branches are not shown on the illustration.

Spinal (Cervical) Nerves

The **spinal (cervical) nerves** originate at the spinal cord. Their branches supply the muscles and scalp at the back of the head and neck, as follows:

15. The **greater occipital nerve**, located in the back of the head, affects the scalp as far up as the top of the head.
16. The **smaller (lesser) occipital nerve**, located at the base of the skull, affects the scalp and muscles of this region.
17. The **greater auricular nerve**, located at the side of the neck, affects the external ears and the areas in front and back of the ears.

18. The **cutaneous colli** (kyoo-**TAY**-nee-us **KOH**-leye) **nerve**, located at the side of the neck, affects the front and sides of the neck, as far down as the breastbone.

The **common carotid arteries** are the main sources of the blood supply to the head, face, and neck. They are located on either side of the neck and divide into internal and external carotid arteries. The internal division of the common carotid artery supplies the brain, eye sockets, eyelids, and forehead. The external division supplies the superficial parts of the head, face, and neck (Fig. 8.3).

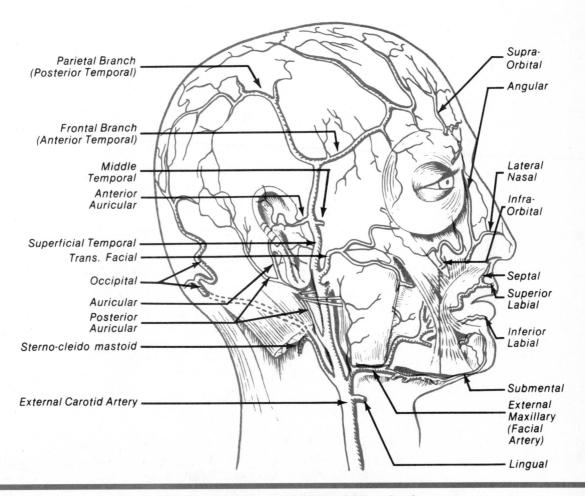

Parietal Branch (Posterior Temporal)
Frontal Branch (Anterior Temporal)
Middle Temporal
Anterior Auricular
Superficial Temporal
Trans. Facial
Occipital
Auricular
Posterior Auricular
Sterno-cleido mastoid
External Carotid Artery

Supra-Orbital
Angular
Lateral Nasal
Infra-Orbital
Septal
Superior Labial
Inferior Labial
Submental
External Maxillary (Facial Artery)
Lingual

8.3 – Diagram of the arteries of the head, face, and neck

The External Maxillary Artery

The **external maxillary**, or **facial artery**, supplies the lower region of the face, mouth, and nose. Some of its branches are:

1. The **submental** (sub-MEN-tahl) **artery** supplies the chin and lower lip.
2. The **inferior labial artery** supplies the lower lip.
3. The **angular artery** supplies the side of the nose.
4. The **superior labial artery** supplies the upper lip, septum (dividing wall) of the nose, and the wings of the nose.

Superficial Temporal Artery

The **superficial temporal artery** is a continuation of the external carotid artery, and supplies the muscles, skin, and scalp on the front, side, and top of the head. Some of its important branches are:

1. The **frontal artery** supplies the forehead.
2. The **parietal artery** supplies the crown and sides of the head.
3. The **transverse facial artery** supplies the masseter.
4. The **middle temporal artery** supplies the temples and eyelids.
5. The **anterior auricular artery** supplies the anterior part of the ear.

The Occipital Artery

The **occipital artery** supplies the scalp and back of the head up to the crown. Its most important branch is the **sterno-cleido-mastoid artery**, which supplies the muscle of the same name.

The Posterior Auricular Artery

The **posterior auricular artery** supplies the scalp, behind and above the ear. Its most important branch is the auricular artery, which supplies the skin in back of the ear.

Veins of the Head, Face, and Neck

The blood returning to the heart from the head, face, and neck flows on each side of the neck in two principal veins: the **internal jugular** and the **external jugular**. The most important veins are parallel to the arteries and take the same names as the arteries.

THEORY OF MASSAGE

Most clients enjoy a properly administered facial or scalp massage for its stimulating and relaxing effects. It produces a glow in the cheeks and a tingling in the scalp. It is important that the barber-stylist understand the principles of massage and acquire a skillful touch.

Massage involves the external manipulation of the face or any other part of the body. This is accomplished with the hands, or with the aid of electrical appliances such as vibrators. Each massage movement is executed in such a way as to obtain a specific result.

The benefits of massage depend upon the type, intensity, and extent of the manipulations used. Massage must be performed systematically. It should never be a casual or irregular process. The condition of the skin and the general physical condition of the client should be considered.

Normal skin may receive soothing, mildly stimulating, or strongly stimulating massage treatments. However, sensitive, inflamed skin could be damaged further by massage. If massage is desired, the manipulations must be gentle and soothing to damaged or sensitive skin. Massage should always be used with judgment and moderation.

Massage should never be recommended or employed when the following conditions are present:

1. Inflammation of the skin
2. Severe skin lesions
3. Pus-containing pimples
4. Client with high blood pressure
5. Skin infection

An understanding of the motor points of the face will result in an effective facial massage (Fig. 8.4 on page 174). A motor point is a point on the skin over a muscle where pressure or stimulation will cause contraction of that muscle.

MOTOR POINTS OF THE FACE

A knowledge of neuro-muscular anatomy is necessary in order to locate the areas overlying muscle motor points and the regions where motor nerves are sufficiently near the surface of the skin to be stimulated.

Trijacial Nerve (Mandibular Division)
Temporalis

Facial Nerve (Temporal Branch)
1. Frontalis
2. Corrugator
3. Orbicularis Oculi

FACIAL NERVE (MAIN TRUNK)

Facial Nerve (Buccal Branch)
4. Nasalis
5. Quad. Labii Sup.
6. Orbicularis Oris

Facial Nerve (Mandibular Branch)
7. Triangularis
8. Quad. Labii Inf.

Cervical Nerve

Brachial Plexus (Erb's Point)

PLATYSMA MUSCLE is cut out to show deeper muscles.

Posterior Auricular Nerve

Occipitalis

Cervical Nerve

Trapezius

BACK VIEW

8.4 – Motor points of the face

When massaging any part of the head, face, or neck, all pressure should be applied in an upward direction. This rule should be followed in all massaging services, whether they are intended to stimulate, relax, or soothe the skin. When applying rotary manipulations, the same rule applies because the pressure should be applied on the upward swing of the movement.

Effleurage

Effleurage (ef-loo-**RAHZH**) (stroking movement). This is a light, continuous movement applied in a slow and rhythmic manner over the skin. No pressure is employed. Over large surfaces, the palm is used; over small surfaces, the fingertips are employed. Effleurage is frequently used on the forehead, face, and scalp for its soothing and relaxing effects.

Position of Fingers for Stroking
Curve the fingers slightly, with just the cushions of the fingertips touching the skin. Do not use the ends of the fingertips for these massage movements. Since the tips of the fingers are pointier than the cushions, the effleurage will be less smooth, and your fingernails are likely to scratch the client's skin. (Figs. 8.5, 8.6)

Position of Palms for Stroking
Hold your whole hand loosely. Keep your wrist and fingers flexible, and curve your fingers to conform to the shape of the area being massaged. (Fig. 8.7)

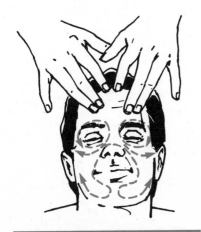

8.5 – Digital stroking of face

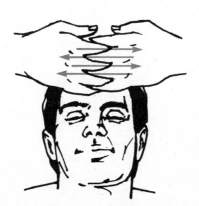

8.6 – Digital stroking of forehead

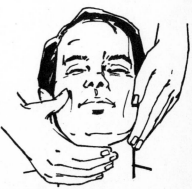

8.7 – Palmar stroking of face

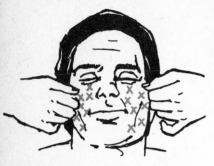

8.8 – Digital kneading of cheeks

Petrissage

Petrissage (pay-tri-**SAHZH**) (kneading movement). In this movement, the skin and flesh are grasped between the thumb and fingers. As the tissues are lifted from their underlying structures they are squeezed, rolled, or pinched with a light, firm pressure. This movement exerts an invigorating effect on the part being treated. Kneading movements give deeper stimulation to the muscles, nerves, and skin glands, and improve the circulation. (Fig. 8.8)

> **NOTE:** Massage movements are directed toward the origin of muscles to avoid damage to muscular tissues.

Friction

Friction (deep rubbing movement). This movement requires pressure on the skin while it is being moved over the underlying structures. The fingers or palms are employed in this movement. Friction has a marked influence on the circulation and glandular activity of the skin. (Fig. 8.9)

Percussion or Tapotement Movement

Percussion (per-**KUSH**-un) or **tapotement** (ta-pot-**MAHN**) (tapping, slapping, and hacking movements). This form of massage is the most stimulating. It should be used with care and discretion. Tapping movements are more gentle than slapping movements. Percussion movements tone the muscles and impart a healthy glow to the part being massaged. (Fig. 8.10)

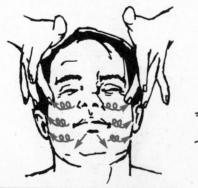

8.9 – Circular friction on face

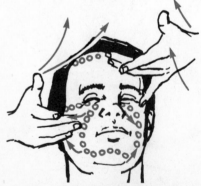

8.10 – Digital tapping on face

In tapping, the fingertips are brought down against the skin in rapid succession, whereas in slapping, the whole palm is used to strike the skin. Hacking movements employ the outer ulnar borders of the hands which are struck against the skin in alternate succession.

In facial massage, only light digital tapping is used.

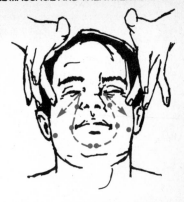

Vibration

Vibration (vye-**BRAY**-shun) (shaking movement). The fingertips or vibrator are used to transmit a trembling movement to the skin and its underlying structures. To prevent over-stimulation, this movement should be used sparingly and should never exceed a few seconds' duration on any one spot. (Fig. 8.11)

8.11 – Vibratory movement of face

PHYSIOLOGICAL EFFECTS OF MASSAGE

Skillfully applied massage influences the structures and functions of the body, either directly or indirectly. The immediate effect of massage is first noticed on the skin. The part being massaged reacts with an increase in its functional activities such as more active circulation, secretion, nutrition, and excretion. There is scarcely an organ of the body that is not affected favorably by scientific massage treatments.

Beneficial results may be obtained by proper facial and scalp massage.

1. The skin and all its structures are nourished.
2. The muscle fiber is stimulated and strengthened.
3. Fat cells are reduced.
4. Circulation of blood is increased.
5. The activity of the skin and scalp glands is stimulated.
6. The skin is rendered soft and pliable.
7. The nerves are soothed and rested.
8. Pain is sometimes relieved.

Electrical appliances most commonly used in giving facial and scalp massage are:

1. Vibrators
2. High-frequency applicators
3. Infrared or ultraviolet lamps, and white or colored bulbs

▼ FACIAL TREATMENT EQUIPMENT

High-Frequency Current

The **high-frequency (Tesla)** current is characterized by a high rate of oscillation, or vibration. It is commonly called the **violet ray**, and is used for both scalp and facial treatments.

The primary action of this current is thermal, or heat-producing. Because of its rapid vibrations, there are no muscular contractions. The physiological effects are either stimulating or soothing, depending on the method of application.

The electrodes for high-frequency are made of glass or metal. (Fig. 8.12) Their shapes vary, the facial electrode being flat and the scalp electrode being rake-shaped. (Figs. 8.13, 8.14) As the current passes through the glass electrode, tiny violet sparks are emitted. All high-frequency treatments should be started with a mild current which is gradually increased to the required strength. The length of the treatment depends upon the condition to be treated. For a general facial or scalp treatment, only about five minutes should be allowed.

Application of High-Frequency Current

For proper use, follow the instructions provided by manufacturer.

There are three methods of using the Tesla current:

1. **Direct surface application.** The barber-stylist holds the electrode and applies it over the client's skin. In facial treat-

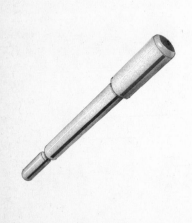

8.12 – Metal electrode attachment for Tesla current

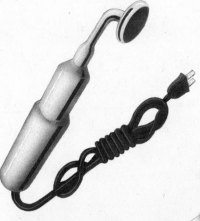

8.13 – Facial electrode using Tesla current

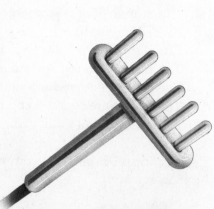

8.14 – Scalp electrode attachment for Tesla current

ments, the electrode is applied directly over the facial cream. (Figs. 8.15, 8.16)

2. **Indirect application.** The client holds the metal or glass electrode while the barber-stylist uses the fingers to massage the surface being treated. At no time is the electrode held by the barber-stylist. To prevent shock, the current is turned on after the client is holding the electrode firmly; current is turned off before removing the electrode from the client's hand.

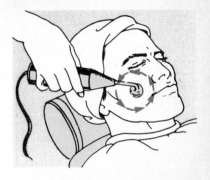

8.15 – Applying high-frequency to face using facial electrode

CAUTION: The client should avoid contact with any metal, such as chair arms, stools, etc. A burn may occur if such contact is made.

3. **General electrification.** By holding a metal electrode, the client's body is charged with electricity without being touched by the barber-stylist.

To obtain relaxing, calming, or soothing effects with high-frequency current, the general electrification treatment is used or the electrode is kept in close contact with the parts treated by the use of direct surface application.

To obtain a stimulating effect, the electrode is lifted slightly from the parts to be treated by using it through the clothing or a towel.

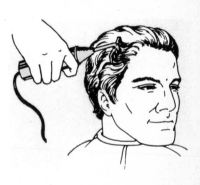

8.16 – Applying high-frequency to scalp using rake electrode

CAUTION: When using high-frequency with skin and scalp lotions, never use a lotion with an alcoholic content. If the use of this type of lotion is necessary, use the electricity first, and apply the lotion after the treatment with electricity has been completed.

Benefits of Tesla High-Frequency

1. Stimulates circulation of the blood.
2. Increases glandular activity.
3. Aids in elimination and absorption.
4. Increases metabolism.
5. Germicidal action occurs during use.

The Tesla current may be used to treat falling hair, itchy scalp, tight scalp, and excessively oily or dry skin and scalp.

The Vibrator

The vibrator is an electric appliance used in massage to produce a succession of stimulating impulses. It has an invigorating effect on muscle tissue, increases the blood supply to the parts treated, is soothing to the nerves, increases glandular activity, and stimulates the skin and scalp.

> CAUTION: **The vibrator should never be used when there is a known weakness of the heart or in cases of fever, abscesses, or inflammation.**

The vibrator may be used by attaching it to the back of the hand. The vibrations are thus transmitted through the hand or fingers to the parts being treated. It is used over heavy muscle tissue such as the scalp, shoulder, and upper back. It is advisable never to use a vibrator on the face or near the eyes.

Steamer or Vaporizer

Steamers or vaporizers are electrical devices applied over the head or face to produce a moist, uniform heat.

The steamer may be used instead of hot towels to cleanse and steam the face. The steam warms the skin, inducing the flow of both oil and sweat. It thus helps to cleanse the skin and soften any scaliness on its surface. The steamer also may be used for scalp and hair reconditioning treatments. When fitted over the scalp, it produces controlled, moist heat. Its action is to soften the scalp, increase perspiration, and promote the effectiveness of applied scalp cosmetics.

Ultraviolet Rays

How applied. Ultraviolet rays are the shortest light rays of the spectrum. The farther they are from the visible light region, the shorter they become. If the lamp is placed from 30 to 36 inches away, practically none of the shorter rays will reach the skin, so that the action is limited to the effect of the longer rays.

The benefits of the shorter rays are obtained when the lamp is within 12 inches of the skin.

CAUTION: Ultraviolet rays are destructive not only to bacteria, but also to tissue, if they are allowed to remain exposed for too long a period of time.

Average exposure to ultraviolet rays may produce redness of the skin, and overdoses may cause blistering. It is well to start with a two- or three-minute exposure, and gradually increase the time to seven or eight minutes. The barber-stylist and client must wear safety goggles to protect their eyes.

Skin and scalp disorders. Ultraviolet rays are used to treat acne, tinea, seborrhea, and to combat dandruff. They also help to promote healing, as well as stimulate the growth of hair.

Infrared Rays

Infrared rays generally produce a soothing and beneficial type of heat that extends for some distance into the tissues of the body.

The effects of infrared rays on exposed area include:

1. heating and relaxing the skin without increasing the temperature of the body as a whole;
2. dilating blood vessels in the skin, thereby increasing blood flow;
3. increasing metabolism and chemical changes within skin tissues;
4. increasing the production of perspiration and oil on the skin;
5. relieving pain.

How applied. The lamp is operated at an average distance of 30 inches. It is placed closer at the start of the treatment and, in order to avoid burning the skin, is then moved back gradually as the surface heat becomes more pronounced. Always protect the eyes of the client during exposure. Place cotton pads saturated with boric acid or witch hazel solution over the client's eyelids. (Fig. 8.17)

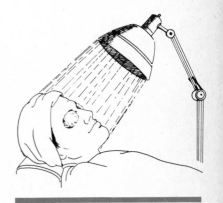

8.17 – Applying infrared rays

CAUTION: Do not permit the light rays to remain on the body tissue more than a few seconds at a time. Move the hand back and forth across the ray's path to break constant exposure. Length of exposure should total about five minutes.

Safety Precautions

1. Disconnect any appliances when they are not being used.
2. Study instructions before using any electrical equipment.
3. Keep all wires, plugs, and equipment in a safe condition.
4. Inspect all electrical equipment frequently.
5. Avoid wetting electric cords.
6. Sanitize all electrodes properly.
7. Protect the client at all times.
8. Do not touch any metal while using electrical appliances.
9. Do not handle electrical equipment with wet hands.
10. Do not allow clients to touch any metal surfaces when electric treatments are being given.
11. Do not leave the room when the client is attached to any electrical device.
12. Do not attempt to clean around an electric outlet when equipment is plugged in.
13. Do not touch two metallic objects at the same time while connected to an electric current.
14. Do not use any electrical equipment without first obtaining full instruction for its care and use.

The protection and safety of the client are the primary concern of the barber-stylist. All electrical equipment should be inspected regularly to determine whether it is in good working condition. Carelessness may result in shocks or burns. The barber-stylist who observes safety precautions will help to eliminate accidents and assure greater satisfaction to all clients.

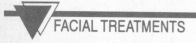

FACIAL TREATMENTS

The barber-stylist does not treat skin diseases, but should be able to recognize various skin ailments and differentiate those that can be serviced in the barber-styling shop from those that should be referred to a physician.

Facial treatments in the barber-styling shop come under two categories:

1. **Preservative**—designed to maintain the health of facial skin by correct cleansing methods, increased circulation, relaxation of the nerves, activation of the skin glands, and increased metabolism.
2. **Corrective**—used to correct skin conditions such as dryness, oiliness, blackheads, aging lines, and minor acne.

The benefits of facial treatments are:

1. They cleanse the skin.
2. They increase circulation.
3. They activate glandular activity.
4. They relax tense nerves.
5. They maintain muscle tone.
6. They strengthen weak muscle tissue.
7. They correct certain skin disorders.
8. They help prevent the formation of wrinkles and aging lines.
9. They improve skin texture and complexion.
10. They help to reduce fatty tissues.

To give the various types of facial treatments, the barber-stylist requires hot and cold water, towels, a vibrator, a therapeutic lamp, and various preparations such as facial creams, ointments, lotions, oils, packs, masks, and powders.

Scientific Rest Facial

The scientific rest facial is a general treatment, beneficial for its cleansing and stimulating action on the skin. It also exercises, as well as relaxes, the facial muscles.

The five causes of wrinkles are:

1. loosening of the elastic skin fibers because of abnormal tension or relaxation of the facial muscles;
2. shrinking of the skin tissue as a result of aging;
3. excessive dryness or oiliness of the skin;
4. facial expressions that continually crease and fold the skin;
5. improper hygiene.

Preparation

Preparation for a scientific rest facial includes:

1. Arrange all the necessary supplies in their proper place.
2. Adjust the chair, linens, and towels.
3. Protect the client's hair by fastening a towel around the head.
4. Recline the hydraulic chair.

All creams and other products should be removed from their containers with a sanitized spatula. Do not dip the fingers into them.

Procedure

The following steps may be followed in giving a scientific rest facial. However, your instructor's routine is equally correct.

1. Apply cleansing cream over the face, using stroking and rotary movements.
2. Remove the cleansing cream with a smooth, warm, damp towel.
3. Steam the face mildly with three towels.
4. Apply tissue cream to the skin with the fingertips.
5. Gently massage the face, using continuous and rhythmic movements. (See **Massage Manipulations** and **Facial Manipulations** in this chapter.)
6. Wipe off any excess cream with a hot towel.
7. Steam the face with hot towels.
8. Follow the steam treatment with a cool towel.
9. Pat astringent or face lotion over the face, then dry it.
10. Apply powder to the face, removing any excess.
11. Raise the hydraulic chair.

Clean-up

1. Discard all disposable supplies and materials.
2. Close containers tightly, clean them, and put them in their proper places.
3. Sanitize all implements used.
4. Wash and sanitize your hands.

Points to Remember in Facial Massaging

1. Have the client thoroughly relaxed.
2. Provide a quiet atmosphere.
3. Maintain supplies in a clean, orderly fashion.
4. Follow a systematic procedure.
5. Give the facial massage properly.

Eleven Reasons Why a Client May Find Fault with a Facial

1. Harming or scratching the skin
2. Excessive or rough massage
3. Getting facial cream into the eyes
4. Using towels that are too hot
5. Breathing into the client's face
6. Not being careful or sanitary
7. Not showing interest in the client's skin problems
8. Carelessness in removing cream, leaving a greasy film behind the ears, under the chin, or in other areas
9. Not permitting the client to relax, either by talking or being tense while giving facial manipulations
10. Leaving the chair to obtain materials or supplies
11. Heavy, rough, or cold hands

Facial Manipulations

In facial manipulations, remember that an even tempo or rhythm induces relaxation. Do not remove the hands from the face after beginning the manipulations. Should it become necessary to remove the hands, they should be feathered off and likewise very gently replaced with feather-like movements.

Each instructor may have developed a particular routine in giving manipulations. The following illustrations merely show

NOTE: Repeat all massage movements three to six times.

the different movements that may be used on the various parts of the face and neck. Follow your instructor's routine. (Figs. 8.18–8.26)

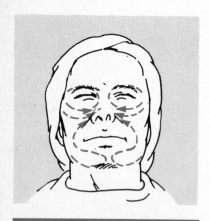

8.18 – Apply cleansing cream lightly over the face with stroking, spreading, and circular movements.

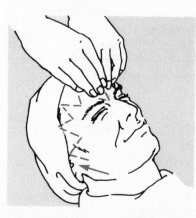

8.19 – Stroke fingers across forehead with up and down movements.

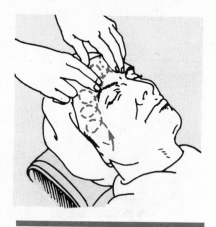

8.20 – Manipulate fingers across forehead with a circular movement.

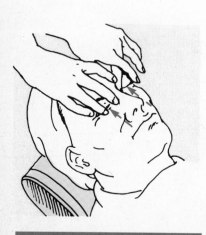

8.21 – Stroke fingers upward along side of nose.

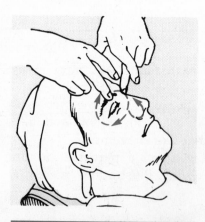

8.22 – Apply a circular movement over side of nose and use a light, stroking movement around the eyes.

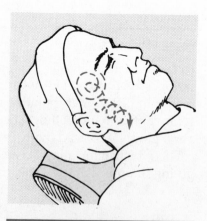

8.23 – Manipulate the temples with a wide circular movement. Also manipulate the front and back of the ears with a circular movement.

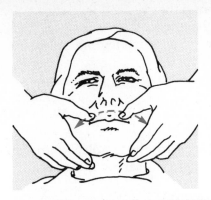

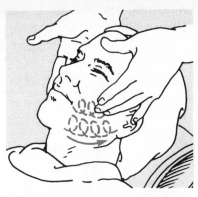

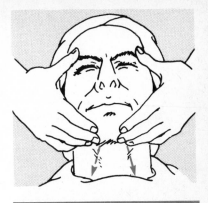

8.24 – Gently stroke both thumbs across upper lip.

8.25 – Manipulate fingers from corners of mouth to cheeks and temples with a circular movement. Manipulate fingers along lower jawbone from tip of chin to ear with a circular movement. Stroke fingers above and below along lower jawbone from tip of chin to ear.

8.26 – Manipulate fingers from under chin and neck to back of ears, and up to temples.

Vibratory Facial

The procedure for a vibratory facial is similar to the scientific rest facial with minor variations. Again we emphasize that the following procedure may be changed to conform with your instructor's routine.

Procedure

1. Prepare the client and steam the face with warm towels.
2. Apply massage cream.
3. Administer the massage, using the vibrator.
4. Apply a little cold cream with light hand manipulations.
5. Remove all the cream with a warm towel and follow with a mild witch hazel steam.
6. Apply one or two cool towels, followed by a face lotion.
7. Dry thoroughly and apply powder.

Massage Movements Using Vibrator

1. Adjust the vibrator on the right hand and place the fingertips on the left nostril. Vibrate the left side of face as follows:
2. Vibrate a few light up and down movements on the left side of the nose.

3. Gently slide the fingers around the eyes and then direct them toward the center of the forehead.
4. Vibrate rotary movement toward the left temple. Pause for a moment.
5. Continue the rotary movements down along the jawline toward the tip of chin.
6. Vibrate from the chin toward the cheek, using wider, firmer movements.
7. Continue with a slow, light stroke at the temple, around the left ear, over the jawbone, toward the center of the neck, and then below the chin.
8. Vibrate rotary movements over the neck, behind the ear, up to the temple, and then toward the center of the forehead.
9. Repeat steps 2 through 8 on the right side of the face.
10. Repeat steps 2 through 8 on the left side and then on the right side of the face.

Rules to Follow in Using Vibrator

1. Regulate the number of vibrations to avoid over-stimulation.
2. Do not use the vibrator for too long in any one spot.
3. Vary the amount of pressure in accordance with the results desired.
4. Do not use a vibrator over the upper lip, as the vibrations may cause discomfort.
5. For soothing and relaxing effects, give very slow, light vibrations for a very short time.
6. For stimulating effects, give light vibrations of moderate speed and time.
7. For reducing fatty tissues, give moderate, fast vibrations with firm pressure.

Rolling Cream Facial

The facial massage formerly identified with the barber-styling shop is the rolling cream facial. For many years, this was the only type of facial service available. However, with the development of new products and techniques, comprehensive facial services have become available. It is advisable, however, to understand the rolling cream facial, its purpose, and its basic procedure.

The rolling cream facial is designed to cleanse and stimulate the skin. Due to the drying qualities of the rolling cream and the application process, this type of facial should be recommended only to clients with normal, oily, or thick skin. It should not be given to clients with very dry skin, acne, tender or sensitive skin, thin skin, or rough or pimpled skin.

Rolling massage cream is pink. It becomes dry and flakes off as it is being massaged over the skin.

NOTE: The following is one of several methods for performing this service. Your instructor may use a different technique which is equally correct.

Procedure

1. Prepare the client.
2. Moderately steam the face with two or three warm towels.
3. Apply dabs of rolling cream to the chin, cheeks, and forehead. Dampen the fingertips of both hands with water and spread the cream evenly over the face and neck with a smooth, stroking movement.
4. Massage the face and neck with uniform, rotary, stroking and rubbing movements with the cushion tips of the fingers, until most of the cream has rolled off.

CAUTION: Be careful not to use rough movements over the skin or permit particles of the cream to get into the client's eyes.

5. Apply a small amount of cold cream to the face and neck, using lighter manipulations. Remove the cream with a warm towel.
6. Apply witch hazel steam to the face and neck with one or more hot towels, following with one or two cold towels to close the pores.
7. Apply astringent lotion. Dry and powder the face and neck.
8. Finish as for a scientific rest facial.

◢ SPECIAL PROBLEMS

Facial for Dry Skin

Dry skin is caused by an insufficient flow of sebum (oil) from the sebaceous glands. The facial for dry skin helps moisturize it. It may be given with or without an electrical current. For more effective results, the use of electrical current is recommended.

Procedure with Infrared Rays

1. Prepare the client as for a plain facial.
2. Apply cleansing cream; remove cream with tissues or with a warm, moist towel.
3. Sponge the face with cleansing lotion.
4. Apply massage cream.
5. Apply lubricating oil, or eye cream, over and under the eyes.
6. Apply lubricating oil over the neck.
7. Cover the client's eyes with cotton pads moistened with witch hazel or boric acid solution.
8. Expose the face and neck to infrared rays for not more than five minutes.
9. Give manipulation three to five times.
10. Remove the massage cream and oil with tissues, or with a warm, moist towel.
11. Apply skin lotion suitable for dry skin.
12. Blot the face dry with tissues or a towel.
13. Complete and clean up as for a plain facial.

> CAUTION: For dry skin, avoid using lotions that contain a large percentage of alcohol. Read the manufacturer's directions.

Procedure with Galvanic Current

The procedure for giving a dry skin facial with galvanic current is similar to the procedure for giving a dry skin facial with infrared rays, with a few changes:

1. Repeat steps 1 through 3 of the procedure used with infrared rays.
2. Apply negative galvanic current for three to five minutes, to open the pores.
3. Repeat steps 4 through 11 of the procedure used with infrared rays.

4. Apply positive galvanic current for three to five minutes, to close the pores.
5. Repeat steps 12 through 13 of the procedure used with infrared rays.

Procedure with Indirect High-Frequency Current

1. Follow steps 1 through 8 of the procedure for a facial with infrared rays.
2. Give manipulations, using the indirect method of applying high-frequency current, for not more than seven minutes. (See Fig. 8.27)
3. Apply two or three cold towels to the face and neck.

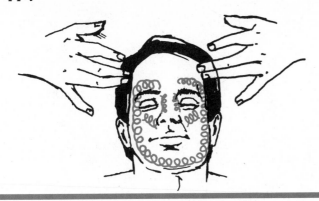

8.27 – High-frequency indirect method. (Client holds electrode.)

4. Sponge the face and neck with skin freshener.
5. Apply a moisturizer.

Facial for Oily Skin and Blackheads (Comedones)

Oily skin and/or blackheads (comedones) are caused by hardened masses of sebum formed in the ducts of the sebaceous glands. Sometimes the client's diet may be a factor. For diet to help minimize oily skin and blackheads, the client should see a physician.

Procedure

1. Prepare the client as for a plain facial. Sanitize your hands.
2. Apply cleansing lotion and remove it with a warm, moist towel, moist cotton pads, or facial sponges.
3. Place moistened eyepads on the client's eyes, then analyze the skin under a magnifying lamp.

4. Steam the face with three or four moist, warm towels, or steam the face with a facial steamer to open the pores.
5. Cover your fingertips with tissue and gently press out blackheads. Do not press so hard as to bruise the skin tissue.

> CAUTION: If it is necessary to cleanse pimples that have come to a head and are open, use rubber or latex gloves. Do not attempt to deal with a skin problem that requires medical attention.

6. Sponge the face with astringent.
7. Cover the client's eyes with pads moistened with a mild astringent.
8. Apply blue light over the skin for not more than three to five minutes.
9. Apply massage cream suitable for the skin condition.
10. Give manipulations.
11. Remove cream with a warm, moist towel, cotton pads, or facial sponges.
12. Moisten a cotton pledget with an astringent lotion. Apply it to the face and neck with upward and outward movements to close the pores.
13. Blot the excess moisture with tissues.
14. Apply protective lotion if needed.
15. Complete and clean up, following proper sanitary procedures.

Whiteheads (Milia)

Milia or **whiteheads** are caused by the formation of sebaceous matter within or under the skin. They usually occur in skin of fine texture. The surface openings of the skin may be so small that the sebum cannot pass out. As a result, it collects under the surface of the skin in small, round, hardened, pearl-like masses that resemble small grains of sand. This condition may be treated under the supervision of a dermatologist.

Facial for Acne

Acne is a disorder of the sebaceous glands; it requires medical direction. If the client is under medical care, the role of the barber-stylist is to work closely with the client's physician to perform facial treatments as prescribed.

Under medical direction, the treatment of acne must be limited to the following measures:

1. reducing the oiliness of the skin by local applications;
2. removing blackheads, using proper procedures;
3. cleansing the skin;
4. using special medicated preparations.

Equipment, Implements, and Materials

- Acne cream or lotion
- Antiseptic lotion
- Cleansing lotion
- Astringent lotion for oily skin
- Towels
- Appropriate mask
- High-frequency magnifying lamp

Procedure

Because acne contains infectious matter, it is advisable to use rubber or latex gloves and disposable materials such as cotton cleansing pads.

1. Prepare all the materials needed for the facial treatment.
2. Prepare the client.
3. Sanitize your hands.
4. Cleanse the client's face.
5. Place cotton eyepads over the client's eyes; then analyze the skin under the magnifying lamp.
6. Apply warm, wet towels to the face to open the pores for deep cleansing.
7. Extract blackheads and cleanse pimples.
8. Cleanse the face with a wet cotton pad that has been sprinkled with astringent.
9. Apply the acne treatment cream. Leave on the eyepads and turn on the infrared lamp for five to seven minutes to enable the treatment cream to penetrate the skin. Or, you can apply high-frequency current with direct application (facial electrode) over the affected area for not more than five minutes. (See Fig. 8.28) Be guided by your instructor.
10. Leave on the eyepads and apply a treatment mask that is suitable for the skin condition. Leave it on the face for eight to ten minutes.
11. Remove the mask with moist towels or cotton pads.

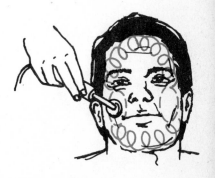

8.28 – Applying high-frequency current with facial electrode

12. Apply astringent to the face with a wet cotton pad.
13. Apply protective fluid or special acne lotion.
14. Complete the cleanup procedures.

Diet for Acne

Modern studies show that acne may be due to both hereditary and environmental factors. It can be aggravated by emotional stress and faulty diet. Acne is not believed to be caused by any particular food or drink, but foods high in fats, starches, and sugars tend to worsen the condition. The client should consult a physician for a prescribed diet. A well-balanced diet, drinking plenty of water, and following healthful personal hygiene habits are recommended.

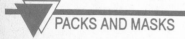

PACKS AND MASKS

Facial packs and masks are popular in the barber-styling shop. They can be used as part of a facial or applied as a separate treatment.

Face packs and masks differ in their composition and usage. Packs are usually applied directly to the skin. On the other hand, masks are applied to the skin with the aid of gauze layers.

High-quality packs and masks should feel comfortable and produce slight tingling and tightening sensations. Whatever product is used, follow the manufacturer's directions for preparation, application, and removal from the skin. It is important that at all times the skin be cleansed before applying a pack or mask.

Depending on their composition, packs can cleanse, soften, smooth, stimulate, and refresh the face. The results obtained, however, are temporary.

Clay Pack

The clay pack is suitable for all except dry skin types. It has a mild tonic effect that prevents undue wrinkling.

Procedure

1. Prepare a warm clay pack according to the manufacturer's directions.
2. Prepare the client by arranging the linen and fastening a towel around the head to protect the hair.
3. Steam the skin with three moderately hot towels.
4. Spread the warm clay pack over the warm skin, using continuous stroking and rotary movements.
5. Cover the eyes with cotton pads moistened with witch hazel.

6. Dry the pack on the skin by exposure to a red dermal lamp.
7. Remove the pack with warm, damp steam towels.
8. (Optional.) Expose the face to soothing blue light for a few minutes.
9. Apply cold cream or tissue cream with a few soothing massage movements.
10. Remove the cream, and apply two cold towels.
11. Apply a mild lotion, dry, and powder.

Hot Oil Mask

The hot oil mask is recommended for extremely dry, parched, and scaly skin, prevalent during dry, hot, or windy weather. It is used to soften, smooth, and stimulate the skin tissues.

Formula for Hot Oil Mask

- 2 tablespoons of olive oil
- 1 tablespoon of castor oil (refined grade)
- ¼ teaspoon of glycerine
- Mix the oils in a small container and warm

Procedure

1. Prepare the client as for a scientific rest facial.
2. Prepare the mask. Saturate cotton pads (4" × 4") or an 18-inch square of gauze with the warm oil mixture.
3. Follow steps 1 through 5 as in scientific rest facial.
4. After the manipulations do not remove the cream, but place the cotton pads or gauze over the face.
5. Adjust the eyepads.
6. Use red dermal light or an infrared lamp for eight to ten minutes.
7. Remove the mask and cream.
8. Finish the facial as in a scientific rest facial.

Commercial Facial Packs and Masks

Available for use in the barber-styling shop are various types of commercial facial packs and masks, such as milk and honey pack, egg white pack, and witch hazel pack. For proper use, the barber-stylist should first read the manufacturer's claims and directions. Judge the merits of the pack or mask before recommending it to a client.

REVIEW QUESTIONS

Muscles

1. Define muscle.
2. What are the three important functions of the muscles?
3. What are the three parts of a muscle?
4. Define: a) origin of muscle, b) insertion of muscle.
5. Name seven sources capable of stimulating muscular tissue.
6. With which muscles of the head, face, and neck is the barber-stylist concerned?
7. Name the scalp muscle and its two parts.
8. What is the function of the frontalis?
9. Which muscle surrounds the eye socket?
10. Which muscle forms a band around the upper and lower lips?
11. Which muscle covers the back of the neck?
12. Which muscle bends the head as in nodding?

Nerves

1. Define nerves.
2. What is the function of nerves?
3. What does stimulation cause the nerves to do?
4. What effect does heat have on nerves? Cold?
5. How may nerve stimulation be accomplished?
6. How many pairs of cranial nerves are there?
7. Which three cranial nerves are the most important in the massaging of the head, face, and neck?
8. Which is the largest cranial nerve?
9. What is the function of the fifth or trifacial nerve?
10. Which cranial nerve controls the muscles of facial expression?
11. Which cranial nerve controls the sense of: a) sight; b) smell; c) hearing?
12. Which region of the head is supplied by the greater occipital nerve?
13. Which cranial nerve supplies the neck muscles?
14. Which branches of the trifacial nerve supply the following regions?
    a) forehead
    b) lower side of nose
    c) skin of upper lip
    d) skin of lower lip
    e) skin above temple
    f) skin of upper part of cheek
15. Which branches of the facial nerve supply the following regions or muscles?
    a) muscles of side of forehead
    b) muscles of chin and lower lip

c) platysma muscle
d) muscle behind ear
e) mouth muscle
f) muscles of upper part of cheek

1. Which main arteries supply blood to the entire head, face, and neck?
2. Name two main divisions of the common carotid arteries.
3. Which branch of the common carotid artery supplies the cranial cavity?
4. Which branches of the common carotid arteries supply blood to various regions of head, face, and neck?
5. Give the common name for the external maxillary artery.
6. Name the artery that supplies the chin.
7. Which artery supplies the forehead?
8. What part of the head does the occipital artery supply?
9. What part of the head does the parietal artery supply? Frontal artery?
10. What artery supplies that part of the scalp that is in back of and above the ear?
11. Name the artery that supplies the eye muscles.
12. Name the principal veins by which the blood from the head, face, and neck is returned to the heart.

1. What is massage?
2. What parts of the body are usually massaged by the barber-stylist?
3. Name five basic movements used in massage.
4. What are the effects of massage on the skin?
5. What is the effect of massage on the blood circulation?

1. What are ten benefits of facial treatments?
2. Which supplies and equipment are required for facial treatments?
3. Why should the barber-stylist know the histology of the skin and the anatomy of the head, face, and neck before giving a facial massage?
4. In giving a plain facial, what attention should the barber-stylist show toward a client?
5. Why should the barber-stylist never lean over the client's face?
6. What preparation should be made before giving a plain facial?
7. Briefly outline the procedure for giving a plain facial.
8. What are five important points to remember in giving a plain facial?
9. Give 11 reasons why a client may find fault with a facial.
10. What is the purpose of a dry skin facial?
11. What are the principal causes of an oily skin?
12. What implement is used to press out blackheads and whiteheads?
13. What is the action of a clay pack on the skin?
14. Which facial treatment requires the guidance of a physician?

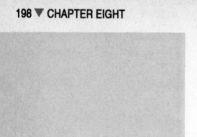

15. In which facial treatments should the eyes be covered with cotton pads?
16. In which facial treatments should an astringent lotion or cream be applied?
17. For what skin condition should a hot oil mask be recommended?

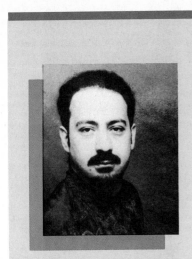

9

Shaving

Learning Objectives

After completing this chapter, you should be able to:

1. *Define the objective of shaving.*
2. *List the factors that should be taken into account before performing a shave.*
3. *Demonstrate the ability to handle the razor in four standard cutting positions and strokes.*
4. *Identify the fourteen shaving areas of the face.*
5. *Demonstrate a neck shave.*
6. *Discuss safety and sanitation procedures and precautions.*
7. *Demonstrate a facial shave.*

Courtesy of: Team Artista, Scarsdale, NY.

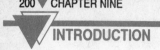

INTRODUCTION

Several decades ago, shaving was one of the services most frequently performed in a barber–styling shop. Today, however, the number of clients desiring to be shaved has declined to a point where shaving is in danger of becoming a lost art. This is due partially to the wide use of safety and electric razors, and also to the fast pace of today's society. It is simply quicker and easier for most men to shave themselves as part of their daily personal hygiene routine.

There are still barber–styling shops, however, where shaves are available for those who wish them. Usually these are either full–service, luxury salons or the more traditional, established shops where the service has been offered for many years. Few chain, unisex, or franchised salons offer shaving services. The art of shaving requires a great deal of attention, skill, and consistent practice.

FUNDAMENTALS OF SHAVING

The object of shaving is to remove the visible part of facial and neck hair without irritating the skin. The professional barber–stylist uses a straight razor and warm lather when shaving a client.

Although there are certain general principles of shaving, there are exceptions. A number of factors need to be considered: hair texture, the grain of the beard, and the sensitivity of the skin. Hot towels should not be used when the skin is chapped or blistered from heat or cold. A person having any infection in the area to be shaved must not be served because of the danger of spreading the infection.

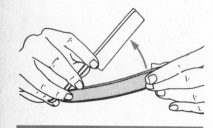

9.1 – Opening razor

> CAUTION: Some states require the stylist to wear protective gloves while shaving a client. Be guided by your instructor about the use of gloves in your state for this procedure.

Four Standard Shaving Positions and Strokes

The correct angle of cutting the beard with a straight razor is called the **cutting stroke**. To achieve the best cutting stroke, the razor must glide over the surface at an angle with the grain of the hair. It should be drawn in a forward movement with the point of the razor in the lead.

Before the student shaves a client, it is necessary to master the fundamentals of handling the razor. (Figs. 9.1 and 9.2)

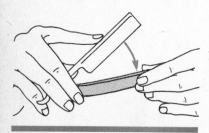

9.2 – Closing razor

To shave the face and neck with ease and efficiency, the following standard positions and strokes should be used:

1. Free-hand position and stroke
2. Back-hand position and stroke
3. Reverse free-hand position and stroke
4. Reverse back-hand position and stroke

Under each of the standard shaving positions and strokes, consideration should be given to:

1. How to hold the razor for each stroke
   a) Position of right hand with razor
   b) Position of left hand
2. How to stroke the razor
3. When to use a particular shaving stroke

Review the proper method of honing and stropping the razor before learning each shaving stroke.

CAUTION: When closing the razor, be careful that the cutting edge does not strike the handle.

Exercise No. 1

Free-Hand Position and Stroke
In the first lesson, the student learns the correct way to perform the free-hand position and stroke. To master this important shaving skill requires regular practice.

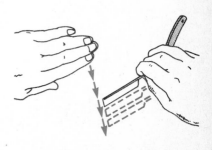

9.3 – Proper way to hold razor for free-hand stroke

1. **How to hold the razor.** The position of the right hand is as follows:
   a) Take the razor in the right hand.
   b) Hold the handle of the razor between the third and fourth fingers, the small fingertip resting on the tang of the razor. Place the tip of the thumb on the reverse side of the shank, close to blade. Rest the fingertips on the back of the shank. (Fig. 9.3)
   c) Raise the right elbow level with the shoulder. This is the position used in the arm movement.

NOTE: Some barber-stylists prefer to use the wrist movement, in which case the elbow is not raised as high.

The position of the left hand is as follows:
a) Keep the fingers of the left hand dry in order to prevent them from slipping on the wet face.
b) Keep the left hand back of the razor in order to stretch the skin tightly under the razor.

Exercise No. 2

Back-Hand Position and Stroke
After learning the free-hand position and stroke, the student is ready to proceed with the back-hand position and stroke.

1. **How to hold the razor.** The position of the right hand is as follows:
   a) Hold the shank of the razor firmly with the handle bent slightly back.
   b) Rest the shank of the razor on the first two joints of the first three fingers. Hold the thumb on the underside of the shank. Rest the end of the tang inside the first joint of the third finger as in Fig. 9.4. The little finger remains idle. For two other ways to hold a razor, see Figs. 9.5 and 9.6.

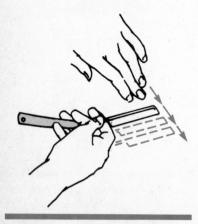

9.4 – First two joints of the first three fingers

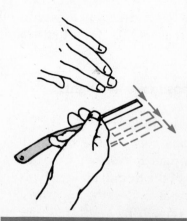

9.5 – First two joints of the first two fingers

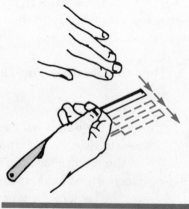

9.6 – Fingers wrapped around handle

c) Turn the back of the hand away from you and bend the wrist slightly downward. Then raise the elbow so that you can move the arm freely. This is the position used for the back-hand stroke with the arm movement.

NOTE: Some barber-stylists prefer to use the wrist movement, in which case the arm is not held as high as for the arm movement.

The position of the left hand is as follows:
a) Keep the fingers of the left hand dry in order to prevent them from slipping.
b) Stretch the skin tightly under razor.

2. **How to stroke the razor.** The back-hand stroke is performed in the following manner:
   a) Use a gliding stroke away from you.
   b) Direct the stroke toward the point of the razor in a forward, sawing movement. (Fig. 9.7)

3. **How to stroke the razor.** The free-hand stroke is performed in the following manner:
   a) Use a gliding stroke, toward you.
   b) Direct the stroke toward the point of the razor in a forward, sawing movement. (Fig. 9.8)

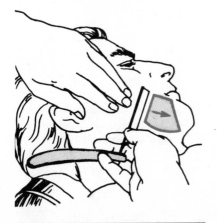

9.7 – Back-hand stroke

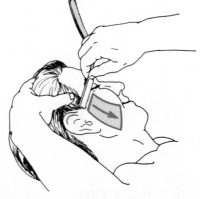

9.8 – Free-hand stroke

4. **When to use the free-hand stroke.** The free-hand position and stroke is used in six of the fourteen shaving areas. See Numbers 1, 3, 4, 8, 11, and 12 shaded on Figs. 9.9, 9.10, and 9.11.

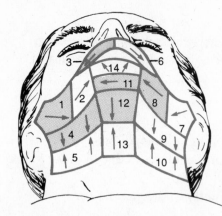

1. Free hand
2. Back hand
3. Free hand
4. Free hand
5. Reverse free hand
6. Back hand
7. Back hand
8. Free hand
9. Back hand
10. Reverse free hand
11. Free hand
12. Free hand
13. Reverse free hand
14. Reverse free hand

9.9 – Diagram of shaving areas for the free-hand stroke

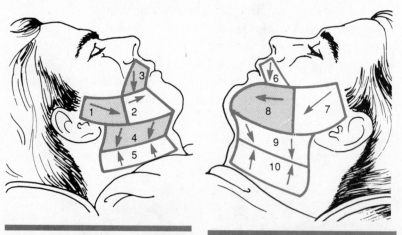

9.10 – Diagram of shaving areas on the right side of the face for the free-hand stroke

9.11 – Diagram of shaving area on the left side of the face for the free-hand stroke

5. **When to use the back-hand stroke.** The back-hand stroke is used in four of the fourteen basic shaving areas. See Numbers 2, 6, 7, and 9 shaded on Figs. 9.12, 9.13, and 9.14.

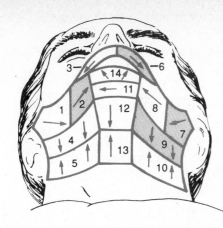

1. Free hand
2. Back hand
3. Free hand
4. Free hand
5. Reverse free hand
6. Back hand
7. Back hand
8. Free hand
9. Back hand
10. Reverse free hand
11. Free hand
12. Free hand
13. Reverse free hand
14. Reverse free hand

9.12 – Diagram of shaving areas for the back-hand stroke

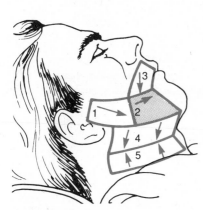

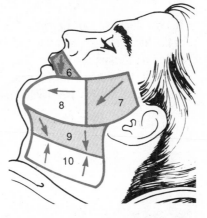

9.13 – Diagram of shaving area on the right side of the face for the back-hand stroke

9.14 – Diagram of shaving areas on the left side of the face for the back-hand stroke

Exercise No. 3

Reverse Free-Hand Position and Stroke

The reverse free-hand stroke and the free-hand stroke are similar in some ways, the main difference being that the movement is directed upward in the reverse free-hand stroke, while the palm of the hand faces the barber-stylist.

1. **How to hold the razor.** The position of the right hand is as follows:

    a) Hold the razor firmly, as in a free-hand position. Turn

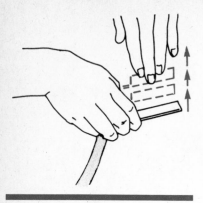

9.15 – Reverse free-hand stroke

the hand slightly toward you so that the razor edge is turned upward. (Fig. 9.15)

The position of the left hand is as follows:

a) Keep hand dry and use it to pull the skin tightly under razor.

2. **How to stroke the razor.** The reverse free-hand stroke is performed in the following manner:

a) Use an upward, semi-arc stroke toward you.

b) The movement is from the elbow to the hand with a slight twist of the wrist. (Fig. 9.16)

3. **When to use the reverse free-hand stroke.** The reverse free-hand stroke is used in four of the fourteen basic shaving areas. See Numbers 5, 10, 13, and 14 shaded on Figs. 9.17, 9.18, and 9.19.

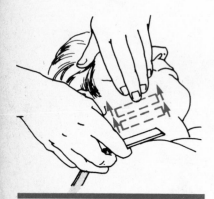

9.16 – Reverse free-hand stroke, shaving area No. 5

> **NOTE:** Because the beard must be shaved at an angle with the grain of the hair, the barber–stylist must determine if the reverse hand positions and strokes are the correct procedure for the individual client. For example: If the hair in cutting area No. 5 grows downward, the free-hand stroke may be used rather than the reverse free-hand stroke.

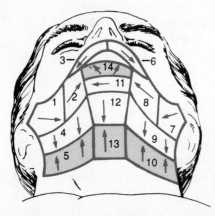

1. Free hand
2. Back hand
3. Free hand
4. Free hand
5. Reverse free hand
6. Back hand
7. Back hand
8. Free hand
9. Back hand
10. Reverse free hand
11. Free hand
12. Free hand
13. Reverse free hand
14. Reverse free hand

9.17 – Diagram of shaving areas for the reverse free-hand stroke

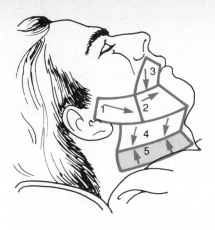

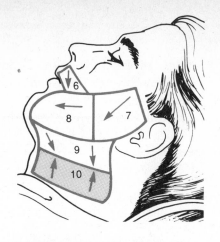

9.18 – Diagram of shaving area on the right side of the face for the reverse free-hand stroke

9.19 – Diagram of shaving area on the left side of the face for the reverse free-hand stroke

Exercise No. 4

Reverse Back-Hand Position and Stroke

The reverse back-hand position and stroke, although not frequently used, require diligent practice in order to master them.

1. **When to use the reverse back-hand stroke.** The reverse back-hand stroke is used for making the left sideburn outline, and for shaving the left side behind the ear while the client is sitting in an upright position. (Fig. 9.20)

2. **How to hold the razor.** The position of the right hand is as follows:
   a) Hold the razor firmly, as in the back-hand position.
   b) Turn the palm of the hand to the right so that it faces upward.
   c) Drop the elbow close to the side.
   The position of the left hand is as follows:
   a) Raise the left arm and hand in order to draw the skin tightly under the razor.

3. **How to stroke the razor.** The reverse back-hand stroke is performed in the following manner:
   a) Use a gliding stroke, directed downward toward the point of the razor in a sawing movement.

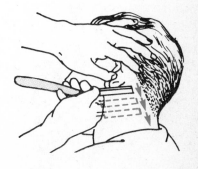

9.20 – Reverse back-hand stroke. Shaving left side of neck below ear.

▼ THE PROFESSIONAL SHAVE

While a professional shave is composed of many individual steps, they all fall under the general classifications: preparation, shaving, and finishing.

The following exercises explain these three classifications in detail.

Exercise No. 5

How to Prepare a Client for Shaving

The stylist's greeting should welcome the client and put the client at ease.

1. Seat the client comfortably in the chair.
2. Ask the client to loosen his collar and drape as for a haircut. Be sure that the towel lies flat and low around the neck area.
3. Change the headrest cover and adjust it to the proper height.
4. Lower, adjust, and lock the chair to the proper height and level.
5. Wash your hands with soap and warm water, and dry them thoroughly.
6. Unfold a clean towel, and lay it diagonally across the client's chest.
7. Tuck the left corner of the towel along the right side of the client's neck, the edge tucked inside the neck–band with a sliding movement of the forefinger of the left hand. (Fig. 9.21) The lower end of the towel is crossed over to the other side of the client's neck and tucked under the neck–band, with a similar sliding motion. (Fig. 9.22)

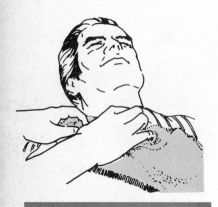

9.21 – Securing the towel on the right side of the client

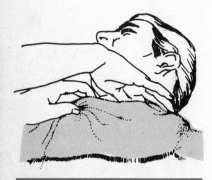

9.22 – Securing the towel on the left side of the client

Exercise No. 6

How to Prepare the Face for Shaving

Lathering and steaming the face are very important steps in preparation for shaving.

Lathering the face serves to:

1. clean the face by dislodging dirt and foreign matter.
2. soften the hair and hold it in an upright position.
3. create a smooth, flat surface over which the razor can glide easily.

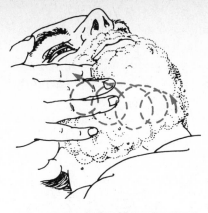

9.23 – Rubbing lather in a rotary movement

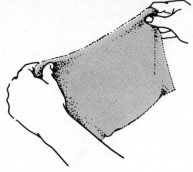

9.24 – Folding a clean towel in half

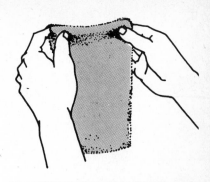

9.25 – Folding towel in half again

Steaming the face helps to:

1. soften the cuticle or outer layer of the hair.
2. provide lubrication by stimulating the action of the oil glands.
3. soothe and relax the client.

CAUTION: Do not use a steam towel if the face is sensitive, irritated, chapped, or blistered.

The face is prepared for shaving as follows:

1. The shaving lather is prepared in the latherizing unit. Transfer a quantity of lather into the hand and spread it evenly over the bearded parts of the face and neck.
2. Rub lather briskly into bearded area with the cushion tips of the right hand, using a circular motion. Rub lather on the right side of the face. (Fig. 9.23) Then gently turn the head with the left hand by lightly grasping the top of the head or the back of the head near the crown. Rub lather on the other side of face. Rubbing time is from one to two minutes, depending on the stiffness and density of the beard.
3. Fold a clean towel once lengthwise. (Fig. 9.24) Then fold it again the short way by bringing together both ends of the towel. (Fig. 9.25)
4. Place the folded towel (Fig. 9.26) under a stream of hot water, allowing it to become thoroughly saturated and heated. (Fig. 9.27)
5. Wring out the towel until it is fairly dry.
6. Bring the steam towel behind the client. Unfold it and hold

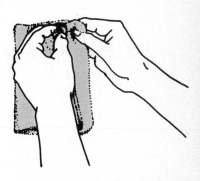

9.26 – Getting ready to place towel under hot water

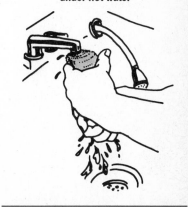

9.27 – Saturating towel thoroughly with hot water

it by the ends. Place the center of towel over the client's mouth, under the chin and the lower part of neck.
(Fig. 9.28) Carefully wrap the towel around the face, leaving the nose exposed. Finally, fold the ends over each other on the forehead, covering the eyes. (Fig. 9.29)

7. While the steam towel is on the client's face, strop the razor

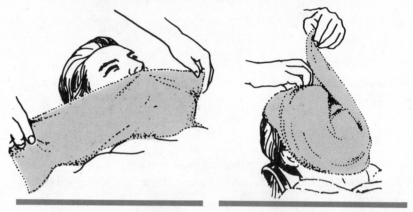

9.28 – Placing towel on client   9.29 – Wrapping towel around client

and immerse it in sanitizing solution. Then wipe the razor dry on a clean towel, and place it in a dry sanitizer until ready for use.

8. Remove the steam towel and wipe the lather off in one operation.

9. Re–lather the beard, then wipe the soap from your hands.

10. Standing on the client's right side, place a piece of clean tissue or paper on the client's chest for wiping lather from the razor. Take the razor out of the dry sanitizer and proceed.

Exercise No. 7

Position and Strokes in Shaving

Razor strokes should be correct and systematic. Proper coordination of both hands is necessary. While the right hand holds and strokes the razor, the fingers of the left hand stretch tightly the skin that is being shaved. A tight skin allows the beard to be cut more easily.

Loose skin tends to push out in front of the razor and can result in cuts or nicks. However, if the skin is stretched too tightly, it will be easily irritated. The skin must be held firmly, neither too loosely nor too tightly, to create a correct shaving surface for the razor. To prevent slipping, use an alum block to help keep the fingers of the left hand dry at all times. (Fig. 9.30)

Shaving Area No. 1

Free-hand stroke. Standing at the right side of chair, gently turn the client's face to the left. With the second finger of the left hand, remove the lather from the hairline. Hold the razor as for a free-hand stroke. Use long, gliding, diagonal strokes, with the point of the razor leading. Beginning at the hairline on the right side, shave downward toward the jawbone. (Fig. 9.31)

Shaving Area No. 2

Back-hand stroke. Remaining in the same position, wipe the razor clean on lather paper. Hold the razor as for a back-hand stroke; use a diagonal stroke with the point of the razor in the lead. Shave all of the beard on the right side of the face. (Fig. 9.32)

Shaving Area No. 3

Free-hand stroke. Keeping the same position, wipe the razor clean. Hold it in the same manner as for a free-hand stroke, shave underneath the nostrils and over the right side of the upper lip, using the fingers of the left hand to stretch the underlying skin. When shaving underneath the nostril, slightly lift the tip of the nose, taking care not to interfere with breathing. To stretch the upper lip, place the fingers of the left hand against the nose, while holding the thumb below the lower corner of the lip. (Fig. 9.33)

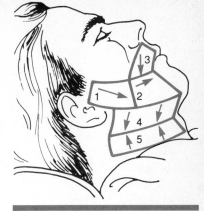

9.30 – Diagram of shaving areas for the right side of the face

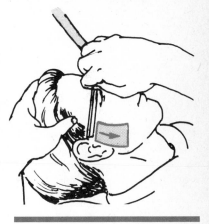

9.31 – Shaving movement No. 1

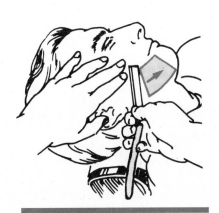

9.32 – Shaving movement No. 2

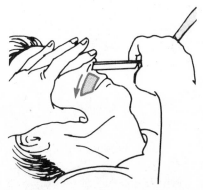

9.33 – Shaving movement No. 3

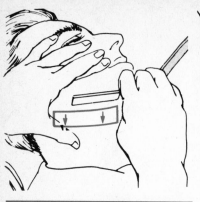

9.34 – Shaving movement No. 4

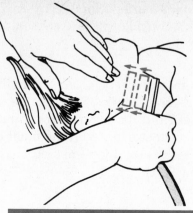

9.35 – Shaving movement No. 5

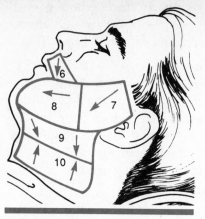

9.36 – Diagram of shaving areas for left side of face

Shaving Area No. 4

Free-hand stroke. Without wiping the razor, start at the point of the chin and shave all that portion below the jawbone, down to the change in the grain of the beard. While shaving, hold the skin tightly between the thumb and fingers of left hand. (Fig. 9.34)

Shaving Area No. 5

Reverse free-hand stroke. Move behind the chair. Hold the razor as for a reverse free-hand stroke. Shave the remainder of the beard upward with the grain. This movement completes shaving of the right side of the face. (Fig. 9.35)

Shaving Area No. 6

Back-hand stroke. (Fig. 9.36) Wipe the razor clean and strop it. Stand to the right side of the client and turn the client's face upward, so that you can shave the left upper lip. Hold the razor as for a back-hand stroke. While gently pushing the tip of the nose to the right with the thumb and fingers of the left hand, shave the left side of upper lip. (Fig. 9.37)

> **NOTE:** Some barber-stylists prefer to shave the upper lip after shaving area No. 8.

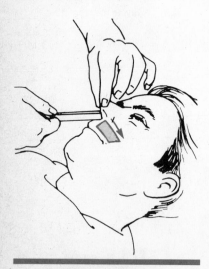

9.37 – Shaving movement No. 6

Shaving Area No. 7

Back-hand stroke. Stand slightly back from the client. Gently turn the face to the right. Re-lather the left side of the face. Clean lather

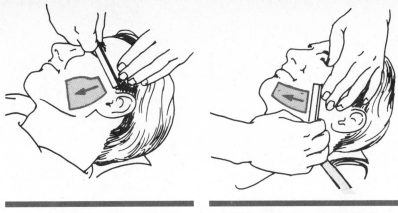

9.38 – Shaving movement No. 7   **9.39 – Shaving movement No. 8**

from the hairline. Stretching the skin with the fingers of the left hand, shave downward to the lower part of the ear, and slightly forward on the face. (Fig. 9.38)

> CAUTION: Be careful to stretch the skin well with the left hand; otherwise the razor may dig in along the ear.

Shaving Area No. 8

Free-hand stroke. Wipe off the razor. Stand to the client's right. Hold the razor as for free-hand stroke. Shave downward on the left side of the face toward the jawbone and point of the chin. (Fig. 9.39)

> NOTE: Some barber-stylists prefer to shave the upper lip at this time. (See Fig. 9.37—Shaving area No. 6.)

Shaving Area No. 9

Back-hand stroke. Wipe off the razor. Keeping the same position, hold the razor as for the back-hand stroke. With the fingers of the left hand tightly stretching the skin, shave downward to where the grain of the beard changes on the neck. (Fig. 9.40)

Shaving Area No. 10

Reverse free-hand stroke. Wipe off the razor. Stand slightly back from the client. Hold the razor as for the reverse free-hand stroke.

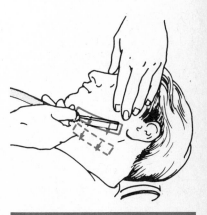

9.40 – Shaving movement No. 9

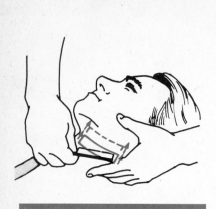

9.41 – Shaving movement No. 10

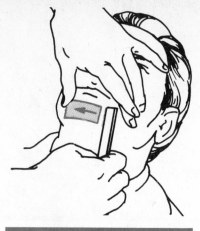

9.42 – Shaving movement No. 11

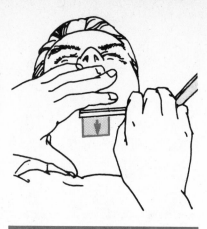

9.43 – Shaving movement No. 12

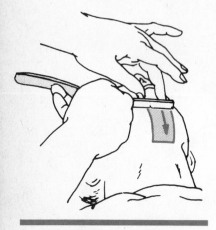

9.44 – Shaving movement No. 12
(alternate method)

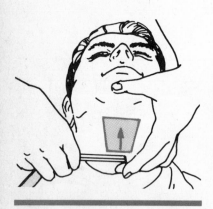

9.45 – Shaving movement No. 13

Stretching the skin tightly with the left hand, shave the left side of the neck upward. (Fig. 9.41)

Shaving Area No. 11

Free-hand stroke. Stand at the client's side and turn the head so the face is pointing up. Holding the razor as for the free-hand stroke, shave across the upper part of the chin. Continue shaving across the chin until it has been shaved to a point below the jawbone. The skin is stretched with the left hand. (Fig. 9.42)

Shaving Area No. 12

Free-hand stroke. Stretch the skin with the left hand and shave the area just below the chin until the change in the grain of the beard is reached. (Fig. 9.43)

Alternate method—some barber-stylists prefer to use the back-hand stroke as shown in Fig. 9.44.

Shaving Area No. 13

Reverse free-hand stroke. Move behind the chair. Hold the razor as for the reverse free-hand stroke. Stretch the skin tightly and shave upward on the lower part of the neck. (Fig. 9.45)

CAUTION: Great care must be taken that the skin over the Adam's Apple is not cut.

Shaving Area No. 14

Reverse free-hand stroke. Remain behind the chair. Shave upward on the lower lip with a few short reverse free-hand strokes. (Fig. 9.46)

Wipe off the razor again, and fold the lather paper in half.

> **NOTE:** When shaving areas No. 13 and No. 14, be careful not to breathe in the client's face. This is annoying and unhealthy.

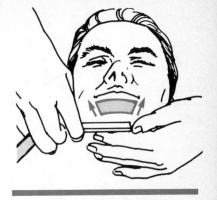

9.46 – Shaving movement No. 14

Close Shaving

The second time over serves to remove any rough or unshaven spots. **Close shaving** is the practice of shaving the beard against the grain of the hair during the **second time over**. This practice is undesirable because it irritates the skin and may lead to infection or ingrown hairs. For this reason, the barber-stylist should be cautious when giving a close shave. However, should the client request it, first remove all traces of lather with a steam towel. Turn the towel over and place it on the face. Strop, sanitize, and close the razor and place it on the work bench. Remove the steam towel and, using a water bottle, sprinkle a little water in the cupped palm of the left hand. (Fig. 9.47) Moisten the bearded part of the face, and proceed with the second time over. Use the free-hand and reverse free-hand strokes in this process.

Stand slightly behind the client. With a free-hand stroke, start to shave the right side of the face. (Fig. 9.48) Stroking the grain of the beard sideways, shave the upper lip and work downward to the

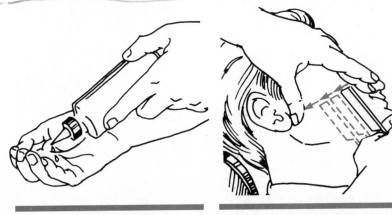

9.47 – Water bottle   9.48 – Shaving right side

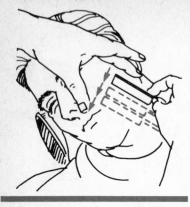

9.49 – Shaving left side

lower jawbone. Shave the lower part of the neck with a reverse free-hand stroke and follow the grain of the beard.

Now, turn the client's face toward you. With a free-hand stroke, start to shave the left side of the face. (Fig. 9.49) Stroking the grain of the beard sideways, shave from the ear toward the tip of the nose. When finished, wipe off the razor on lather paper and discard it.

Once Over Shave

The **once over** shave takes less time for a complete and even shave. For a once over shave, give a few more strokes across the grain when completing each shaving movement. This will assure a complete and even shave with a single lathering.

Exercise No. 8

Final Steps in Face Shaving

The final steps in face shaving require attention to a number of important details.

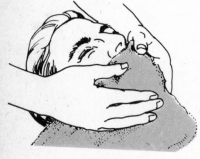

1. Apply face cream with massaging motions.
2. Prepare a steam towel and apply it over the face. A facial treatment may be done at this time.
3. Remove the steam towel from the face.
4. Apply finishing lotion with several facial manipulations.
5. Remove the towel from the client's chest.
6. Position yourself behind the chair.
7. Spread the towel over the client's face. First dry the lower part, then the upper part of the face.
8. Move to the right side of the chair.
9. Wrap the towel around your hand as described in Exercise No. 9.
10. Thoroughly dry the face. (Fig. 9.50)
11. Select a dry spot of towel and fold it around the hand.
12. Sprinkle talcum powder over the dry towel.
13. Apply powder evenly to the face.
14. Raise the chair to an upright position.
15. Shave the neckline, if necessary, as described in Exercise No. 10.

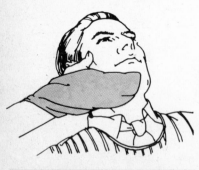

9.50 – Drying client's face

16. Comb the hair neatly as desired.
17. With the neck towel, wipe off loose hair, lather, or powder from the face and clothing.
18. Remove linen.
19. Hand the client the check for services rendered and thank him courteously.

Mustache trimming must be done before applying a steam towel (Step 2) or after Step 17.

Exercise No. 9

Wrapping a Towel Around the Hand

A properly trained barber-stylist knows how to wrap a towel around the hand with ease and skill for the purpose of:

1. Cleansing and drying the face.
2. Applying powder to the face.
3. Removing all traces of powder, lather, and any loose hair from the face, neck, and forehead.

The student should practice the following methods. Figs. 9.51–9.53 show one method of wrapping a towel around the hand and Figs. 9.54–9.59 (next page) show an alternate method.

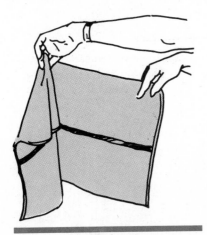

9.51 – Hold towel the long way and grasp it.

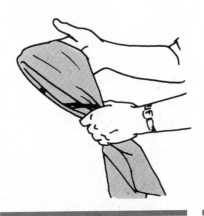

9.52 – Holding the right hand in front of you, draw the upper edge of the towel across the palm of the right hand. Then grasp the towel and draw it toward the right arm.

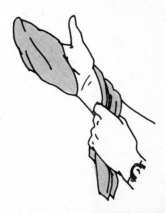

9.53 – Holding the towel in this position, twist it around the outside of the wrist and hold the ends of the towel to keep them from flapping in the client's face.

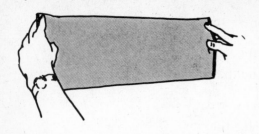

9.54 – Use linen or paper towel, usually 16 × 24 inches. Fold the towel in half lengthwise.

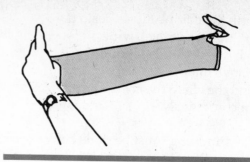

9.55 – Fold towel again in half lengthwise.

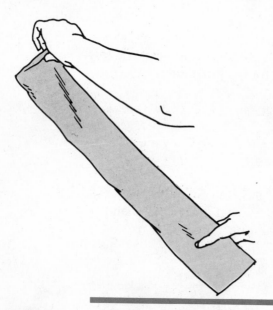

9.56 – Grasp the towel between the index and middle fingers.

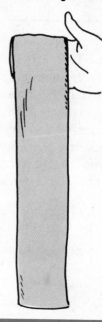

9.57 – Bring the towel around to cover the palm.

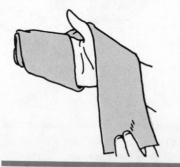

9.58 – Bring the towel around the back of the hand and twist it forward around the thumb.

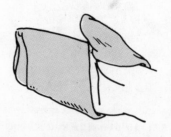

9.59 – The towel is folded neatly; therefore, the end will not flap in the client's face.

Exercise No. 10

Neck Shave

The neck shave, as part of the regular shave, involves shaving the neckline on both sides of the neck below the ears.

Raise the chair slowly to an upright position, tuck the towel around the back of the neck, and apply lather. Shave the neckline, first at the right side using a free-hand stroke, and then at the left side using a reverse back-hand stroke, as described in Exercise No. 4. (Figs. 9.60 and 9.61)

The lather from the razor may be transferred to the palm or base of the left thumb or a strip of tissue, a corner of which is tucked under the towel.

Clean the shaven part of the neck with your palm and fingers, moistened with witch hazel, antiseptic, or warm water. Remove the towel from around the neck and dry thoroughly. (This is the time to suggest a scalp treatment or hair tonic.)

Position yourself behind the chair, replace the towel around the client's neck, and comb or style the hair as desired by the client.

Releasing the Client

Take the towel from the back of the neck and fold it around the right hand. Remove all traces of powder and any loose hair. Discard the towel and remove the chair cloth from the client. Make out the price check and thank the client as it is handed to him.

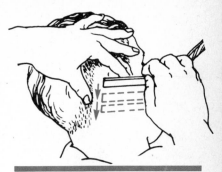

9.60 – Shaving right side of neck using free-hand stroke

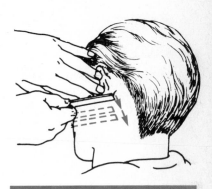

9.61 – Shaving left side of neck using back-hand stroke

Points to Remember in Shaving

1. Always use a forward sawing movement with the point of the blade leading.
2. The experienced barber-stylist will observe the hair slope and shave with it—never against it.
3. A heavy growth of beard requires careful lathering and special razor technique.
4. The lather should not be scattered carelessly over the face.
5. The fingers of the left hand should be kept dry in order to grasp and stretch the skin and hold it firmly.
6. Hot towels should not be used on excessively sensitive skin, nor should they be used when the skin is chapped or blistered from cold or heat.
7. Take special precautions in shaving, especially beneath the

lower lip, lower part of the neck, and around the Adam's Apple, as these parts of the face and neck are usually the most tender and sensitive, and are easily irritated by very close shaving.

Nine Reasons Why a Client May Find Fault with a Shave

1. Dull or rough razors.
2. Unclean hands, towels, or shaving cloth.
3. Cold fingers.
4. Heavy touch.
5. Poorly heated towels.
6. Lather that is either too cold or too hot.
7. Glaring lights over head.
8. Unshaven hair patches.
9. Scraping the skin and close shaving.

REVIEW QUESTIONS

Shaving

1. What three points should the barber-stylist know about the client's skin and hair when shaving?
2. What are nine requirements of a good shave?
3. How should the client be prepared for shaving?
4. How should the beard be prepared for shaving?
5. Which five sanitary precautions should be observed by the barber-stylist?
6. What is the most effective way to rub lather into the beard?
7. What action does the lather have on the beard?
8. What is the purpose of steaming the face?
9. When should a hot towel not be applied to the face?
10. Name the four standard positions and strokes used in shaving.
11. How should the razor be used for the free-hand stroke?
12. How should the razor be used for the back-hand stroke?
13. How should the razor be used for the reverse free-hand stroke?
14. What should be the direction of the shaving strokes in respect to the grain of the hair?
15. When are the reverse back-hand position and stroke usually used?
16. How many shaving areas are there in shaving the first time over?
17. Which side of the face is shaved first and which stroke is used first?
18. How is a once over shave given?

19. What part of the neck is shaved with the standard or regular shave?
20. What are the final steps after shaving?
21. When should a facial be suggested to the client?
22. When should a hair tonic or scalp treatment be suggested to the client?
23. Give nine reasons why a client may find fault with a shave.
24. How is a close shave produced?
25. Why is a close shave undesirable?

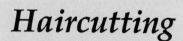

Haircutting

Learning Objectives

After completing this chapter, you should be able to:

1. *Discuss the art of haircutting.*
2. *Demonstrate an understanding of the term envisioning.*
3. *Discuss the client consultation and explain its importance.*
4. *Identify the sections of the head as applied to haircutting.*
5. *Discuss the principles of facial shapes.*
6. *List and define the fundamental terms used in haircutting.*
7. *Demonstrate the following: finger and shear cut, shears over comb cut, clipper cut, and razor cut.*
8. *Demonstrate a neck shave.*

Courtesy of: Hair: Joico International USA Team. Photo: Havriliak.

The art of haircutting involves individualized and precise designing, cutting, and shaping of the hair. In order to perform the art of haircutting successfully, the barber–stylist must be at ease using a variety of implements, techniques, and methods.

A good haircut is the foundation of all hairstyles. The importance of this cannot be stressed enough. Thorough instruction in the proper way to cut, blend, and taper the hair using clippers, shears, and razors, and continual practice under an instructor's guidance are necessary to achieve and refine professional skills. The barber–stylist needs to acquire facility in the skill of haircutting in order to create attractive, easy–to–manage hairstyles for clients.

The hairstyle chosen should accentuate the client's strong features and minimize the weaker ones. The client's head shape, facial contour, neckline, and hair texture must be taken into consideration. The barber–stylist also should be guided by the client's wishes, personality, and lifestyle.

ENVISIONING

Just what is the desired result and how does the barber–stylist achieve it? A client expects a well-blended, evenly cut, and attractive hairstyle. The length and design will vary with the individual.

It is essential for the barber–stylist to be able to envision what the client wants. The stylist must also envision the finished haircut before beginning to cut. You can learn a client's preferences and expectations during the initial consultation. A client may describe a new style, or may have a style in mind but ask for your suggestions. If no information is volunteered, you must ask questions regarding the frequency with which the client's hair is cut, whether the current style is satisfactory, and if the client has any special problems of which you should be aware. With experience and practice, the barber–stylist learns what questions to ask.

The specifics of the cut will also be discussed during the consultation.

The ability to visualize haircutting sections will assist the barber–stylist in developing individual cutting patterns, help to eliminate technical mistakes, prevent getting lost or confused during the haircutting process, and enable the stylist to easily check his or her work. In the designing and cutting of hair, the barber–stylist should envision the hair in sections . (Figs. 10.1–10.3)

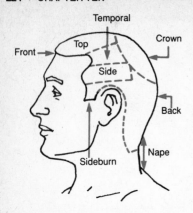

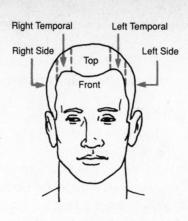

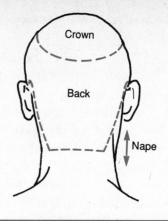

10.1 – Diagram of sections of head—side view

10.2 – Diagram of sections of head—front view

10.3 – Diagram of sections of head—back view

 BASIC PRINCIPLES OF HAIRSTYLING

Which Hairstyle Shall It Be?

Before beginning to cut, the barber-stylist studies the client's features and offers suggestions as to what kind of hairstyle is most suitable.

The barber-stylist must perfect the skill of haircutting. Each haircut should represent a work of art. Hairstyling has been defined as the artistic cutting and dressing of hair to best fit the client's physical needs and personality. Try to give a haircut that emphasizes the proper contour lines of the head.

Facial Types

The facial type of each person is determined by the position and prominence of the facial bones. There are seven facial types: oval, round, triangular, square, pear–shaped, oblong, and diamond. To recognize each facial type and be able to give correct advice, the barber–stylist should be acquainted with the outstanding characteristics of each.

While no amount of exercise will change the basic facial shape, hairstyles can complement facial shape in much the same way as certain clothes flatter the body.

NOTE: When recommending a hairstyle for a face shape, keep in mind the limitations of the individual, like hair type, hair line (receding, growth pattern, etc.), age of client, etc.

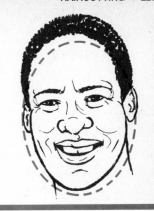

10.4 – Oval face

The following facial types should constitute a guide for choosing an appropriate style.

Oval Facial Type
The oval–shaped face is generally recognized as the ideal shape. Any hairstyle is suitable. Try changing the part. Experiment—keeping in mind elements such as lifestyle, comfort, and ease of maintenance. (Fig. 10.4)

Round Facial Type
The aim here is to slim the face. Hair that is too short will emphasize fullness. An off-center part and some waves at eye level will help lessen the full appearance. Beards should be styled to make the face appear oval. (Fig. 10.5)

Triangular Facial Type
The potential problems with this facial shape are over-wide cheekbones and a very narrow chin. Keep the hair close to the crown and temples and longer and fuller in back. A full beard helps to fill out a narrow jaw. (Fig. 10.6)

Square Facial Type
To minimize the angular features at the forehead, use wavy bangs that blend into the temples. This softens the square forehead and draws attention to a strong jaw. If a beard is worn, it should be styled to slenderize the face. (Fig. 10.7)

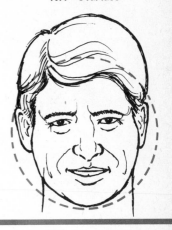

10.5 – Round face

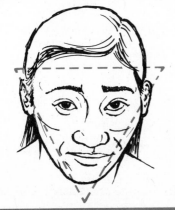

10.6 – Triangular face

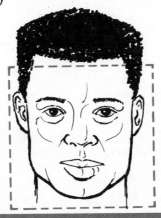

10.7 – Square face

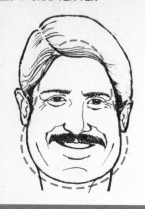

10.8 – Pear-shaped face

Pear-Shaped Facial Type

This shape is narrow at the top and wide on the bottom. Volume and fullness at the crown and temples are necessary to provide balance. Short, full styles are best, ending just above the jawline. A good perm could be another way to achieve width at the top. If a beard is worn, it should be styled to slenderize the lower jaw. (Fig. 10.8)

Oblong Facial Type

The long face needs to be shortened, the angularity hidden, the hairline never exposed. Blown bangs can provide a solution. A layered cut is best. A mustache helps to shorten a long face. (Fig. 10.9)

Diamond Facial Type

The aim here is to fill out the face at the temples and chin and keep hair close to the head at the widest points. Deep, full bangs give a broad appearance to the forehead and a one-length cut in the back adds width. A full, square, or rounded beard would also be appropriate. (Fig. 10.10)

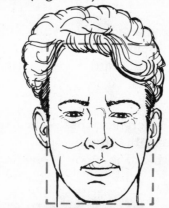

10.9 – Oblong face

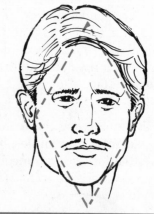

10.10 – Diamond face

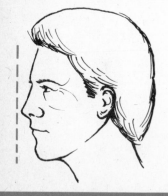

10.11 – Straight profile

Profiles

Always look at a client's profile. When creating a hairstyle, the profile can be a good indicator as to the correct shape of hairstyle to choose.

Straight

All hairstyles usually are becoming to the straight profile. (Fig. 10.11)

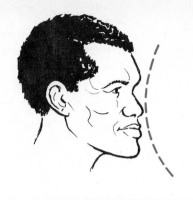

10.12 – Concave profile (prominent forehead and chin)

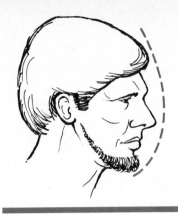

10.13 – Convex profile (receding forehead, prominent nose, and receding chin)

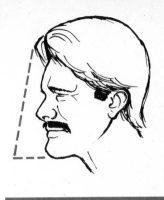

10.14 – Angular profile

Concave

Requires close hair arrangement over the forehead to minimize the bulge of the forehead. (Fig. 10.12)

Convex

To conceal a short, receding forehead, arrange the top front hair over the forehead. A beard minimizes a receding chin. (Fig. 10.13)

Angular

Hair that is drawn forward conceals a receding forehead. A short beard and mustache help to minimize a protruding chin. (Fig. 10.14)

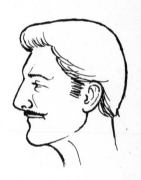

10.15 – Prominent nose

Nose

Nose shapes are closely related to profile. When studying a client's face, the nose must be considered both in profile and in full face.

Prominent Nose

A hooked nose, a large nose, or a pointed nose all come under this classification. To minimize the prominence of the nose, bring the hair forward at the forehead and back at the sides. (Fig. 10.15)

Turned-Up Nose

Comb the hair down over the forehead and back at the sides. (Fig. 10.16)

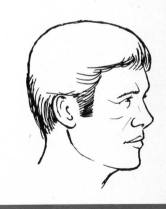

10.16 – Turned-up nose

Neck

The length of the neck should also be a factor in determining the overall shape of the hairstyle. The length, height, fullness, and partings of the hair should be considered when deciding which style would best complement the client's neck size.

Long Neck

Leave the hair full or longer at the neck to minimize the length. (Fig. 10.17)

Short Neck

Leave the neck exposed to create an appearance of length. (Fig. 10.18)

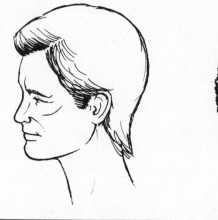
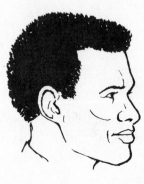

10.17 – Long neck   **10.18 – Short neck**

▼ FUNDAMENTAL PRINCIPLES OF HAIRCUTTING

The fundamental principles of haircutting should be thoroughly understood. The same general techniques are used in cutting, shaping, tapering, and blending men's and women's hair. Differences arise in the overall design line, contour, or shape (which includes the volume) and the styling.

Fundamental Terms Used in Haircutting

The **design line** is the outer perimeter line of the haircut and may act as a **guide line** depending on the design. A guide line is a cut that is made by which another section of hair will be cut. Guide lines are classified as being either **stationary** or **traveling**. Both types may originate at either the outer perimeter (design line) of the hair, or at an interior section, usually the crown area. Most haircuts are achieved by using a combination of the two types of guide lines.

The stationary guide line is used for overall, one-length haircut designs for a solid form or for maintaining the length of one section while hair is brought from another section or parting to meet it.

The traveling guide moves along a section of hair as each cut is made. Once the traveling guide has been cut, a parting is taken from in front of it, combed with the guide, and cut. A new parting is then taken, combed with the second parting of hair, and cut against the new guide line. Care must be taken not to re-cut the original or subsequent guides as the stylist moves along the section. When performed properly, the traveling guide line ensures even layering and blending.

A **parting** is a smaller section of hair, usually one-quarter to one-half inch, parted off from a larger section for the purpose of cutting the hair. Partings may be held horizontally or vertically, depending on the desired effect.

Degrees are angles at which the hair is held while cutting. **Elevations** are the levels at which hair is cut.

When the hair is cut at a 0–degree angle, it is held straight down while cutting and is considered to be a low elevation. A stationary guide line is used to achieve an overall one–length or blunt cut effect.

A 45–degree cut is held at a 45–degree angle. Cutting the hair at 45 degrees means that the hair is held either vertically or horizontally at approximately 45 degrees from the head. Holding the hair horizontally at 45 degrees and using a stationary guide line will achieve a stacked effect, while use of a vertical angle will produce a layered effect. Haircuts at or below the nape area, cut at 45 degrees, are considered low elevation cuts.

The 90–degree angle is probably the most common used in haircutting. It can produce layering, tapering, and blending effects. When using the 90-degree angle, the hair is held straight from the head from where it grows. This requires a traveling guide line in order to move around the entire head. Lengths on various sections of the head can vary, but the hair will still be blended overall and considered to be a high elevation cut.

The term **uniform** is used to denote a haircut that is cut at equal lengths throughout the sections of the hair. It is achieved with a traveling guide line.

Layering is produced by cutting the interior sections of the hair and can originate from the crown, the perimeter, or the design line. Layering can be angled (shorter on top and longer at the perimeter), uniform (even throughout), or full-tapered (longer on top and shorter at the perimeter), and can create fullness or a feathered effect.

Tapered or **tapering** means that the hair conforms to the shape of the head, usually shorter at the nape and longer in the crown and top areas. Blending of all of the hair lengths is extremely important in tapering.

Weight line refers to the heaviest perimeter area of a 0- or 45-degree cut. It is achieved by use of a stationary guide line and may be cut in at a variety of levels on the head, depending on the style. Most often, a weight line is used in combination with a tapered nape area.

Texturizing is performed after the overall cut has been completed. Thinning or notching shears are used to create wispy or spikey effects.

Thinning refers to removing excess bulk from the hair.

Outlining means marking the outer perimeter of the haircut in the front, over the ears, and at the sides and nape of the neck.

Hairstyling involves arranging the hair in a particular style, appropriately suited to the cut, and often requires the use of hair styling aids such as hair spray, gel, or mousse.

> **NOTE:** Almost all hairstyles require a combination of haircutting degree angles, which can be used on all hair types and are suitable for both genders.

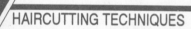

HAIRCUTTING TECHNIQUES

The methods in which implements are used are classified as: finger and shear, razor, shear-over-comb, and clipper techniques. It is important to note, however, that almost every haircutting procedure requires the use of a combination of techniques and implements. The following exercises illustrate standard and updated techniques for men's and women's cuts for several classifications. Now it is time to take your implements in hand and begin your practical training in haircutting and hairstyling.

Finger and Shear Technique

The technique of finger and shear cutting is the most frequently used method. This is where the ability to envision the sections plays an important role. Although the hair is not literally sectioned off in most men's haircutting, unless the length of the hair warrants it, there are two areas when a hair clip may be necessary: on the sides, just above the ears; and at the nape, when cutting a guide line.

When cutting hair with the finger and shear technique, a parting is held between the index and middle fingers of the left hand with just enough tension to produce a straight, even cut. The comb and shears are held in the right hand until the parting is ready for cutting, at which time the comb is palmed in the left hand between the thumb and index finger. The hair should be clean and damp to produce the most precise cut.

> **NOTE:** The following method is one way to perform finger and shear technique. Remember, your instructor's method is equally correct.

Procedure for Side Part

Start finger and shear work on the top of head. Then proceed to the right side and finish on the left side. To perform finger technique on top, start at the front part of the head and work toward the crown.

To perform finger technique on the top and right side of head, stand behind the client.

1. Hold the shears and comb as follows:
   a) Hold the shears by inserting the third finger in the grip and placing the little finger on the brace.
   b) Grasp the comb with left hand.
2. Start just above the right temple, palm the shears in the right hand, (Fig. 10.19) and comb a strand of hair two or three inches in width toward the back of the head.
3. Raise the comb sufficiently to permit the first and second fingers of the left hand to grasp the hair underneath the comb. The fingers holding the hair should bend to conform with the shape of the head.
4. Place the comb between the thumb and index finger of the left hand.
5. Cut the hair at a proper length to blend well with the shorter hair on the side of head. (Fig. 10.20)
6. Hold on to the cut hair, palm the shears, transfer comb from the left to right hand, and comb through the hair held in the fingers of the left hand.
7. Release the fingers, sliding the comb and picking up underneath hair beyond the cut just made, and cut the hair.
8. Comb the hair at that point again and repeat the same cut-

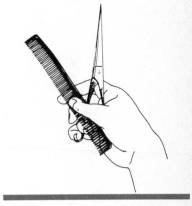

10.19 – Proper way to hold comb and shears

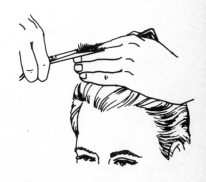

10.20 – Make cut over fingers.

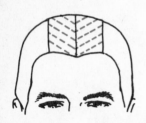

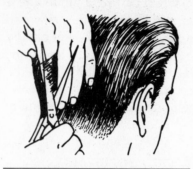

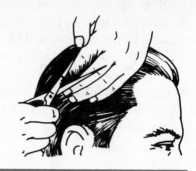

10.21 – Diagram for finger and shear technique

10.22 – Finger and shear technique on back part of head

10.23 – Finger and shear technique on right side of head

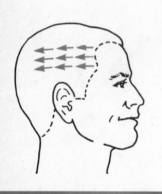

10.24 – Diagram for right side of head

ting movements until the back of the head is reached. (Fig. 10.21)

9. Start again at the front of the head, continue to comb and cut until the back of the head is reached again. (Fig. 10.22)

10. Continue to comb and cut, going a little lower each time until the side of the head is reached. (Figs. 10.23 and 10.24)

Left Side of Head

To perform finger technique on the left side of the head, stand to the left of the client. The finger technique for the left side of the head is performed in the same way as on the right side, with the exception that the barber-stylist stands to the side in front of the client, and the hair is combed away. (Figs. 10.25–10.27)

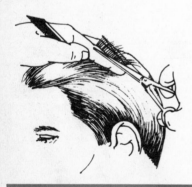

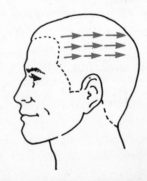

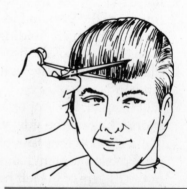

10.25 – Finger and shear technique on left side of head

10.26 – Diagram for left side of head

10.27 – If required, trim hair to desired length.

Procedure for Center Part and Pompadour

Center part. Do finger and shear work on the top right side first, and then the left side. For a pompadour (layered) hairstyle, part the hair in the center, then follow the same procedure for the center part.

> **NOTE:** Some barber-stylists prefer to do the finger and shear work from the top to the sides, whereas others find it more convenient to work from the sides to the top. Follow your instructor's directions.

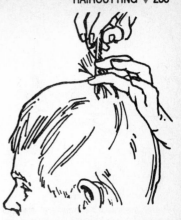

10.28 – Parting at the forward part of the crown

Updated Finger and Shear Technique

Procedure

1. Client consultation.
2. Drape the client for wet service.
3. Shampoo.
4. Remove the waterproof cape and replace it with a haircutting chair cloth.
5. Face the client toward the mirror and lock the chair.

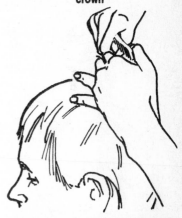

10.29 – 90-degree parting to establish top guide line

Step 1

1. Comb the hair down in front, sides, and back. Standing behind the client, take a one–quarter to one–half inch parting (depending on the density of the hair) at the forward–most part of the crown. (Fig. 10.28)
2. Comb the parting straight up at 90 degrees and hold it between the fingers of the left hand. (Fig. 10.29)
3. Bend the parting from right to left to determine at what length the hair will bend (bending point) to lie down smoothly (usually between two and three inches). When this length has been determined, re-comb the parting and, using the fingers of the left hand as a level, cut the hair that extends beyond the fingers. This cut establishes the traveling guide line for the top section. (Fig. 10.30)
4. Pick up a second parting, retaining the guide line, comb, and cut. (The guide line should be visible and parallel to the top of the fingers.) A rhythm will soon develop: part hair for parting; comb hair in front of parting forward (so it doesn't interfere with first parting); comb parting, retaining previous guide; and, cut hair that extends past the guide line.

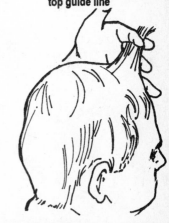

10.30 – Traveling guide, forward top position

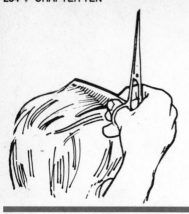

10.31 – Comb top section back.

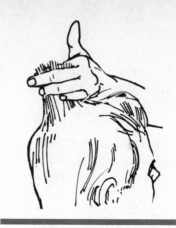

10.32 – Holding original guide from side position

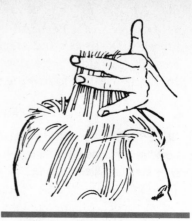

10.33 – Following arc of head

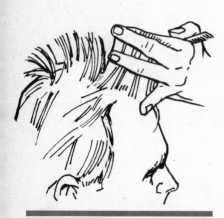

10.34 – Following the arc for the front top section

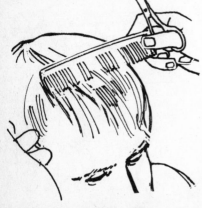

10.35 – Comb hair forward.

5. Complete the top section of hair, moving forward with each parting and cut. Remember to hold each parting at a 90–degree angle from where it grows.

Step 2

1. Comb the top section back. (Fig. 10.31) Move to the client's left side. Starting at the forehead, part off the top section of hair, front to back, with the thumb and middle finger.
2. Hold the original guide line and a one-half inch parting at the crown at 90 degrees, and cut. This establishes the guide for the crown and back sections. (Fig. 10.32)
3. Work forward, still maintaining a side-standing position. Following the arc and contour of the head, even off any length that does not blend with the traveling guide. (Fig. 10.33) If Step 1 was performed correctly, no more than one-quarter of an inch should need to be evened. Step 2 is a checkpoint for your work on the top section. (Fig. 10.34)

Step 3

1. Comb the hair forward and move in front of the client. (Fig. 10.35) Holding the front hair section between the fingers of the left hand at 0 degrees, begin in the middle and cut to the desired length. Cut right, and then left of the center to the ends of the width of the eyebrows, or to include the temporal area. The front and temporal design line has just

been completed and will act as a traveling guide for the temporal area. (Fig. 10.36)

Step 4

1. Move behind the client.
2. Beginning on the client's right, pick up the front hair of the temporal region. A small amount of the top hair previously cut should be visible.
3. Hold the hair at 90 degrees and cut to the top guide line. (Fig. 10.37)
4. Continue the procedure, working back to the middle of the crown area. (Fig. 10.38) Cut hair only from the temporal region; do not pick up side hair. When approaching the crown area, reposition yourself so as to move toward the client's left, but not as far as the side of the client.

Step 5

1. Repeat Step 4 procedure on the left side of the client's hair. Parting cuts will be made from the top guide through the temporal region, rather than to the top guide. If the front design line was cut correctly, the excess hair in the front temporal region should not exceed one inch. The crown hair should meet upon completion of Step 5. (Fig. 10.39)
2. Top, temporal, and crown areas are now cut.
3. Comb the hair for Step 6.

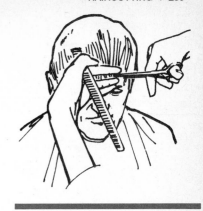

10.36 – Cutting front section, center, right, then left

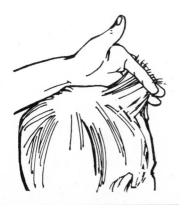

10.37 – Right temporal region—working toward crown

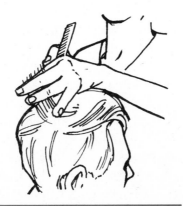

10.38 – Cutting middle of crown area

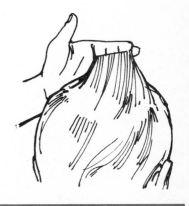

10.39 – Cutting left side temporal area, meeting at crown

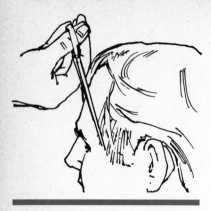

10.40 – Cutting side area—left side pictured to show back-hand technique

Step 6

1. Moving to the right of the client, comb the hair straight down on the sides.
2. Take a one–half inch horizontal parting at the hairline, from the top of the ear to the sideburn area, and an angled one–half inch parting from the right temple to the sideburn. (Fig. 10.40)
3. Comb back the remaining hair or secure it with a hair clip. (Fig. 10.41)
4. Cut the inside design line either to cut around the ears or to cover part of the ears at the desired length. (Fig. 10.42) If cutting around the ear, gently bend or slightly tug the ear down, out of the way.

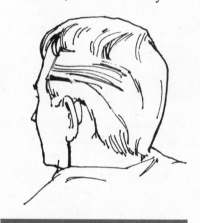

10.41 – Hair combed back

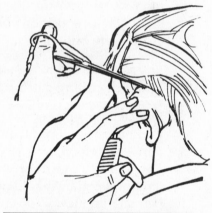

10.42 – Arching around ear

5. Move toward the front of the client, facing the temporal and side areas.
6. Using the front and side design lines (which are acting as guide lines), cut the hair between these two points at 0 degrees against the skin, cutting along the natural hair line.
7. Holding the hair between the fingers at 0 degrees, check the design line cut.
8. Proceed with the rest of the side hair, repeating the partings as the density of the hair requires.
9. Move behind the client. Pick up the hair in vertical partings, holding it straight out to the side. The design/guide line should be visible at the tips of the fingers when working on the right side of the client's head.

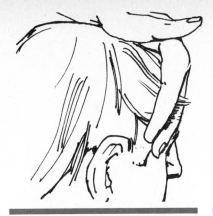

10.43 – Vertical partings; note hair visible between fingers. (Hair is cut on the outside of the fingers.)

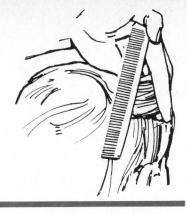

10.44 – Following side contour of head to meet with temporal region

10. Make a straight, vertical cut from the guide line, cutting off any hair that extends past the guide.
11. Continue cutting partings of hair while following the contour of the head until reaching the temporal region. (Figs. 10.43, 10.44) The hair should meet. Check the procedure by checking the blend of hair from the side design/guide line to the top section guide.
12. Proceed until all the side hair is cut. Stop at the topmost point behind the ear. Repeat for the left side. You may be positioned facing the client in order to work from the design/guide line up when blending the hair, or may prefer to remain behind the client.
13. The top, temporal, crown, and side areas are now cut.

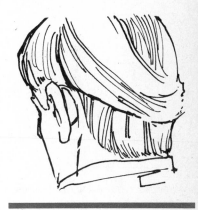

10.45 – One-half inch horizontal parting at nape

Step 7

1. Move behind the client. Make a one–half inch horizontal parting at the nape of the neck. (Fig. 10.45) Secure excess hair with a clip.
2. Starting in the center of the nape, cut the hair to the desired length; cut left and then right, to the corners of the nape area. (Fig. 10.46) Check the design line cut.
3. Move to the right of the client, cutting hair in a downward direction, from side hair to right nape corner.
4. Comb and check the cut. Repeat for the left side. A reverse

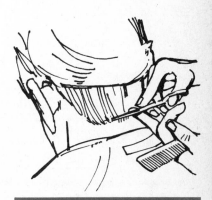

10.46 – Cutting design line

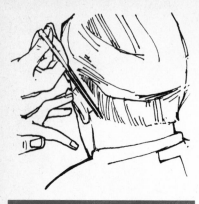

10.47 – Downward direction from ear area design line to nape corner area on left side of client

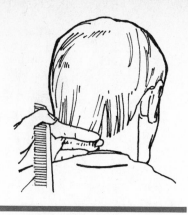

10.48 – Cutting design line at 0 degrees

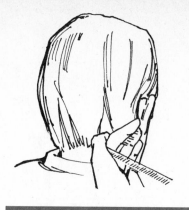

10.49 – Behind the ear 0-degree line cut and check

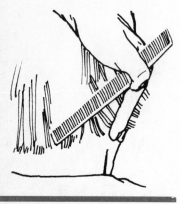

10.50 – Vertical partings blending from design/guide line

shear cutting method is required to cut downward on the client's left side. (Fig. 10.47)

5. Drop down and comb the remaining hair as density allows. Holding the design/guide line between the fingers, cut hair at 0 degrees. (Fig. 10.48) Complete 0–degree cutting at the nape and behind the ear areas. (Fig. 10.49)
6. Pick up the hair in vertical partings and cut up to the crown area, meeting the guide line there. (Fig. 10.50)
7. Proceed until the entire back section is cut.
8. Check the entire haircut by combing the hair up in 90–degree sections, making sure that the hair blends from one section to another. (Figs. 10.51–10.53)

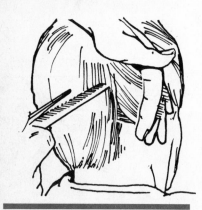

10.51 – Vertical partings following contour of head

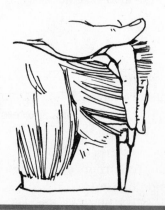

10.52 – Vertical partings following contour of head

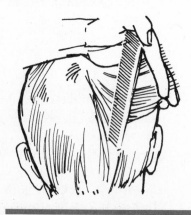

10.53 – Vertical partings following contour of head

Step 8

1. Dry the client's hair in a free–form style. This method requires the stylist to move the dryer briskly from side to side while drying the hair. Begin at the nape, using the brush in the left hand to hold mid–section hair out of the way while drying underneath hair first. The nozzle of the dryer should be pointing downward, 6 to 10 inches away from the hair. As the hair is dried, check the cut for blending qualities. Proceed to dry the sides and top.

2. Brush the hair into place using a directional nozzle, if needed. (Fig. 10.54)

3. Use a trimmer (outliner) to clean up sideburns, sides (in around-the-ear styles), and nape. (Figs. 10.55–10.57) Check the behind-the-ear area for any difference in hair length or design.

4. Recomb into the finished style.

5. Consult with the client regarding the use of hair spray.

6. The haircut and style is now complete. Dust or vacuum stray hairs, making sure none remain on the client's face or neck.

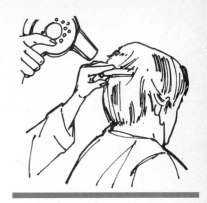

10.54 – Free-form blow-drying

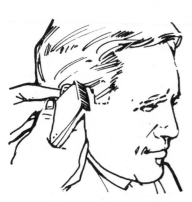

10.55 – Outlining and trimming around ear

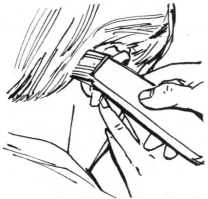

10.56 – Behind the ear outlining and cleaning up

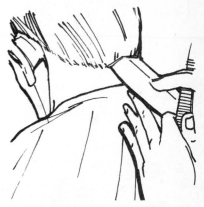

10.57 – Outlining and cleaning up the nape area

NOTE: If the client does not want hair spray but needs a fixative, a dab of light hair gel or conditioner on the stylist's palms, passed lightly over the hair, will calm down any static electricity, stray hairs, or excess fullness.

▼ WOMEN'S HAIRCUTTING

The art of cutting women's hair is important in the barber-stylist's professional development. As in the exercise of any other personal skill, differences of opinion exist with reference to the proper procedure to be followed.

The Basic Haircut

A basic haircut means different things to different people. However, this term is primarily used to describe an all-purpose haircut. A basic haircut is one that can be shaped or molded easily into a wide variety of finished hairstyles.

The techniques described in this chapter present only one method of performance. Your instructor may have another method that may be equally correct.

Preparation

1. Drape the client for wet service.
2. Shampoo.
3. Drape the client for a haircut.
4. Examine the head shape, facial features, and hair texture.
5. Comb and brush the hair free of tangles.
6. Divide the hair into four or five main sections.

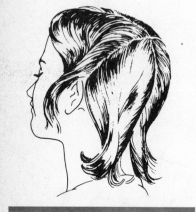

10.58 – Four-section parting

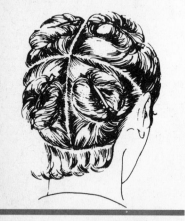

10.59 – Four sections with guide line

Sectioning the Hair for Cutting

There are several correct ways to section the head for cutting. The following are two accepted methods. Your instructor's method is equally correct.

Four Section Parting

The hair should be sectioned as shown in Fig. 10.58. Pin up, as in Fig. 10.59, leaving the nape hair to use as length guide.

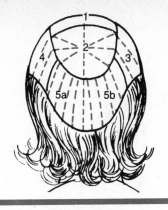

10.60 – Back view

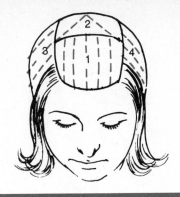

10.61 – Top view (section No. 1 shown with vertical partings)

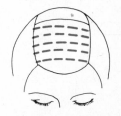

10.62 – Top view (section No. 1 shown with horizontal partings)

Five Section Parting

Five section parting, with sub-parting panels: Section and pin up the hair in the order shown in Figs. 10.60–10.63.

The back section (No. 5) may be divided into Sections No. 5a and No. 5b for easier handling.

The top section (No. 1) may be sub-parted in two ways, as shown in the above figures, with partings running in either a horizontal or vertical direction.

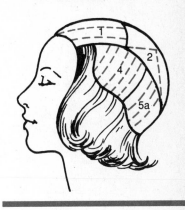

10.63 – Side view

Procedure

1. Divide the hair into five sections.
2. Determine the length of the guideline hair, the section that will serve as a length guide for the cut. (Fig. 10.64)
3. **Blunt cut** (cutting hair straight, without slithering) the guideline strand of nape hair.
   a) Blunt cut the strand on the left side, closest to the earlobe, using the earlobe as a guide. (Fig. 10.65)

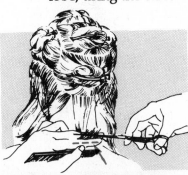

10.64 – Cut strand at center nape to desired length.

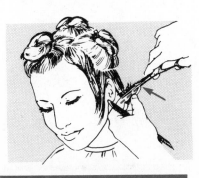

10.65 – Use ear lobe as guide on left side.

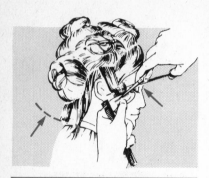

10.66 – On right side follow same procedure.

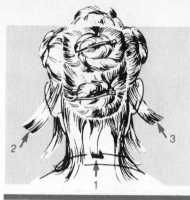

10.67 – Shows three strands of guideline hair cut to desired length.

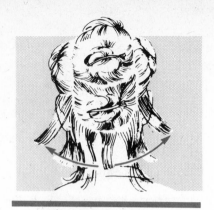

10.68 – Follow up by cutting all remaining guideline hair.

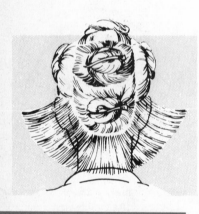

10.69 – Guideline hair properly cut

b) Blunt cut the strand on the right side to match the left side. (Fig. 10.66)

c) Blunt cut from the back center to left front. (Fig. 10.67)

d) Blunt cut from the back center to the right front to complete the guide line. (Figs. 10.68, 10.69)

4. Let down section No. 5 and divide it into two equal parts (No. 5a and No. 5b). Match the length with the guideline hair. Either the left or right side may be done first. (Fig. 10.70) Hold the hair panels out from the head while cutting. Continue cutting sections No. 3 and No. 4 in the same manner.

Crown section No. 2. Hold pre-cut strands out from the head. Match the length by picking up strands from the section already cut. Continue around the head, matching lengths with the sides and back hair. (Fig. 10.71)

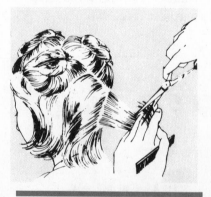

10.70 – Cutting section No. 5b

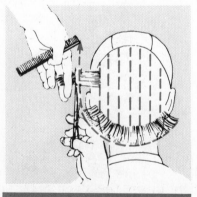

10.71 – Cutting hair on the back side of the hand

Divide section No. 1 into two parts. Pick up hair from the middle of the section, using previously cut hair as a guide. Maintain the hand movements in a 45-degree arc. Proceed to cut both parts of section No. 1 in the prescribed manner.

If bangs are to be cut, move directly in front of the client for even cutting. Test the hair for bounce (elasticity), then determine the desired length. If bangs are to be short, use the bridge of the nose as a guide. If they are to be long, shape the strands to blend into the length of the sides.

Thinning. To complete the shaping of the hair, excess bulk should be removed with thinning or regular shears. It is recommended that all hair be checked for proper length. (Fig. 10.72)

Hair that has been correctly cut and tapered is easily adaptable to many different styles. (Fig. 10.73)

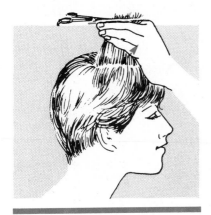

10.72 – Thinning the hair

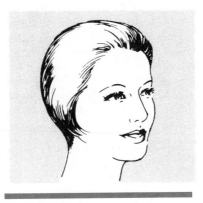

10.73 – Head completely cut

Completion

Remove the neck strip, towel, and hair cloth or plastic cape. Thoroughly remove all hair clippings from the hair cloth or cape, client's clothing, and the work area. Release the client or proceed with the next professional service desired.

Helpful Hints on Women's Short Cuts

Regardless of the prevailing hair fashion, there will always be a number of clients who want their hair cut or molded short. To satisfy these clients you must know how to shingle the hair. The illustrations on page 244 show how shingling is accomplished by using the regular shears and comb.

> **NOTE:** In shingling, the blade of the shears is held parallel with the comb; only the top blade moves and does the cutting.

Shingling procedure. Start at the nape line, shingling the hair upward in a graduated effect. After reaching the top of the section being cut, turn the comb downward and comb the hair. Proceed, section by section, until the entire back of the head is shingled in a smooth, uniform manner. (Figs. 10.74–10.77)

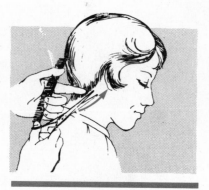

10.74 – Outlining neckline

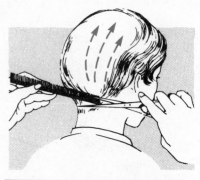

10.75 – Shingling the back of head

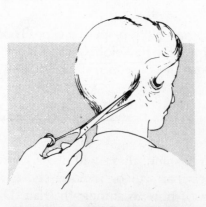

10.76 – Cleaning neck with points of shears

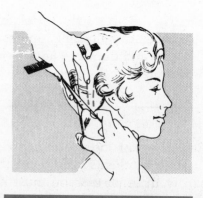

10.77 – Clipping hair ends

Style cutting is the art of cutting the hair to facilitate the development of waves by tapering or shaping the hair to conform with the formation of a wave. The hair would be cut slightly deeper in the trough or indentation of the wave, and more shallowly at the crest. This method facilitates the formation and durability of a hair wave.

The Use of Trimmers

The use of the trimmers to clean the neckline does not make the hair grow in more thickly. The amount of hair can only be as great as the number of hair follicles, and these are not increased by the use of trimmers or any other implement.

Correcting Split Hair Ends

Trichoptilosis (tri-kop-ti-**LOH**-sis) is the technical term for split hair ends. When the hair becomes dry and brittle, the hair ends split. Temporary relief for this condition may be obtained by cutting the hair ends.

Clipper and Comb Technique

It is best to practice tapering with the blade guard of a disconnected electric clipper before actually cutting any hair.

To learn to handle clipper properly, the student should practice the following exercises.

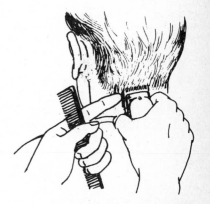

10.78 – Tapering the hair with a clipper; steady clipper with left hand.

1. **How to hold clipper and comb.**
   a) Pick up the clipper with the right hand.
   b) Place the thumb on the left side and fingers on the right side of the electric clipper. Hold it lightly to permit freedom of wrist movement.
   c) With the left hand comb hair down.
   d) With the left hand steady the clipper. (Fig. 10.78)
2. **How to use clipper and comb.**
   a) Use a clipper blade that gives a longer cut before using a clipper blade that gives shorter cut. (Fig. 10.79)
   b) For a gradual, even taper, tilt the blade as you clip so that the clipper rides on the heel of the bottom blade.
   c) Do not move the clipper into the hair too fast. It will have a tendency to jam the clipper blades and pull the hair.
   d) After tapering one strip of hair, comb it down, smooth it, and start tapering the next strip.

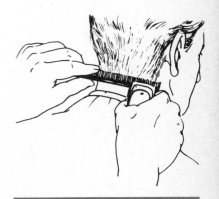

10.79 – Tapering the hair with clipper over the comb

Be guided by your instructor as to where to begin the clipper cut. Some barber-stylists prefer to start in the middle of the nape area, while others work from right to left or left to right. As long as the hair is tapered evenly all methods are equally correct.

When Hand Clipper Is Used

While the electric clipper is used by most barber-stylists, it is advisable to learn to use a hand clipper as well. It can be used to taper the hair in the same manner as the electric clipper. The hand clipper is a much slower cutting implement.

Standard Method of Clipper Haircutting

Cutting and tapering the hair with the clipper can be accomplished in the following ways:

1. Clipper cutting against the grain is accomplished by cutting the hair in the opposite direction from which it grows. Taper the hair by gradually tilting the clipper, until it rides on its heel. (Fig. 10.80)
2. Clipper cutting with the grain means the cut is in the same direction in which the hair grows. (Fig. 10.81)
   When using a clipper on hair that has a tight curl formation, try to cut with the grain. Cutting tight, curly hair against the grain clogs up the clipper blades.
3. When cutting across the grain with clippers, the hair is cut neither with nor against the grain. It is usually done on the sides of the head. (Fig. 10.82)

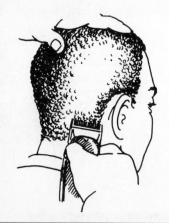 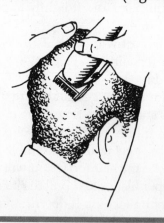 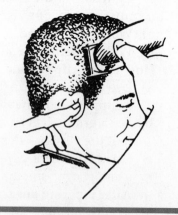

10.80 – Clipper cutting against the grain   10.81 – Clipper cutting with the grain   10.82 – Clipper cutting across the grain

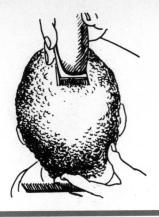

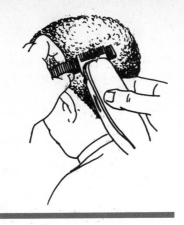

10.83 – Hair that grows in a whirlpool; taper against the grain in a circular movement.

10.84 – Clipper cutting over the comb

4. Cutting the hair in a circular motion using clippers is advisable in whorl areas, or in places where the hair does not grow in a uniform manner. (Fig. 10.83)
5. Clipper cutting over a comb is a method of cutting in which the hair may be cut with a minimum change of clipper blades. (Fig. 10.84)

Clipper Over Comb Technique

Figs. 10.85–10.91 show one way in which clipper over comb technique is accomplished. Remember your instructor's method is equally correct.

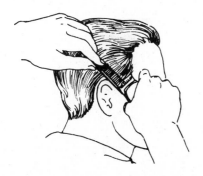

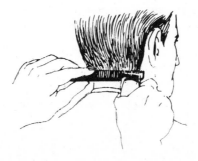

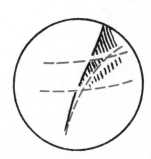

10.85 – Tapering sideburn and over ear

10.86 – Starting taper at base of neck

10.87 – In tapering with a clipper, be sure to tilt the comb away from the head in order to form a uniform taper for medium or longer cut.

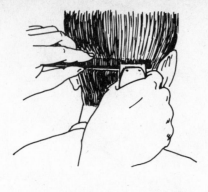

10.88 – The top of taper usually is no higher than the top of the ear.

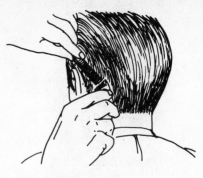

10.89 – Tapering the left side to match with the right side

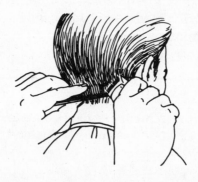

10.90 – Clipping hair across the teeth of comb

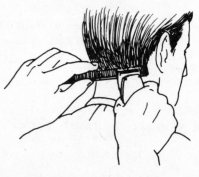

10.91 – Tapering the nape area

Arching with a Clipper

Many barber-stylists prefer to use a clipper constructed with a small head having a fine cutting edge, for squaring off sideburns and making the outline around the ears and sides of neck. This method of arching is more efficient and precise due to the maneuverability of the smaller cutting head. (Figs. 10.92–10.96)

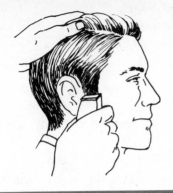

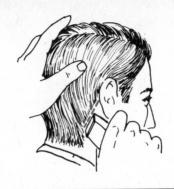

10.92 – Squaring off right sideburn and arching; turn clipper over on its cutting edge.

10.93 – Outlining right side of neck

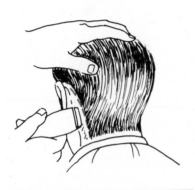

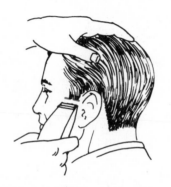

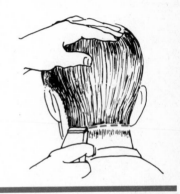

10.94 – Outlining left side of neck

10.95 – Squaring off left sideburn

10.96 – To produce a square nape line turn clipper over on its cutting edge.

Short Layered Cut

The short layered cut denotes a short hairstyle in which the hair is combed back without a part or to either side depending on the direction of hair growth.

Hair texture. Coarse hair is the most desirable for a short layered cut or brush cut. Fine hair is acceptable if it is thick enough and the client's head is properly shaped. Fine, thin hair is the least desirable.

Crew Cuts

Many barber-stylists refer to the crew cut as a short pomp or brush cut. The length of hair on the sides and back of the head usually determines the crew cut style, as in the list that follows.

1. Short sides and back—short crew cut.
2. Semi-short sides and back—medium crew cut.
3. Medium sides and back—long crew cut.

Generally, the edging and siding are done first, the top area last. However, the topping can be done with the clipper and then the shears and comb are used to smooth out any uneven spot or area.

The top hair should be graduated in length from the front hairline to the back part of the crown. The top hair, from side to side, should form a slight curve to conform with the general contour of the head.

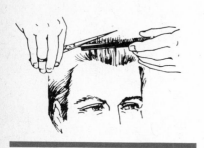

10.97 – Standing in back using shear and comb

Flat Tops

The sides and back areas of the flat top are similar to that of a crew cut, with the following exceptions:

1. The top area—the emphasis is on flatness.
2. The sides at top—appearance is square.

Suggested Procedure

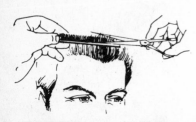

10.98 – Standing in front using shear and comb

1. Stand behind the client. The hair at the crown is cut flat to about one-quarter to one-half inch in length, one inch in depth, and two to three inches in width.
2. Standing in front of the client, the front center hair is cut down flat about two inches in length and one inch in depth, then straight across both sides. It is important that the hair in the center and the sides are the same height.
3. Ask the client if the front hair is the desired length. If it is not, then cut the hair to the desired height.

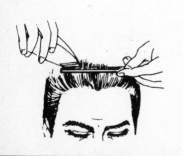

10.99 – Standing in back using clipper over comb

The clipper or shears and comb may be used in cutting the flat top. (Figs. 10.97–10.99)

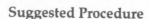

Brush Cut

The brush cut is popular with boys as it requires the least attention. Some men, too, desire this style for the same reason. (Figs. 10.100, 10.101)

Procedure

The sides and back areas are cut as for a short crew cut. The top hair is cut the same length, about one-quarter to one-half inch all over the top, following the contour of the head.

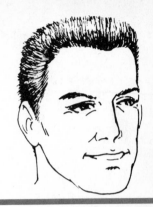

10.100 – Brush cut for man

Shaving Neck and Outlined Areas

Preparation for a Neck Shave

The neck shave contributes to the appearance of the finished haircut. Shaving the outlined areas of the sideburns, around the ears, and the sides of the neck below the ears gives the client a clean appearance. If the haircut requires a round or square outline at the nape of the neck, the free-hand stroke should be used at the back of the neck.

To prepare for a neck shave follow these steps:

1. Remove all cut hair from around the head and neck with a clean towel, tissues, or hair vacuum.
2. Loosen the chair cloth and neck strip carefully so that no cut hair will fall down the neck or shirt.
3. Discard the cut hair at the base of the chair by picking up the chair cloth at the lower edge and bringing it up to the upper edge. Remove the chair cloth carefully so that no cut hair will fall on the client. Drop the upper edge of the chair cloth, giving a slight shake to dislodge all cut hair.
4. Replace the chair cloth as before. It should be left a few inches away from the neck so that it does not come in contact with the client's skin.
5. Spread a face or paper towel straight across the shoulders, then tuck it into the neckband.

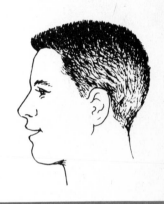

10.101 – Brush cut for boy

Applying Lather for Neck Shave

1. Prepare lather in the same manner as for the beard.
2. Apply a light coating of lather at the hairline, around and over the ears, to the sideburns, and down the sides of the

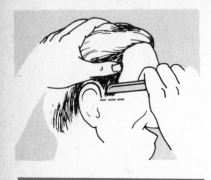

10.102 – Shaving right sideburn to proper length

neck. If the back of the neck is to be shaved, apply lather to the back of the neck up to the hairline.

3. Rub the lather in lightly with the balls of the fingers or thumb.

Shaving Outlined Areas

The purpose of this exercise is to shave the outlined areas of the ears, neck, and sideburns.

1. **Shaving right side**
   a) Hold the razor as in the free-hand stroke.
   b) Place the left thumb on the scalp above the point of the razor and stretch the scalp under the razor.
   c) Shave the sideburn to the proper length. (Fig. 10.102)
   d) Shave around the ear at the hairline and straight down the side of the neck, using the free-hand stroke with the point of the razor. Be careful not to shave into the hairline at the nape of the neck. (Fig. 10.103–10.105)

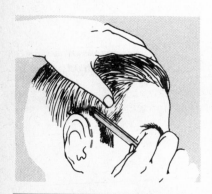

10.103 – Shave over ear.

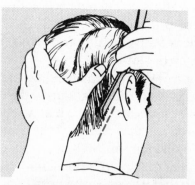

10.104 – Shave outline below ear.

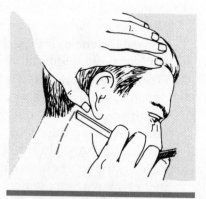

10.105 – Clean neck below ear.

> **NOTE:** The ear should be protected when using the razor around or behind it. The thumb of the left hand can be used to bend the ear out of the way, while the index finger acts as a leverage brace against the client's head. The remaining three fingers should be positioned against the top side section of the head.

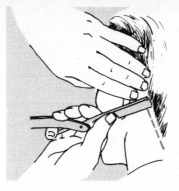

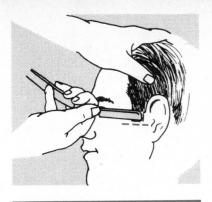

10.106 – Shave left sideburn to proper length using reverse back-hand stroke.

10.107 – Shave left side of neck using back-hand stroke.

2. **Shaving left side**

   a) Hold the razor as in the reverse back-hand stroke.

   b) Place the left thumb on the scalp above the razor point, and stretch the skin under the razor.

   c) Shave the sideburns to the proper length. (Fig. 10.106)

   d) Shave around the ear at the hairline, using the free-hand stroke.

   e) Shave the neck below the ear, using the reverse back-hand stroke with the point of the razor. (Fig. 10.107) Hold the ear away with the fingers of the left hand. If the stroke is done with one continuous movement, a straight line will be formed down the side of the neck.

   f) If necessary shape the nape area round, square, or tapered. (Figs. 10.108–10.111)

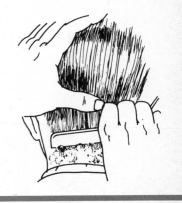

10.108 – To achieve a square or round shaped hair style, shaving or precision outlining is required.

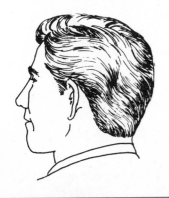

10.109 – Round

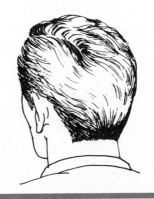

10.110 – Square

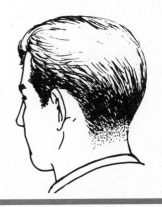

10.111 – Tapered

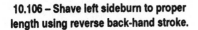

3. Provided the client does not specify otherwise, shave the neck outline straight down the side of the neck behind the ears.

▼ FOUR BASIC PATTERNS FOR CUTTING SIDES AND BACK

To simplify haircutting procedures, edging and siding have been divided into four basic patterns: short, semi-short, medium length, and trims and long haircuts.

A variety of hairstyles can be developed or created from these basic haircut patterns to suit the client's tastes and desires.

Short Haircut Styles

Short haircuts are required in the armed forces, where neatness and uniformity are important.

Starting with the coarse clipper blade at the left sideburn, proceed upward to the hatband, then gradually tilt the heel of the clipper back as you proceed up the head until it runs off the side of the head. Repeat this movement as you proceed toward the back of the head.

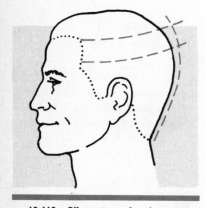

10.112 – Clipper taper for short cut

> **NOTE:** It is important to remember that an even, gradual taper, giving a smooth, blended appearance, is the object. There must not be any ridges left, from either the shears or the clipper.

Use the fine clipper blade to taper the left sideburn. Proceed in the same manner on the back and right side of the head.

To gradually blend the fine clipper taper with the coarse clipper taper, tilt the heel of the clipper. (Fig. 10.112)

Semi-Short Haircut Styles

Semi-short styles are similar to short haircuts with the following exceptions:

1. The coarse clipper starts tilting back at the top of the ears instead of at the hatband, producing a slightly longer hairstyle.

2. The length of the hair on the back is longer than on the sides. The coarse clipper goes up the head to about the top of the ears and then starts to taper out.

3. In using the fine clipper blade, remove only the sideburn lines. When going around the ears, remove about one-half inch from the hairline. (Fig.10.113)

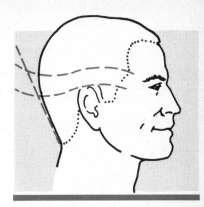

10.113 – Clipper taper for semi-short haircut

Medium-Length Haircut Styles

Medium-length styles do not give a scalped appearance.

The coarse clipper may be used on the sideburns. However, as soon as the teeth of the clipper start cutting into the hair the clipper is tilted on its heel, ending the clipper taper about even with the top of the ears. The coarse clipper is not used around the ears. In this style the fine clipper blade is not used on the sides at all.

On the back of the head, the coarse clipper proceeds up the head to a point at about the middle of the ears. Then the clipper is tilted back as you proceed upward, and the taper ends by the time the top of the ears is reached.

The fine clipper blade is used to remove the hairline at the nape of the neck. (Fig. 10.114)

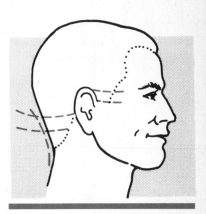

10.114 – Clipper taper for medium haircut

Trim and Long Haircut Styles

Hair trims and long haircuts require considerable skill and artistic sense. Some professional barber-stylists refer to these haircut styles as *shear-trim* or *clippers in the nape area and shears on the side*. When a client asks for a trim, it usually means a cut that matches the length of the last haircut.

For best results, the barber-stylist must consider the color and texture of the hair and the client's facial characteristics.

With these styles the coarse clipper is started at the hairline of the nape and the clipper is tilted at the bottom of the ears. The rest is done with shears and comb. The fine clipper blade is used to taper the hairline and also to remove the fine hair at the nape, below the ears.

For sideburns and over the ears, the hair is shortened with the shears and comb. The outline around the ears is kept to the natural hairline. (Fig. 10.115)

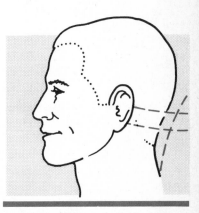

10.115 – Clipper taper for long trim

▼ VARIATIONS OF STYLES

The Fade

The fade is quite popular with teenagers and young adults. Its name derives from the fact that the hair at the nape and sides is cut extremely close, becoming gradually longer in the temporal region and lower crown area and longest at the top. Hence, it fades to nothing at the hairline.

Starting at the center of the back of the nape, begin with Size 1 clipper blades. If the hair is not short enough, go to the next smallest size. The hair is clipper-cut to the crest of the occipital or hatband area. Cut the sides to the temporal region using the next longer clipper blade, or one that will taper in the hatband area to the top section. Trim the top section.

To gradually blend the fine clipper taper with the longer clipper taper, tilt the heel of the clippers. (Fig. 10.116)

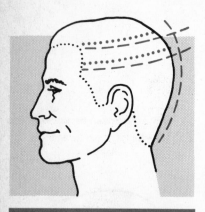

10.116 – Clipper taper for the *fade*

Bi-Level

The bi-level cut is most often achieved with clippers and shears. However, clippers are being used to cut sections of hair held between the fingers and may be used in this haircut if a texturized or layered look is desired. The clipper is used to cut the nape and sides to the desired length. The top is either layered and texturized, or cut to one length using a weight line. The weight line may vary in style lengths.

For a medium-length style, section off the top, crown, and temporal area hair and secure with a hair clip. Proceed with clipper cutting, stopping midway in the back area. Clipper cut the sides. Take a horizontal parting of secured hair and establish a design/guide line. Cut the hair at 0 degrees until all the partings are cut. If the top is to be layered, proceed with a 45- or 90-degree cut, using the guide line.

Clipper cutting for a shorter length, bi-level style usually requires cutting higher into the temporal region with slight blending to the top section. (Fig. 10.117)

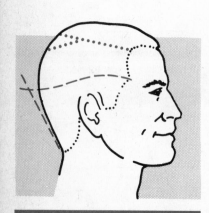

10.117 – Clipper taper for the bi-level cut

Updated Clipper Cut

Procedure

1. Drape the client for wet service.
2. Shampoo.
3. Drape the client for haircut service.

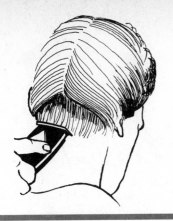

10.118 – Start by blunt cutting the guide line in the neck.

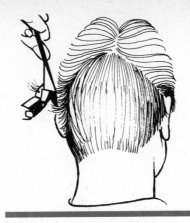

10.119 – Attach a one-half inch guide comb and proceed to remove the bulk in the back of the head.

4. Establish a design line at the nape using the clipper to cut the hair at 0 degrees. (Fig. 10.118)
5. Attach a one-half inch comb attachment, and using the clipper-over-comb technique, remove excess bulk from the back section. (Fig. 10.119)
6. Cut the sides to the base of the temporal region. (Fig. 10.120)
7. Blend the top and sides by holding the hair at 90 degrees and cutting against the fingers with the clipper. (Fig. 10.121)

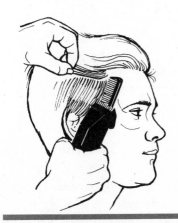

10.120 – Proceed to the sides using a horizontal sectioning.

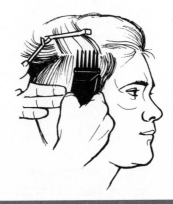

10.121 – Use the one-half inch guide comb while cutting the sides.

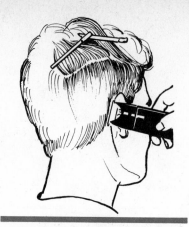

10.122 – Outline behind the ears and sideburns.

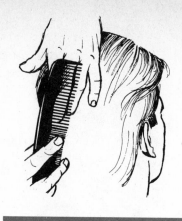

10.123 – Blend the sides by projecting the hair with fingers.

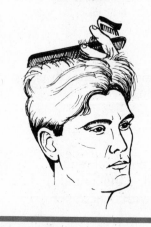

10.124 – Blend the top by projecting the hair with fingers.

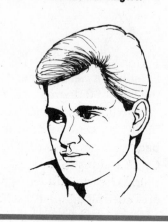

10.125 – Finished style

8. Complete trimming and outlining work. Check the haircut. (Fig. 10.122–10.125)

Women's Clipper Cut

Procedure

Steps 1 through 3 are the same as those for an updated clipper cut.

4. Section the top, side, and back hair, leaving a one-half inch parting around the perimeter to establish a guide line.
5. Clipper cut the nape design line. Using clippers against the fingers, cut the side design line at a 0-degree level. Use the clipper-over-comb technique for the nape and back areas.

Finish cutting the sides at 90 degrees using horizontal partings. Cut the bangs and use them as a guide line for the top section, blending back to the crown. (Figs. 10.126–10.130)

6. Style high at the crown and swept up and back at the sides. (Fig. 10.131)

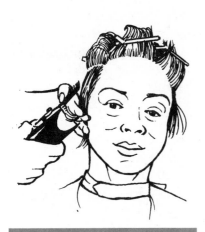

10.126 – Starting at the side, cutting first section against your finger

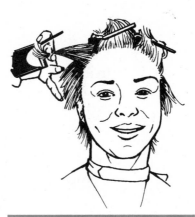

10.127 – Next section will be cut at a 90-degree angle. Continue working up.

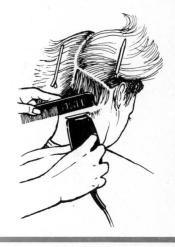

10.128 – To begin sectioning the back, take a diagonal parting, cutting the hair with a point in the back.

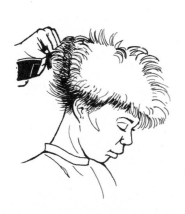

10.129 – Use clipper-over-comb technique on the neckline.

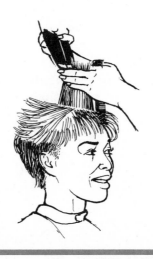

10.130 – Using the bang as a guide line, cut the hair shorter in the crown, blending the top and back.

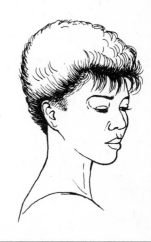

10.131 – Finished style

SHEAR-AND-COMB TECHNIQUE

The shear-and-comb technique is used to cut the ends of the hair and even up the clipper taper, usually after the clipper work is completed.

To learn the shear-and-comb technique, practice of the following exercises is recommended.

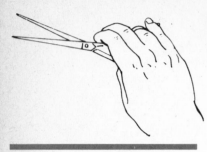

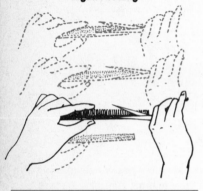

10.132 – Proper way to hold shears for regular cutting

1. **How to hold shears and comb.**
   a) Pick up the shears firmly with the right hand and insert the thumb into the thumb grip. Place the third finger into the finger grip and leave the little finger on the finger-brace of the shears. (Fig. 10.132)
   b) Pick up the comb with the left hand and place the fingers on top of the teeth with the thumb on the backbone of the comb. (Fig. 10.133) (For the student, start with the coarse teeth of the comb. After sufficient skill is developed, use the fine teeth of the comb.)
      To comb the hair downward, turn the comb toward the client's head, as in turning a key, by using the thumb and the first two fingers. (Fig. 10.134)
   The positions of both hands are as follows:
   a) Hold the shears and comb slightly to your right front.
   b) Hold the comb parallel with the still blade of the shears, as in Fig. 10.133.

10.133 – Holding comb and shears

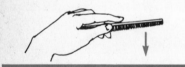

10.134 – Turning the comb downward

2. **How to use shears and comb.** (Fig. 10.135)
   a) Keep one blade still while moving the other blade with the thumb. Master this technique before attempting to do an actual haircut.
   b) While manipulating the shears, move both shears and comb slowly upward at the same time.
   c) Turn the teeth of the comb down when combing the hair down. (Fig. 10.134)
   d) Finish one vertical strip at a time before proceeding with the next strip to the left. Working from right to left gives a better view of the work.

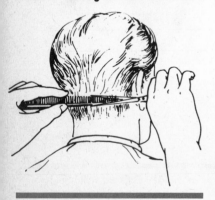

10.135 – Using shears and comb

Suggestions on the Use of the Shears and Comb

The procedures given here may be changed to conform with the instructor's routine. (Figs. 10.136–10.144)

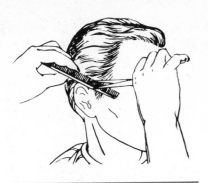

10.136 – Right sideburn

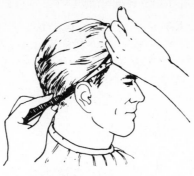

10.137 – Over and back of ear

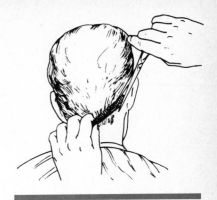

10.138 – Side of neck

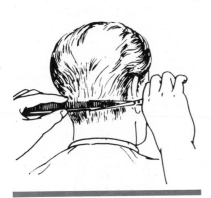

10.139 – From nape to as high as necessary

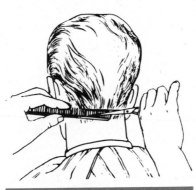

10.140 – Even up clipper taper.

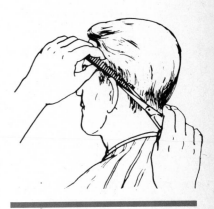

10.141 – Side of neck and over ear

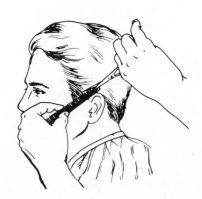

10.142 – Front of ear and left sideburn

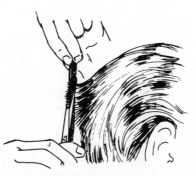

10.143 – Using comb and shear to blend hair at back of head

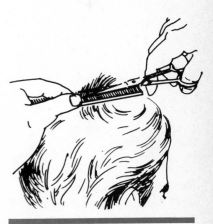

10.144 – Up and over comb and shear technique on top of head

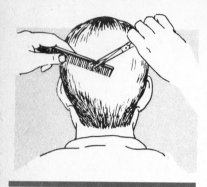

10.145 – Shear-point tapering ragged or choppy areas

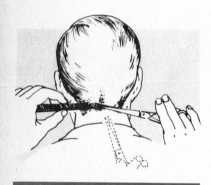

10.146 – Shear-point tapering depression in nape

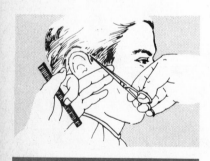

10.147 – Outlining in front of and over the ear

Shear-Point Tapering

Shear-point tapering is a useful technique for thinning out difficult heads of hair caused by hollows, wrinkles, and creases in the scalp, and by whorls of hair on the scalp. Dark and ragged hair patches on the scalp can be minimized by this special technique. The shear-point taper is performed with the cutting points of the shears. Only a few strands of hair are cut at a time and then combed out. Continue cutting around the objectionable spot until it becomes less noticeable and blends in with the surrounding outline of the haircut. (Figs. 10.145, 10.146)

CAUTION: Do not cut the hair close to the skin in the hollows or wrinkles, as it will cause unevenness and nicks to appear.

Arching Technique

The arching technique is a way of marking the outer border of the haircut in front, over the ears, and on the side of the neck. This outlining is accomplished with the points of the shears and is usually performed while doing the shears and comb work.

To learn arching technique the student should practice the exercise diligently.

As with all techniques, the following is one method of arching. Other methods may be equally correct. Be guided by your instructor.

1. **How to hold the shears with the right hand.**
   a) Pick up the shears and insert the thumb in the thumb grip. Place the third finger into the finger grip and little finger on the brace of the shears.
   b) Use the most convenient fingertip of the left hand to steady the point of the shears. (Fig. 10.147)
2. **How to arch the right side.**
   a) Always make an outline around ear as close to the natural hairline as possible.
   b) Start in front of the ear and make a continuous out-

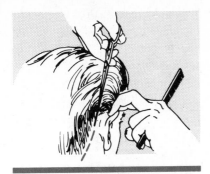

10.148 – Outlining the right side of neck downward

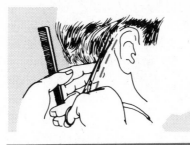

10.149 – Outlining the right side of neck upward

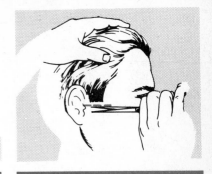

10.150 – Squaring off the right sideburn

line around the ear and down the side of the neck. (Fig. 10.148)

c) Reverse the direction of arching back to the starting point. (Fig. 10.149)

d) Continue arching around the ear until a definite outline is formed.

e) Square off the length of the right sideburn. (Fig. 10.150)

NOTE: Some barber-stylists prefer to square off the sideburn before arching the right side.

---

3. **How to arch the left side.**

Starting in front of the left ear, make a continuous outline with the shears over the left ear and down the side of the neck. (Fig. 10.151); then reverse the direction of the shears and return to the starting point. The squaring off of the left sideburn to match the right sideburn is done last. (Fig. 10.152)

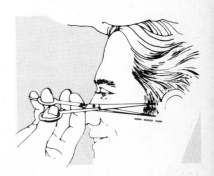

10.151 – Outlining the left side of neck downward

Hair Thinning

Hair thinning reduces the bulk of the hair. Thinning (serrated) shears or regular shears can be used for this purpose.

Plan of thinning the hair. The barber-stylist stands behind the client, combing away the front hair that does not require thinning. The hair is then thinned on both sides of the head, strand by strand

10.152 – Squaring off left sideburn

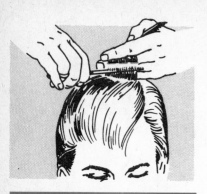

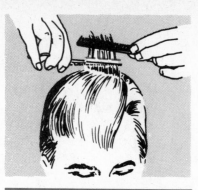

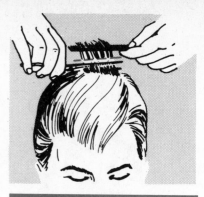

10.153 – Thinning hair with thinning shears—holding hair between index and middle finger

10.154 – Thinning hair with thinning shears—holding hair with comb facing away from barber-stylist

10.155 – Thinning hair with thinning shears—holding hair with comb facing barber-stylist

as required, and the loose cut hair is combed out. The top part is done last.

1. **Thinning with serrated shears.** The hair strand is combed and the spread hair held between the index and middle fingers. (Fig 10.153) Then the hair is cut about one inch from the scalp. If another cut is necessary it should be made about one inch from the first cut. Do not cut twice in the same place. To shorten the hair use the regular shears.

2. **Thinning with serrated shears and comb.** Instead of the index and middle fingers, the comb may be used to hold the hair. (Figs. 10.154, 10.155) The thinning is done in the usual manner.

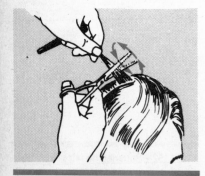

10.156 – Thinning hair—using regular shears

CAUTION: Do not cut the hair too closely to the scalp or thin out too much hair, as it will cause short hair ends to protrude and light spots to appear.

Back-combing. Combing the short hair of the parting or section first, toward the scalp, guards against thinning out too much hair. Thin hair using regular shears. (Fig. 10.156)

3. **Thinning with regular shears.** Hold a small strand of hair between the thumb and index finger. Insert the strand in

the shears. Slide the shears up and down the strand, closing them slightly each time they are moved toward the scalp. Slither enough to allow the hair to lie close to the scalp wherever needed.

MEN'S RAZOR HAIRCUTTING

Razor haircutting provides a wide range of opportunity for the barber-stylist to express artistic and professional talent. It provides an additional technique for achieving the ultimate objective: to design a hairstyle that enhances the client's appearance.

Competence in this technique requires thorough training, dedication, and long practice. It is not a skill that is easily or quickly acquired. It demands painstaking care, careful concentration, and constant effort. The technique of handling a razor should be mastered completely before attempting to use it to cut or style a client's hair.

Razor haircutting is especially suitable for thinning and shortening, tapering and blending, wisping or feathering specific areas (for example, neckline, around ears, bangs, etc.), making resistant hair more manageable. As always, the barber-stylist must consider the client's styling wishes; the client's features, head shape, and facial contour; and hair texture.

Razor Stroking and Combing

Proper stroking of the razor and combing during the tapering process are of utmost importance in razor haircutting. It is better to taper a little at a time than to taper too much. Remember, after the hair is cut it cannot be replaced.

Arm and Hand Movements

Some barber-stylists prefer the arm movement, in which the razor stroking and combing is done with stiff arms, using the elbows as a hinge. Others use both wrist and arm movements. This is a matter of preference. The barber-stylist should develop a technique best suited to the individual, which gives the desired results.

Razor Taper-Blending

Razor cutting is the best technique to use for taper-blending of the hair. The cutting action of the razor permits a smoother blend than that usually accomplished with scissors and/or clippers.

Light taper-blending. The razor is held almost flat against the surface of the hair. Note the small amount of hair that is cut when

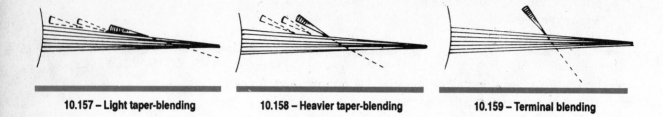

| 10.157 – Light taper-blending | 10.158 – Heavier taper-blending | 10.159 – Terminal blending |

the blade is only slightly tilted. (Fig. 10.157) Very little pressure is used.

Heavier taper-blending. The razor is held up to 45 degrees from the surface of the hair strand. As the razor is tilted higher, the depth of the cut increases. (Fig. 10.158) Usually a little more pressure is used than in light tapering.

Terminal blending. The angle of the razor blade is increased to almost 90 degrees. (Fig. 10.159) Short sawing strokes are used. Other terms used for terminal blending are hair-end tapering and blunt cutting.

Razor and Comb Coordination

Razor stroking and combing are done in a continuous movement. The razor tapers while the comb removes the cut hair and recombs the hair for the next stroke or strokes.

Tapering Coarse, Thick (Bulky) Hair

The use of a razor with a safety guard is recommended for the beginner. After gaining proficiency, a razor without a safety guard may be used, under the guidance of the instructor.

More strokes and heavier tapering are required for coarse, thick hair. The first strip of hair usually is combed first, followed by three razor strokes and followed again with the comb. The comb removes the cut hair and recombs the hair, allowing you to see how much hair has been cut. It also creates a guide to use for tapering the next strip. (Figs. 10.160–10.165)

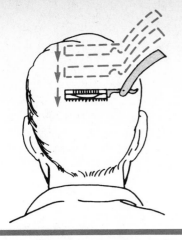

10.160 – Crown area—three long strokes are to be used.

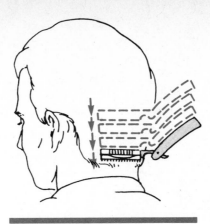

10.161 – Nape area—four short strokes should be used.

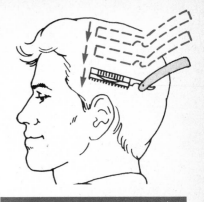

10.162 – Left and right sides of head—three strokes may be used.

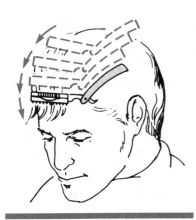

10.163 – Top area—consideration must be given to the hair style to be created. The stroking and the pressure of the razor largely depend upon the amount of hair to be removed to achieve the finished hairstyle.

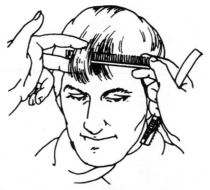

10.164 – Front hair—to equalize the length of long and uneven front hair, pick up the hair with the comb in the right hand. Hold the hair straight out between the middle and index fingers of the left hand.

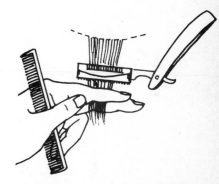

10.165 – Transfer the comb to the left hand. Hold the razor at an angle, and with short, sawing strokes cut the hair to the desired length.

Tapering Normal Texture (Average) Hair

Hair of normal texture—neither coarse nor fine—is considered average hair. Razor stroking this type of hair requires fewer strokes

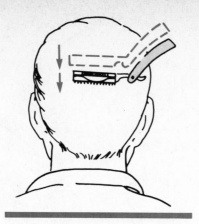

10.166 – Crown area—two long strokes are used.

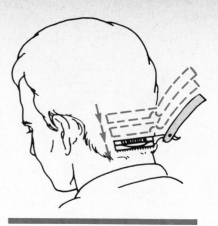

10.167 – Nape area—three short strokes are used.

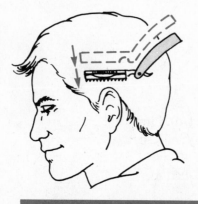

10.168 – Left and right sides of head—two short strokes may be used.

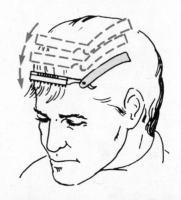

10.169 – Top of head—the stroking and pressure of the razor in this area are the same as for the sides and back areas.

and lighter pressure than does coarse, thick (bulky) hair. (Figs. 10.166–10.169)

Fine Hair

With fine hair, there is usually no bulk to remove. However, the razor may be used to blend hair ends to achieve a particular hairstyle.

Stroking of the razor is usually lighter than for normal (average) hair.

Hair Sectioning for Razor Haircutting

Short hair or hair that is cut regularly usually does not require any sectioning. However, in razor haircutting sectioning the head is usually necessary.

There are several good ways to section the head. Your instructor's method may be equally correct.

The head may be sectioned in any of the following ways:

1. **Umbrella effect.** Before sectioning the hair, it is advisable to comb it first in an umbrella effect. Starting at the crown, comb the hair in all natural directions, similar to the spokes of a wheel. (Fig. 10.170)
2. **Two sections.** First, part the hair from ear to ear across the crown. All hair in front of the part is combed forward. All hair behind or below the part is combed down. (Fig. 10.171)
3. **Three sections.** First, part the hair from ear to ear across the crown. All top and side hair is combed forward. Then make a vertical part from the crown to the nape. Each of these subsections is combed toward the sides. In the nape area where there is no part, comb the hair down. (Fig. 10.172)
4. **Four sections.** Add one more section to the previous three sections. Make a top center part. On each side comb the hair down. (Fig. 10.173)
5. **Four sections (alternate method).** First, part the hair from ear to ear across the crown. Second, section the right side from the center of the right eyebrow to the crown and comb down. Make another section on the left side from the center of the left eyebrow to the crown and comb down. Comb all back hair down. (Fig. 10.174)

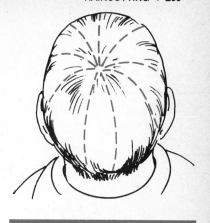

10.170 – Umbrella effect

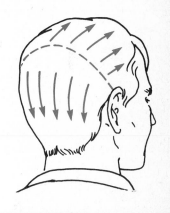

10.171 – Two sections

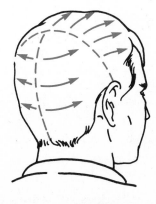

10.172 – Three sections

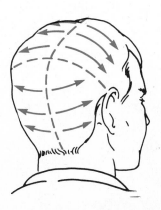

10.173 – Four sections

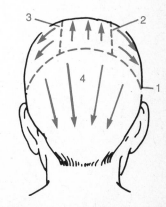

10.174 – Four sections (alternate method)

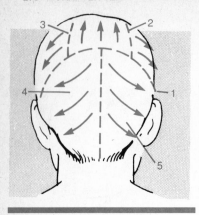

10.175 – Five sections

6. **Five sections.** Sectioning is the same as Number 5, except that the back section is divided in two and combed as indicated by the arrows. (Fig. 10.175)

Procedure for a Basic Razor Haircut

The method used for razor haircutting should follow a basic plan that can be varied for different hairstyles. No two artists will follow the same procedure. In this text, one basic plan is followed. Other procedures may be different, but equally correct. Two plans are outlined here: one followed in this text, and an alternate plan.

Pattern 1 — Used in this Text

1. Back part of head (Fig. 10.176)
   a) Downward
   b) Top right to left-downward
   c) Top left to right-downward
2. Right side of head (Fig. 10.177)
   a) Downward
   b) Toward the back
   c) Toward the face
3. Left side of head (Fig. 10.177)
   a) Downward
   b) Toward the back
   c) Toward the face
4. Top hair (Fig. 10.178)
   a) Crown to forehead
   b) Top left side
   c) Top right side

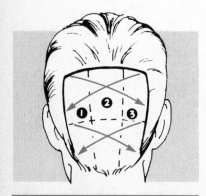

10.176 – Back

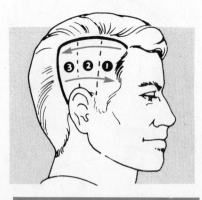

10.177 – Sides

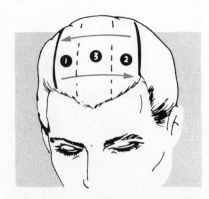

10.178 – Top

Pattern 2 — Alternate Method

1. Right side of head
   a) Downward
   b) Toward the back
   c) Toward the face
2. Left side of head
   a) Downward
   b) Toward the back
   c) Toward the face
3. Back part of head
   a) Downward
   b) Top right to left-downward
   c) Top left to right-downward
4. Top hair
   a) Top left side
   b) Top right side
   c) Crown to forehead

Razor Cutting for Back of Head

Some barber-stylists prefer to razor cut the back of the head first, then the sides. This is a matter of preference.

1. Section the hair into three vertical partings or subsections. (Fig. 10.179)
2. Taper the hair, one strip at a time in a downward direction, blending it with hair previously trimmed. (Fig. 10.180) Use short, even razor strokes. Be careful to avoid ridges, lines, or any appearance of unevenness (choppiness).
   a) **First strip.** Start at the upper left side, below the crown (pivot area) and taper downward.

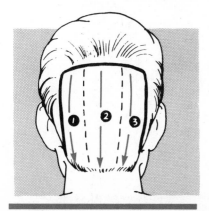

10.179 – Back area subdivided into three strips

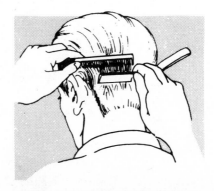

10.180 – Taper to blend with nape hair.

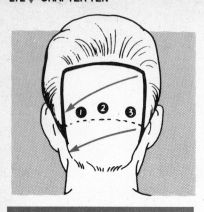

10.181 – Comb back hair from right top toward left, downward.

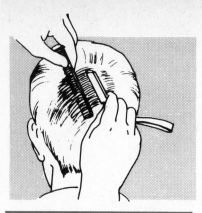

10.182 – Top section—taper lightly from right top, downward toward the left.

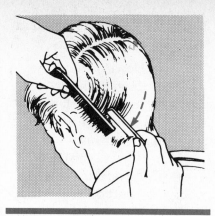

10.183 – Lower section—blend with nape hair, right to left.

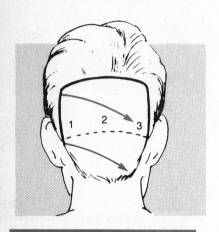

10.184 – Comb hair from top left to right, downward.

b) **Second strip.** Start below the crown (pivot area) and taper downward toward the center of the nape.

c) **Third strip.** Start at the upper right side below the crown, and taper downward.

3. Comb the hair from the top-right side toward the left downward. (Fig. 10.181) Taper the hair into two sections.

a) **Top section.** Taper lightly from right to left. (Fig. 10.182)

b) **Lower section.** Taper to blend with the nape hair from the right to the left side. (Fig. 10.183)

4. Comb the hair from the top-left side toward the right downward. (Fig. 10.184)

a) Taper the upper and lower sections downward toward the right in the same manner as previously explained. (Figs. 10.185, 10.186)

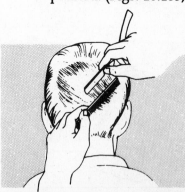

10.185 – Upper section—start at the top left, and taper toward right downward.

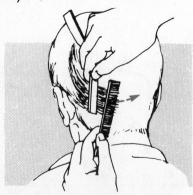

10.186 – Lower section—taper the lower back section toward the right.

Important Reminder

For best results in razor cutting the barber-stylist must:

1. Avoid tapering too close to the hair part.
2. Avoid thinning the hair too close to the scalp.
3. Avoid over-tapering the hair. It is better to cut less hair than too much. Cut hair cannot be replaced.
4. Cut hair that is sufficiently damp.
5. Cut clean hair (no interference from sprays, gels, debris, etc.).

NOTE: Proper angle of razor/hair ratio is very important. If razor is flat, damage on ends will occur; if razor is too straight (angle) cut will be too clean (comparable to a shear cut).

Razor Cutting for Right Side

Some barber-stylists prefer to start razor cutting on the right side of the head; others prefer to start on the left. This is a matter of preference—either way is correct.

1. **Pattern for Right Side**
   a) Comb the hair downward and subdivide it into three vertical partings. (Fig. 10.187)
   b) Taper downward, Sections 1, 2, and 3.
   c) Comb the hair toward the back.
   d) Taper lightly toward the back.
   e) Comb the hair toward the face.
   f) Taper lightly toward the face.
2. **Downward Direction**
   a) **Vertical partings.** With the comb in the right hand, use the index finger of the left hand to section the hair into three vertical partings. (Fig. 10.188)

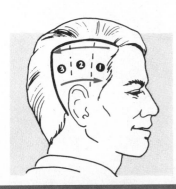

10.187 – Right side pattern

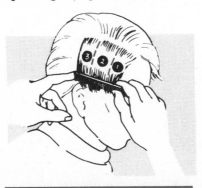

10.188 – Part hair into three vertical sections.

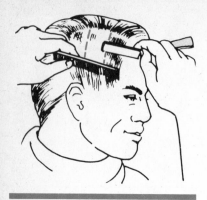

10.189 – Taper the first section.

b) **Section 1.** Start about three-quarters of an inch from the part and taper downward. (Fig. 10.189) Cut off uneven hair ends. (Fig. 10.190)

c) **Section 2.** Repeat the same tapering procedure as for Section 1.

d) **Section 3.** Repeat the same tapering procedure as for Section 1.

CAUTION: Be sure to protect the ear with the comb.

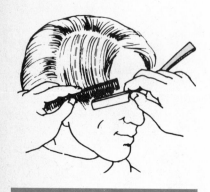

10.190 – Remove uneven hair ends.

3. **Toward the Back**

   a) Comb the hair away from the face toward the back of the head. (Fig. 10.191)

   b) Taper hair. Start tapering slightly back from the hairline (Fig. 10.192) and continue to taper lightly toward the back of the head.

4. **Toward the Face**

   a) Comb the hair forward and downward toward the face. (Fig. 10.193)

   b) Taper the hair, starting at the upper back corner. (Fig. 10.194)

   c) Continue to taper toward the front hairline.

   d) If necessary, cut off extra long hair at the hairline.

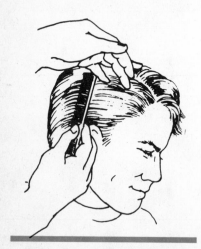

10.191 – Comb hair toward the back.

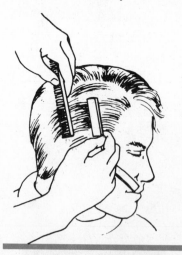

10.192 – Taper toward the back.

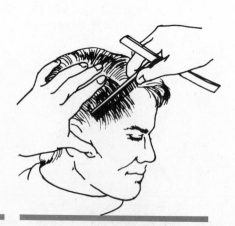

10.193 – Comb hair toward face.

Razor Cutting for Left Side

Follow exactly the same procedure as that outlined for the right side of the head.

1. Comb the hair downward and subdivide the left side into three vertical sections. (Fig. 10.195)
2. Taper Sections 1, 2, and 3 downward.
3. Comb and taper the hair lightly toward the back.
4. Comb and taper the hair lightly toward the face.

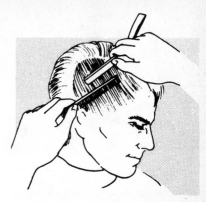

10.194 – Taper toward face.

Razor Cutting for Top of Head

In razor cutting, the top part of the head is of utmost importance. Usually this is the area where most creative skill is required to achieve the desired hairstyle. How much to taper depends on the style and the amount of hair. The order in which tapering is done is a matter of preference.

1. **Top hair forward.** Usually this step in razor cutting is done first. Comb the hair forward evenly. (Fig. 10.196)
   a) **Top right side.** Start to taper just forward of the crown and proceed toward the forehead. (Fig 10.197) How much to taper depends upon the desired hairstyle.
   b) **Top left side.** Repeat on the left top side in the same manner.
   c) **Top center** is usually done last. Be careful not to taper too much hair.
   d) **Front section.** Insert the comb in the hair to pick up

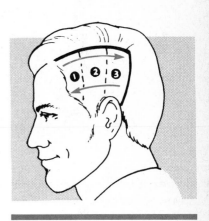

10.195 – Left side pattern

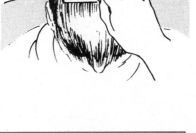

10.196 – Comb hair forward.

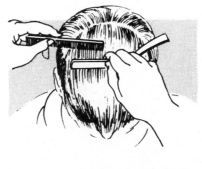

10.197 – Taper top right side toward forehead.

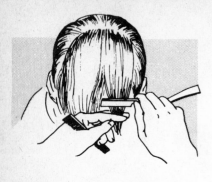

10.198 – After tapering top left side, taper front hair.

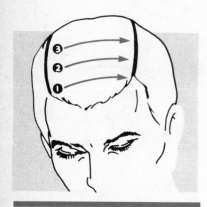

10.199 – Comb top hair evenly to left side.

the left half of the front section; hold the hair firmly between the middle and index fingers.

1) Taper the hair. (Fig. 10.198) Comb the hair forward again and remove any unevenness.

2) Repeat this procedure until all front hair has been tapered.

2. **Top left side.** Comb and distribute the top hair evenly to the left side of the head. (Fig. 10.199)

   a) **Start at top front.** Lightly taper the top hair downward to blend with the side hair. If necessary, trim uneven hair along the hairline. (Fig. 10.200)

   b) **Middle top area.** Proceed in the same manner as above.

   c) **Back top area.** Continue to taper in the same manner. It is of utmost importance that the hair over the ear blend with the back hair.

CAUTION: Be sure that the ear is protected with the comb when tapering this area.

3. **Top right side.** After the left side is completed, comb and distribute the hair to the right side of the head. (Fig. 10.201)

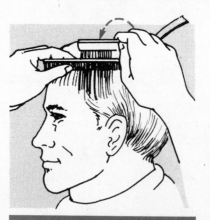

10.200 – Taper the right side from front to back, to blend with previously tapered hair.

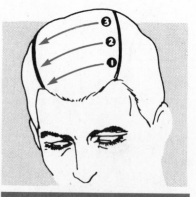

10.201 – Comb top hair evenly to right side.

a) **Start at top front.** Follow the same procedure for tapering the right side of the head as that outlined for the left side of the head. (Fig. 10.202)

> CAUTION: The same precaution must be taken to protect the ear from injury by protecting it with the comb, and extreme caution must be taken that the hair blends with the back hair.

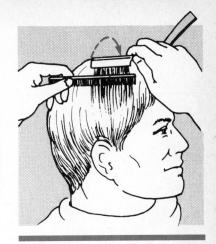

10.202 – Taper top front hair to blend with previously tapered hair.

Completion

Shave the neckline and under the ears if required. Be sure to cut very low without attempting any further tapering.

If the client wishes to have the arch shaved around the ears do so, but remember to keep as close to the ears as possible.

Clean up around the neck and ears. If special styling such as air-waving, etc., is desired, it should be done at this time. Otherwise the haircut is completed. Part and comb the hair. Wipe off loose hair with a towel, tissue, or hair vacuum. Remove the towel or neck strip and chair cloth, and release the client in the usual manner.

Clean-up. Put everything in proper order and place used implements in a container to be sanitized. Wash your hands.

Safety Precautions and Reminders for Razor Haircutting

1. Wash the hands before and after working on a client.
2. Examine the client's scalp and hair before razor cutting. Look for unusual conditions or disorders such as growths, depressions, rashes, abrasions, or balding spots.
3. Analyze the client's head shape, facial contour, neckline, and hair texture.
4. Buy and use only good quality haircutting implements.
5. Scissors and razors must be kept sharp at all times. Have implements sharpened when necessary. A dull cutting edge may cause pain or discomfort to your client.

CAUTION: **Do not test sharpness of implements with your fingers.**

6. Extend scissors (handles first) to persons receiving them. Protect the skin by guiding the scissor blades with the fingertips of the left hand or with a comb. Avoid nipping the skin or digging points of scissors into a client's neck or scalp.

7. Replace or resharpen dull razor blades. Place discarded blades into a closed container. A dull razor will pull the hair and cause pain or discomfort to the client. To avoid injury, use a razor with a guard until you are proficient in razor cutting.

8. Section the hair before virgin hairstyling or before cutting long hair.

9. Wet hair before using a razor to cut, taper, or thin.

10. Tapering the hair too closely to the hair part will cause coarse or medium-textured hair ends to stand up and make the part look ragged. Thinning coarse hair too closely to the scalp will create short, stubby hair ends that will protrude through the top layer. Avoid over-tapering the hair; it is impossible to correct a haircut after too much hair has been removed.

11. Do not leave implements exposed. Avoid dropping them to the floor, since this may cause damage to cutting surfaces, or knock implements out of line which may cause injury.

12. Clean and sanitize implements after each use. Store them in a dry sanitizer until they are to be used again.

13. Protect implements after each use. Place scissors in their case and keep razors closed.

14. Combs made of hard rubber are the most durable and are popular with barber-stylists. A variety of sanitized combs must be available to perform the various phases of haircutting. Combs must be cleaned and sanitized after each use.

15. Keep clippers clean and lubricated. Hair must be removed and clipper blades must be cleaned and sanitized after each use. Avoid dropping the detachable clipper blades to the floor, since this may cause damage to the cutting surface and/or may cause injury.

16. To avoid injury, do not annoy or distract anyone who is in the process of cutting hair.

Women's Razor Cutting

Preparation

1. Seat the client; adjust the neck strip and plastic cape.
2. Analyze the head shape, facial features, and hair texture.
3. Decide on a suitable haircut with the client.
4. Comb and brush the hair free of tangles.
5. Shampoo and cut the hair while it is wet.

Procedure

1. Divide the hair into five sections.
2. Determine the length of the nape guideline hair.
3. Blunt cut a guideline strand of nape hair. (Fig. 10.203)
   a) Blunt cut a strand on the left side; use the earlobe as a guide.(Fig. 10.204)
   b) Blunt cut a strand on the right side to match the left side. (Fig. 10.205)

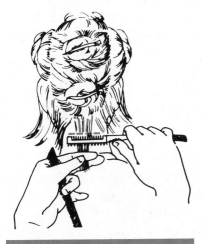
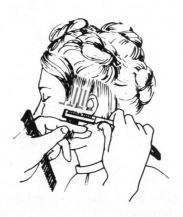
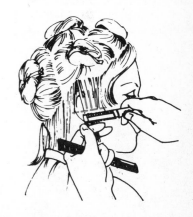

10.203 – Blunt cut a strand at center nape for desired hair length.

10.204 – On the left side, use ear lobe as a guide for measuring desired length.

10.205 – On the right side, follow same procedure as for the left side.

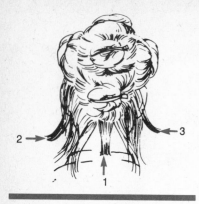

10.206 – Placement of cut guide line strands

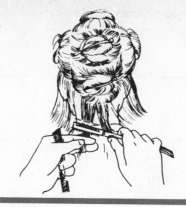

10.207 – Guideline hair—cut guideline hair from center to left, matching length of previously cut strands.

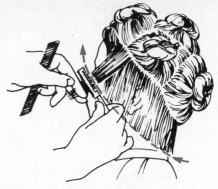

10.208 – Continue to cut and blend the remainder of hair on the left side.

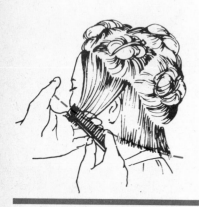

10.209 – Left side guide line completed—length evenly matched

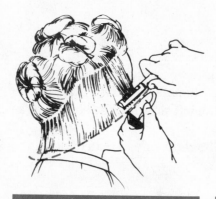

10.210 – The same procedure used on the left side is continued on the right side.

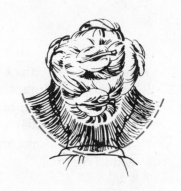

10.211 – Guideline hair completely cut

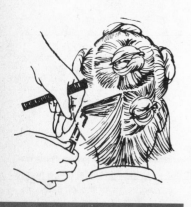

10.212 – Shaping section No. 5a

c) Use guideline hair to cut from the back center to the left front and back center to the right front. (See Figs. 10.206–10.210)

d) Complete guide line. (Fig. 10.211)

Divide section No. 5 into two parts (sections No. 5a and No. 5b). From the center of section No. 5a, pick up horizontal strands. Pick up the guideline strand for length. When the guideline hair falls away, cut the hair—moving the hands out and upward into a 45-degree arc. (Fig. 10.212) Proceed to cut to the left into section No. 4 in the same manner. Return to section No. 5b and cut this section, moving to the right into section No. 3, always lifting the hands in an upward 45-degree arc as the hair is cut. Measure carefully with guide line. Next, proceed to cut section No. 2 (crown) using previously cut hair as a guide.

Top Section

Divide section No. 1 into two parts. Pick up hair from the middle of the section, using previously cut hair as a guide. Maintain the hand movements in the 45-degree arc. Proceed to cut both parts of section No. 1 in the prescribed manner. (Figs. 10.213, 10.214)

If bangs are to be cut, move directly in front of the client for even cutting. Test the hair for bounce (elasticity); then determine the desired length. If bangs are to be short, use the bridge of the nose as a guide. If they are to be long, shape strands to blend into the length of the sides.

To complete the shaping of the hair, excess bulk should be removed by thinning with a razor, thinning shears, or scissors. All hair should be checked for proper length.

Hair Properly Razor Cut

The barber-stylist should strive for proficiency in women's razor cutting. If the hair is cut uniformly all over the head, the client will have no problem in combing and styling the hair. (Figs. 10.215—10.217) If the hair is cut in different lengths, the client may encounter difficulty in combing and styling it.

Completion

Remove the neck strip and plastic cape. Thoroughly clean all hair clippings from the cape, clothing, and work area.

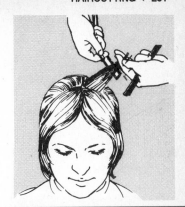

10.213 – Shaping top section

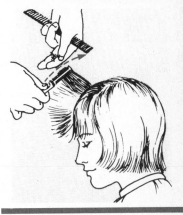

10.214 – Alternate method of shaping top section

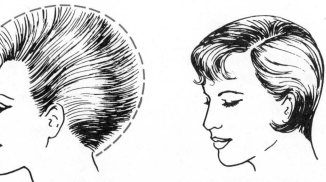

10.215 – Correct uniform razor cutting

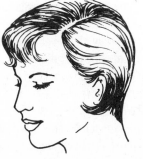

10.216 – Completed razor cutting with bang effect and/or off-face style

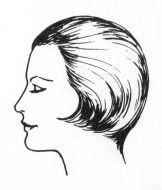

10.217 – Hair razor cut for a straight back style

Helpful Hints in Women's Haircutting

There are as many ways to cut women's hair as there are barber-stylists. The following suggestions will help to achieve special results.

1. To develop a soft pompadour effect, hair is parted parallel to the hairline and directed off the face for cutting. This technique positions the hair properly for cutting the ends underneath, giving lift and softness to the hair.
2. For a side-angled bang, direct the hair parallel to the forehead. Shorten the hair to a point that is approximately level with the outer ends of the eyebrow.
3. To create an off-the-face style, direct the hair back from the hairline in vertical partings. Start cutting the hair about three inches from the hairline at the face, and shorten it as previously planned.
4. A lifted nape effect can be accomplished by sectioning the hair vertically across the crown, downward. The lengths are graduated in a blended taper from about three inches to two inches at the nape.

One of the objectives in hairstyling is to minimize and draw attention away from the client's less attractive features. This can be done either by partially concealing less attractive features, or by counteracting them by drawing attention away from them. The above suggestions should be of help in planning a haircut that achieves these goals.

REVIEW QUESTIONS

Haircutting Principles

1. What does the haircutting process involve?
2. A good haircut is_____.
3. How may stylists achieve attractive, easy-to-manage hairstyles?
4. What should a hairstyle accomplish?
5. What four physical considerations help to determine the best haircut and style for the client?
6. What ability does the barber-stylist need to perfect in order to determine what a client wants in a haircut?
7. Name 11 haircutting areas used in men's hair.
8. What are the fundamental principles of haircutting?
9. Name 16 terms used in haircutting.
10. What degree angle is probably the most commonly used?
11. Name the four methods used in haircutting.

12. In what condition should the hair be to achieve the most precise finger and shear cut?

1. To get a better view of shears and comb work, what procedure should be followed?
2. What is the proper position of the shears and comb in haircutting?
3. What is the purpose of finger work in haircutting?

1. What preliminary facial analysis should be performed before cutting the hair?
2. Why is it important that the barber-stylist have an understanding of facial types?
3. Which is considered the perfect facial type?

1. Where is clipper work generally started and finished on the client's head?
2. How should the clipper be used in tapering the hair?
3. For upward tapering, what is the proper position of the shears and comb?
4. To get a better view of shears and comb work, what procedure should be followed?
5. What plan is followed in shaving the neck outline?
6. Name the shaving strokes used: a) over the right side of the neck; b) left side of the neck.
7. List four important final steps of a haircut.

1. What should be considered before giving the client a razor haircut?
2. For what three purposes can the barber-stylist use a razor haircut?
3. Name two types of razors used in haircutting.
4. Which two hand positions can be used in holding the razor?
5. Name three ways to taper-blend the hair with a razor.
6. Which method of taper-blending requires the least amount of pressure with the razor?
7. Describe the coordination of razor and comb movements.
8. What kind of stroke and pressure is employed to taper: a) coarse, bulky hair; b) normal (average) hair?
9. Why should the client's scalp and hair be examined before razor cutting?
10. For best results, what should the barber-stylist avoid when giving a razor cut?
11. To prevent accidents, what three precautions should be followed by the barber-stylist?

Women's Haircutting

1. Name the main implements used in haircutting.
2. What purpose is served by thinning the hair?
3. Why may fine hair be cut closer to the scalp than coarse hair?
4. About how close to the scalp should: a) fine hair; b) medium hair; c) coarse hair be thinned?
5. In which areas is it advisable not to thin the hair?
6. Why is it not advisable to thin hair in the hair part?
7. Why should you avoid removing too much hair during the thinning process?
8. Why should the hair be damp for razor shaping?
9. What is meant by back-combing?
10. What is meant by slithering the hair?

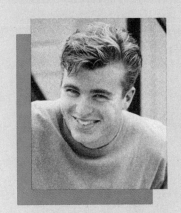

Hairstyling

Learning Objectives

After completing this chapter, you should be able to:

1. Define hairstyling.
2. Demonstrate free-form blow-drying techniques.
3. Demonstrate styling the hair with the blow-dryer, comb, and brush.
4. Demonstrate a shadow wave and air-curling.
5. Identify the parts of a curling iron.
6. Demonstrate curling iron techniques.
7. Demonstrate a finger wave.

Courtesy of: Hair: ABBA of PA. Photo: Jack Cutler.

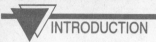

▼ INTRODUCTION

Hairstyling is the art of arranging the hair into an appropriate style following a haircut or shampoo. Today, many haircuts require minimal hairstyling techniques due to the quality of the cuts and the availability of effective styling aids such as gels, mousses, and freeze sprays. Some haircuts, on the other hand, require more styling attention, be it blow-drying, curling iron work, or finger waving. It is important for the barber-stylist to be proficient in such techniques.

▼ BLOW-DRYING

Free-Form Blow-Drying Technique

Free-form blow-drying is a quick, easy method of drying the client's hair. It can build fullness into the style and allows the hair to fall into the natural lines of the cut. Some advantages of free-form blow-drying are:

1. It shows the client how to duplicate the hairstyling method.
2. It demonstrates the quality of the haircut.
3. It speeds up the blow-drying service.
4. It allows the stylist to check the accuracy of the work.

Procedure

After the haircut is complete, begin at the nape area, holding the hair out of the way with a brush in one hand. As the hair underneath is dried, the brush releases the next area. The dryer should be held 6 to 10 inches from the area being dried, at an angle with the nozzle pointing downward on the hair, and should be moved briskly from side to side as it dries the hair. The sides may be dried in the same manner. The top should be dried loosely and then brushed in to the desired style, followed by the dryer. (Figs. 11.1–11.4)

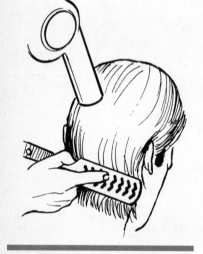

11.1 – Blow-drying the back of the head

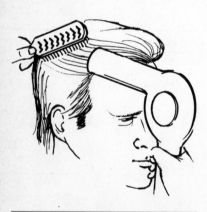

11.2 – Blow-drying the right side of the head

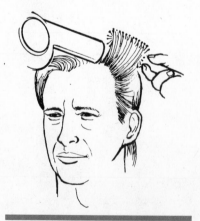

11.3 – Blow-drying the left side of the head

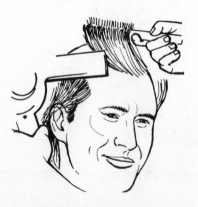

11.4 – Blow-drying the top of the head

Comb and Blower (Dryer) Technique

After the hair has been shampooed and left damp, a styling lotion is applied and combed through the hair.

Procedure

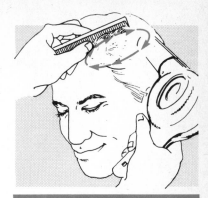

11.5 – Lift for height along left side part.

1. **Lift along the left hair part.** To create a lift or a little height along the left hair part, start at the front of the head and work toward the crown. Insert the hand comb about one and one-half inches from the part and draw the comb a little to the back and toward the part simultaneously. This will create a ridge. (Fig. 11.5) Adjust the blower to hot and direct the hot air back and forth until a soft ridge has been formed. Repeat, following these instructions, for the second and third sections.

> CAUTION: Direct the hot air at the ridge and not at the scalp.

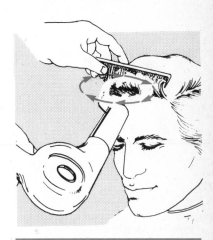

11.6 – Create a high front.

2. **High forward front.** Insert the hand comb from one-half to two inches from the front, depending upon the height of the front hair desired. Draw the comb a little to one side and toward the forehead to create a high ridge. (Fig. 11.6) Direct hot air from the blower back and forth along the forehead until a high soft ridge has been created.
3. **Lift along the right hair part.** Hold the hand comb with the right hand and the blower with the left hand. The procedure is the same as previously outlined for creating a lift for the left side part. (Fig. 11.7)
4. **Final steps.** Brush and comb the hair into the desired style.

Shadow Wave with Comb and Blower

A shadow wave is the same as a regular wave with low ridges. To accomplish it, a hand comb and blower may be used. Hair that has a natural wave will respond more readily to shadow waving than hair that is straight. Shadow waving is recommended for the front and sides of the head.

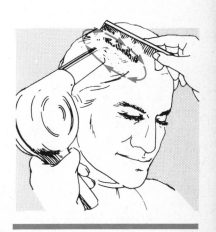

11.7 – Lift for height along right side part.

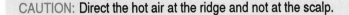

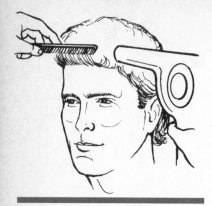

11.8 – Shadow waving—creating a shallow wave

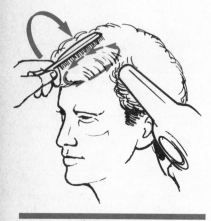

11.9 – Fullness—top side of part

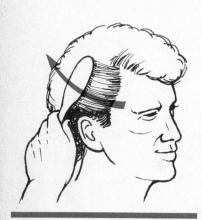

11.10 – Fullness—right side of head

Procedure

1. Shampoo, towel dry, and comb the hair in the desired direction. Apply a small amount of styling lotion; add more as needed. Warm water may be used instead of styling lotion.

2. Insert a hand comb about two to two and one-half inches from the hairline and draw the comb forward, a little to one side, so that the hair will form a shallow wave. (Fig. 11.8) If the wave does not form readily, the hair can be guided into a wave by pressing it with the index finger or middle finger of the right hand. After the wave has been formed, apply hot air from the blower in a rotating motion. Maintain this position until the wave has formed.

3. After waving, adjust a styling hair net, dry, and finish the hairstyle in the usual manner.

Brush and Blower Technique

The use of a narrow brush and a blower is another method of styling the hair. At times the stylist will prefer to use a brush instead of a comb to achieve a certain effect.

Create Fullness

In areas where fullness is desired, or to give contour to the head, the hair is first lifted with a brush, with hot air from the blower directed at the lifted hair. The hair is then molded softly with the comb or brush into the hairstyle desired.

Before beginning styling, shampoo and towel dry the hair, leaving it damp. Then apply styling lotion, comb through the hair, and proceed with the styling.

Fullness at Top Side of Part

Brush the top hair away from part. Then, with a twist of the wrist, draw the brush slightly toward the part, creating a slight directional ridge. Blow hot air along the ridge, moving the blower back and forth. Avoid blowing hot air on the scalp. Repeat section by section, working from front to back. (Fig. 11.9)

Fullness on Right and Left Side of Head

Right side. To create fullness at the right side of the head, brush the hair slightly toward the back. (Fig. 11.10) Then, with a twist of the wrist, turn and push the brush forward, creating a lift. (Fig. 11.11) Blow hot air on the area until the hair is set in position.

Left side. Repeat the same procedure as for right side of head. (Fig. 11.12)

Fullness for the Front Hair

A brush may be used to create a high lift at the front hairline. Draw the brush underneath the hair, and with a quick turn of the wrist turn the brush upward. Use the blower in a back and forth movement until the hair is partially dry. Remove the brush by drawing it outward. The hair is then combed so that the hair ends blend with the rest of the hairstyle. A shadow wave may be created with the hair ends behind the lifted hair. (Fig. 11.13)

Crown Swirl

Comb the crown hair in a swirl effect, with the grain or in the desired direction. Then brush the hair slightly forward in the direction previously followed with the comb. While brushing, twist the wrist inward and draw the hair slightly in reverse, thus creating fullness in the area. (Fig. 11.14) Blow hot air on the area with a rotating motion, until the desired fullness has been achieved. Direct the hot air through the hair, avoiding hot air application directly to the scalp. Repeat this procedure on various parts of the crown until the swirl effect has been achieved. To achieve swirl effects on the top and front areas of the head, the same procedure may be followed. (Fig. 11.15)

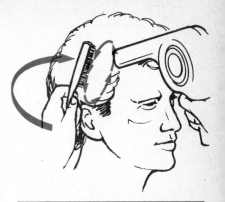

11.11 – Creating a lift with the brush

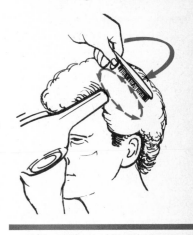

11.12 – Fullness—left side of head

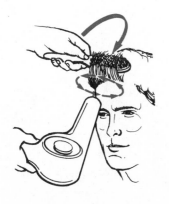

11.13 – Fullness—for front hair

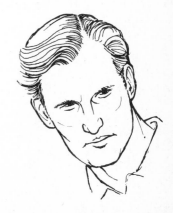

11.14 – Swirl fullness in the crown area

11.15 – Swirl effects on the top and front areas

AIR-WAVING WOMEN'S HAIR

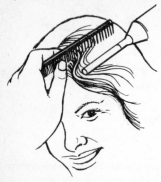

The hair is styled after it has been cut, shampooed, and towel dried, using an electric air-waver comb and styling comb. To achieve ridges and waves on various parts of the head, the hair must be slightly damp. Apply styling lotion lightly to assist in creating the desired hairstyle.

It is important to locate the natural wave formation of the hair, as this will help to establish the natural hair growth pattern. (Fig. 11.16) Comb the hair in the direction of the planned hairstyle, using an air-waver, until it is dry enough to hold a wave.

11.16 – Combing hair in direction of wave desired

Procedure

Right side part. Starting at the front of the head, insert the styling comb into the hair about one and one-half inches from the part. Draw the styling comb toward the back. Insert the air-waver under the comb and draw the air-waver comb toward the face to form a ridge. Hold both combs in this position until a firm ridge has been formed. (Fig. 11.17) Continue toward the crown until the entire length of the ridge is completed.

Form the second ridge starting at the crown and working toward the front. The ridge and shaping is made just the reverse of the first ridge. (Fig. 11.18) Support the completed ridgeline with the styling comb while the air-waver comb lifts and designs the pattern.

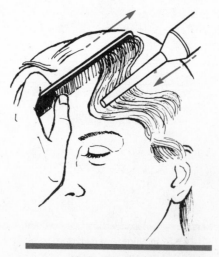

11.17 – Forming ridge

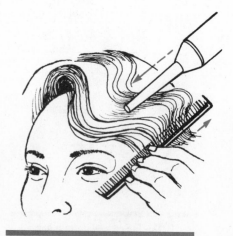

11.18 – Forming second ridge

Left side part. The procedure is exactly the same as that for the right side part, except that the hand comb is held in the right hand and the air-waver is controlled by the left hand. However, the waving should start at the crown and work forward, toward the face.

A finished wave is formed with the air-waver comb and styling comb, taking advantage of the natural waving pattern of the hair. (Fig. 11.19)

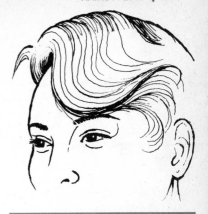

11.19 – Finished style

AIR-CURLING

Air-curling is most successful on hair that is naturally curly or has received a permanent wave. The basis for all successful air-curling styling is carefully planned hair cutting. In order to receive air-curling properly, hair should be cut with tapered ends. Successful air-curling is extremely difficult on hair with blunt-cut hair ends. (Fig. 11.20)

The following technique is offered as one method of creating a natural looking, easy-to-wear, informal style with a brush and blower.

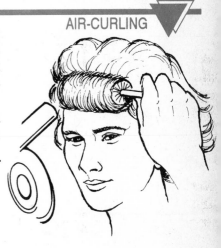

Procedure

1. Shampoo and towel dry the hair.
2. Properly cut the hair, leaving tapered ends.
3. Apply styling lotion and/or conditioner.
4. Pre-plan the style. Start at the crown or top of the head, as desired. Section the hair, pick up a wide strand, and comb through. (Figs. 11.21 and 11.22)

11.20 – Air-curling with round brush

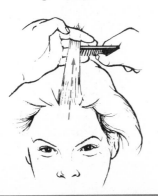

11.21 – Section a wide strand of hair for air-curling.

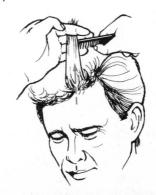

11.22 – Section a wide strand of hair for air-curling

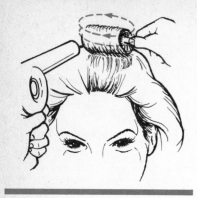

11.23 – Air-curling women's hair

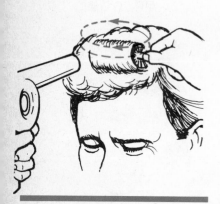

11.24 – Air-curling men's hair

5. Bring the comb out to the hair ends and insert the brush. Brush through the strand, bringing the brush out to the ends.

6. Roll the hair with the brush, making a complete downward turn, away from the face, until the brush rests on the scalp. Maintain this position and start the blower. Direct the blower very slowly through the curl, using a back-and-forth movement. (Fig. 11.23 and 11.24) When the hair section is completely dry, release the brush with a rounded movement. Use clippies to secure each curl as it is completed and to hold it in place until it is cooled off.

7. Continue making curls in the same manner across the crown and back of the head. Clip each curl as completed. Shape the neckline curls with a comb, or make pin curls at the nape for a finished, close-to-the-head look.

In air-curling it is essential that the scalp be thoroughly dry. The hairstyle will not hold if the scalp is damp.

Complete the styling with a light application of lacquer to give shine and holding power to the hair. (Figs. 11.25–11.28)

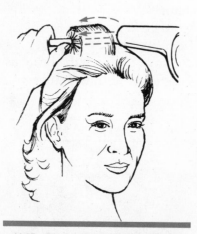

11.25 – To give the crown hair a slight lift, a small round brush is used. The dryer is kept on the move from side to side, along the curl. Secure each curl with clippies as it is completed.

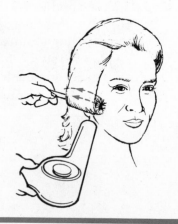

11.26 – To create a page boy effect, curl hair under with a brush and blow dry.

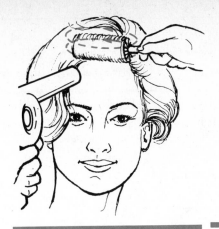

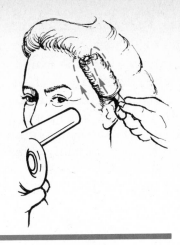

11.27 – To create a smooth top with flip, the hair ends are lifted by placing brush close to scalp. Rotate brush. As the brush rotates, the hot air is directed to the base within the cupped area.

11.28 – Side hair lift

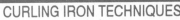

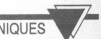

CURLING IRON TECHNIQUES

The use of curling irons is in great demand in the modern shop. The mastery of this technique is a basic requirement for success as a barber-stylist.

Implements

Thermal curling iron styling requires the use of three implements in addition to the regular barber-styling tools: a metal comb, an electric dryer, and electric curling irons.

1. Metal combs are preferred because they can withstand and retain heat.
2. The hand dryer is used to prepare the shampooed hair for styling and, in conjunction with a styling brush or comb, can help form the base design of a style very quickly. Curling irons and combs are then used to complete the style.
3. The curling irons must be made of the best quality steel to hold an even temperature. The curling or styling portion of the iron is composed of two parts: the rod (prong), and the shell (groove or bowl). The rod is solid steel and perfectly round. The shell also is perfectly round, with the inside grooved so that the rod can rest in it when the irons are closed.

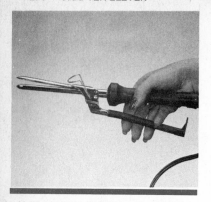

11.29 – Use the little finger to open the clamp.

Heat Testing Irons

Before discussing the manipulative techniques, a word of caution must be offered. Always heat test the irons before applying them to the hair. Clamp the heated iron over a tissue neck strip and hold it for five seconds. If the paper scorches or turns brown, the iron is too hot. Decrease the temperature before using. It should be noted that fine, lightened, or badly damaged hair can withstand less heat than normal hair. Use pressing cream or oil on African-American black hair to help prevent breakage or scorching.

Curling Iron Manipulations

The following is a series of basic movements for the use of heated curling irons. Most other movements employed are adaptations or derivations of these.

The method of holding the iron is a matter of personal preference. The technique chosen should provide ease, comfort, and facility of movement. The surrounding photo series shows a grip with only the little finger used for opening the clamp. Some barber-stylists prefer to use the little finger plus the ring finger for this purpose. Either method is equally correct. (Fig. 11.29–11.36)

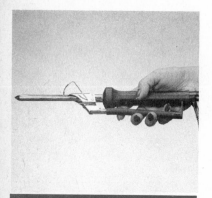

11.30 – Use three middle fingers to close and manipulate irons.

> **NOTE:** Those barber-stylists who use stove-heated curling irons will find that the techniques are very similar to those presented here for electric curling irons.

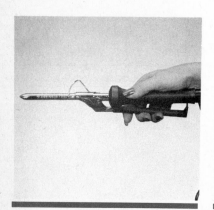

11.31 – Shift the thumb when manipulating the irons.

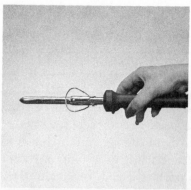

11.32 – Close clamp and make a one-quarter turn downward.

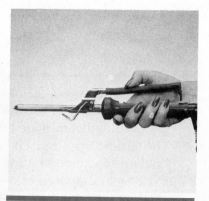

11.33 – Irons have made a one-half turn. Use the thumb to open clamp and relax hair tension.

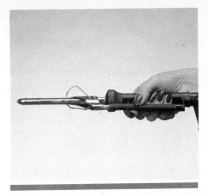

11.34 – Rotate irons to three-quarters of a complete turn.

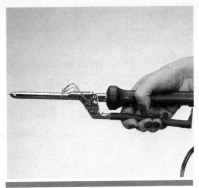

11.35 – Full turn

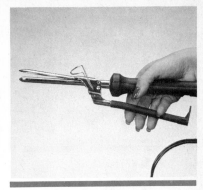

11.36 – Alternate method—use little and ring fingers to open clamp.

Constant Practice Required

Practice is required in order to develop any degree of efficiency in manipulating curling irons. Three exercises must be repeated until perfected.

1. To develop a smooth rotating action, practice turning the iron while opening and closing it at regular intervals. Dexterity must be developed in rotating the irons both downward and upward. (Fig. 11.37)
2. It is important to practice releasing the hair to prevent binding. Open and close the irons in a quick, clicking action to prevent binding.
3. Practice guiding the hair strand into the center of the curl as you rotate the iron. This exercise results in the end of the strand being firmly in the center of the curl. (Fig. 11.38)

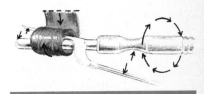

11.37 – Rotating movement while opening and closing the irons

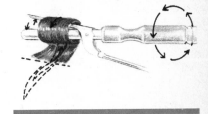

11.38 – Guiding the hair strand into the center of the curl while rotating the irons

Thermal-Iron Curling Techniques on Short Hair

The method set forth should be used in iron-curling of short hair only.

The base of each curl is formed by sectioning and parting to conform with the size of the curl desired. It is important to consider hair length, density, and texture. The base is usually about one and one-half to two inches in width, and approximately one-half inch in depth.

After the base is sectioned off, the hair in the curl section must be combed smoothly straight out from the scalp, in order for the heat

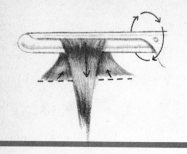

11.39 – Form a base.

and tension to be the same for all hairs in the section. Loose hairs may result in an uneven and ragged curl.

1. Insert the iron with the rod down, close the shell, and hold it at the base for approximately five seconds. Slide the iron up approximately one inch from the scalp. (Fig. 11.39)
2. Hold the ends of the hair strands with the thumb and two fingers of one hand, with a medium degree of tension. Turn the iron downward (toward the practitioner) with the other hand. (Fig. 11.40)
3. Open and close the iron rapidly, as you turn, to prevent binding and creases in the hair caused by the shell. Guide the ends of the strand into the center of the curl as you rotate the iron. (Fig. 11.41)
4. The result of this procedure will be a smooth, finished curl with the ends firmly fixed in the center. (Fig. 11.42)

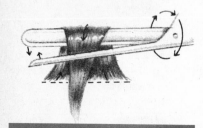

11.40 – Turn irons downward.

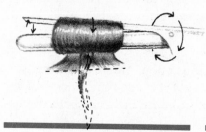

11.41 – Rotate irons and guide ends of strand into center.

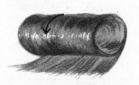

11.42 – Finished curl

Thermal-Iron Curling—Medium Hair

Section and form the base of the curl as described earlier.

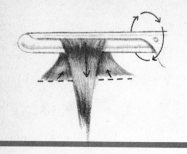

11.43 – Insert the hair into open irons at the scalp.

1. The hair is inserted into the open iron at the scalp; the hair is pulled over the rod in the direction of the curl, and the shell is closed. Hold in this position for about five seconds. Then slide the iron up about one inch from the scalp. The shell must be on top. (Fig. 11.43)
2. The iron is rotated downward one-half revolution. Pull the end of the strand over the rod to the left and direct it toward center of the curl. (Fig. 11.44)

3. Complete the revolution of the iron and continue directing the ends toward the center. (Fig. 11.45)

4. Make another complete revolution of the iron. The entire strand has been curled with the exception of the end. Enlarge the curl by opening the shell. Insert the end of the curl in the opening created between the shell and the rod. (Fig. 11.46)

5. Close the shell and slide the iron toward the handle. This technique will move the ends of the strand into the center of the curl. Rotate the iron several times to even out the distribution of the hair in the curl. (Fig. 11.47)

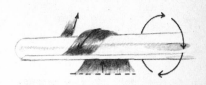

11.44 – Turn irons downward one-half revolution.

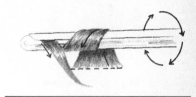

Removing the Curl from the Iron

During the curling process the comb is used to protect the client's scalp from possible burns.

When the curl is formed and the ends are freed from between the rod and the shell, one complete revolution of the iron is made inside the curl. This final revolution is made to smooth the ends and to loosen the hair from the iron. The comb is then used in conjunction with the iron to remove the curl. The iron is drawn in one direction while the comb holds the curl steady and slowly and carefully draws it in the opposite direction. Thus the curl is removed from the iron. (Fig. 11.48)

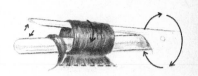

11.45 – Complete the revolution of the irons.

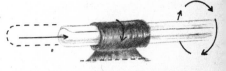

11.46 – Make another complete revolution.

Volume Thermal-Iron Curls

In order to create volume or lift in the finished hairstyle, the barber-stylist develops volume curls. The degree of lift desired will determine the type of volume curls being used.

Volume Base Curls—developed to provide maximum lift or volume since the curl is placed very high on its base.

Section off the base in the manner previously described. Hold the curl strand up at a 135-degree angle. Slide the iron over the strand about one-half inch from the scalp. Wrap the strand over the rod with medium tension. Maintain this position for approximately five seconds to heat the strand and set the base. Roll the curl in the usual manner and place it firmly, forward and high on its base.

Full Base Curls—designed to provide strong curls with full lift.

Section off the base as described. Hold the hair strand at a 125-degree angle. Slide the iron over the hair strand about one-half inch

11.47 – Close the shell and slide irons toward the handles.

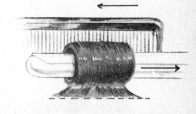

11.48 – Removing the curl using the comb as guide

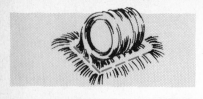

11.49 – Full base

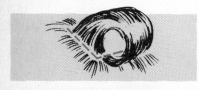

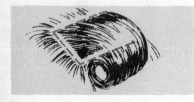

11.50 – One-half off base

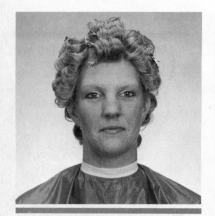

11.51 – Off base

from the scalp. Wrap the strand over the rod with medium tension. Maintain this position for about five seconds to heat the strand and set the base. Roll the curl in the usual manner and place it firmly in the center of its base. (Fig. 11.49)

Half Base Curls—designed to provide strong curls with moderate lift.

Section off the base as described. Hold the hair at a 90-degree angle. Slide the iron over the hair strand about one-half inch from the scalp. Wrap the strand over the rod with medium tension. Maintain this position for about five seconds to heat strand and set base. Roll the curl in the usual manner and place it half off its base. (Fig. 11.50)

Off Base Curls—designed to provide strong curls with only slight lift.

Section off the base as described. Hold the hair at a 70-degree angle. Slide the iron over the hair strand about one-half inch from the scalp. Wrap the strand over the rod with medium tension. Maintain this position for about five seconds to heat the strand and set the base. Roll the curl in the usual manner and place it completely off its base. (Fig. 11.51)

Finished Thermal Curl Settings

For best results when giving a thermal setting, clip each curl in place until the whole head is complete and ready for styling. (Figs. 11.52–11.54)

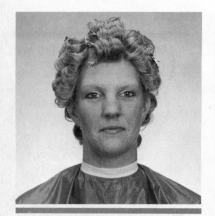

11.52 – Front view completely curled

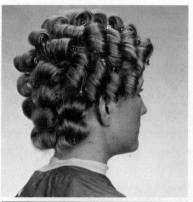

11.53 – Side view

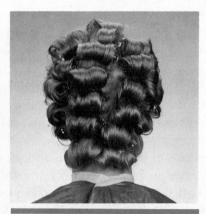

11.54 – Back of head completely curled

Styling the Hair After a Thermal Curl or Wave

After thermal-waving or curling, style the hair according to the client's wishes. Brush the hair working up from the neckline; push the waves and curls into place as you progress over the entire head. If the hairstyle is to be finished with curls, do the bottom curls last. (Fig. 11.55–11.58)

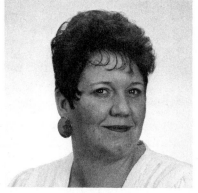

11.55 – Finished thermal style for short hair

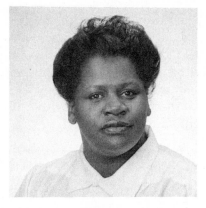

11.56 – Finished thermal style for short hair

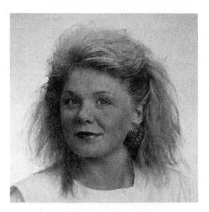

11.57 – Finished thermal style for medium length hair

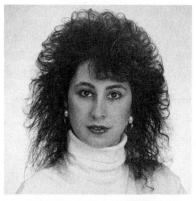

11.58 – Finished thermal style for long hair

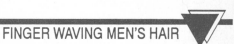

FINGER WAVING MEN'S HAIR

Finger waving is the technique of creating hairstyles with the aid of the fingers, comb, waving or styling lotion or gel, hairpins or clips, and a styling hair net.

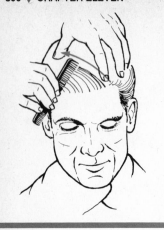

11.59 – Shaping top area

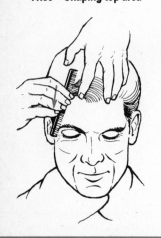

11.60 – Shaping first ridge

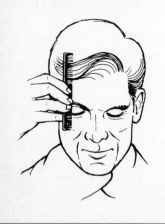

11.61 – Flatten comb against head.

The best results in developing soft, natural waves are obtained in hair that either has a natural or a permanent wave. It is more difficult to properly finger wave straight hair. A finger wave should harmonize with the shape of the client's head, as well as with facial features.

Styling Lotion and Comb

The use of a good styling lotion makes the hair pliable and keeps it in place. The proper choice of styling lotion or gel should be governed by the texture and condition of the client's hair. A good styling lotion is harmless to the hair; it should not flake after it has dried.

Hard rubber combs with both fine and coarse teeth are recommended for finger waving.

Preparation

Drape the client with a clean towel and a shampoo cape. After the client's hair is shampooed, towel-blot the hair.

The hair is then parted, combed smooth, and arranged to conform to the desired hairstyle. Styling lotion is applied with an applicator, or pump-sprayed on to the hair and distributed with the comb. Avoid using excessive amounts of styling lotion.

To locate the direction of natural hair growth, comb the hair away from the face and push it forward with the palm of the hand.

The finger wave may be started on either side of the head. In this presentation, the work begins on the right top side.

Shaping the Top Area

Shape the top hair with a comb, using a circular movement, starting at the front hairline and working toward the back until the crown has been reached. (Fig. 11.59)

Forming the First Ridge

The index finger of the left hand is placed directly above the position for the first ridge.

With the teeth of the comb pointing slightly upward, the comb is inserted directly under the index finger. Draw the comb forward about one inch along the fingertip. (Fig. 11.60)

With the teeth still inserted in the ridge, flatten the comb against the head in order to hold the ridge in place. (Fig. 11.61) Remove the left hand from the head and place the middle finger above the ridge and the index finger on the teeth of the comb. Emphasize the ridge by closing the two fingers and applying pressure. (Fig. 11.62)

CAUTION: Do not try to increase the height of the ridge by pushing or lifting it up with the fingers. This will distort and move the ridge formation off its base.

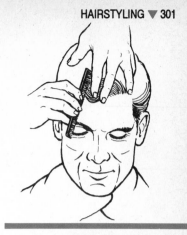

11.62 – Emphasize first ridge of the wave.

Without removing the comb, turn the teeth down and comb the hair in a right semicircular motion to form a dip in the hollow part of the wave. (Fig. 11.63) This procedure is followed section by section until the crown has been reached. (Fig. 11.64)

The ridge and wave of each section should match evenly without showing separations in the ridge and hollow part of the wave.

Forming the Second Ridge

The formation of the second ridge is begun at the front of the crown area. (Fig. 11.65) The movements are the reverse of those followed in forming the first ridge. The comb is drawn back from the fingertip, thus directing the formation of the second ridge. All movements are followed in a reverse pattern until the hairline is reached, thus completing the second ridge. (Fig. 11.66)

Third ridge. If an additional ridge is required, the movements are the same as for the first ridge.

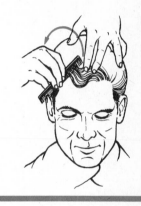

11.63 – Hair is combed in a semi-circular effect to form first wave.

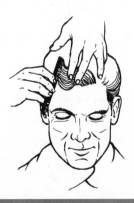

11.64 – Completing the first ridge at the crown

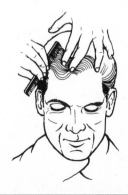

11.65 – Beginning of the second ridge

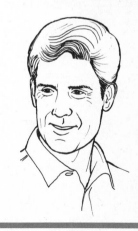

11.66 – First and second ridges completed

Completing the Finger Wave

1. Place a net over the hair, and if a pedestal dryer is used, safeguard the client's forehead and ears with cotton gauze or paper protectors.
2. Adjust the dryer to medium heat and allow the hair to dry thoroughly; otherwise the wave will comb out.
3. After the client's hair is completely dried, remove the hair net. Remove clips and pins from the hair.
4. Comb the hair into natural waves.

Shadow Waving

Shadow waving is recommended for the sides, and sometimes the back, of the head. The wave is made in exactly the same manner as in finger waving, except that the ridges are kept low.

Reminders and Hints on Finger Waving

1. Avoid the use of an excessive amount of styling lotion.
2. Before finger waving, locate the natural wave in the hair.
3. To emphasize the ridges of a finger wave, press and close the fingers, holding the ridge against the head.
4. To create a longer-lasting finger wave, mold the waves in the direction of the natural hair growth.
5. Before combing it out, the hair should be thoroughly dried.
6. A styling hair net is placed over the hair to protect the setting while the hair is being dried.
7. To hold the finger wave in place longer, lightly apply a hair spray.
8. Lightened or tinted hair that tangles or snarls is easier to comb if a cream rinse is used.

SAFETY PRECAUTIONS AND REMINDERS

1. Move moderately hot air back and forth on the hair and away from the scalp. Avoid holding the dryer in one place for too long.
2. To avoid scalp burns, keep the teeth of a heated metal comb away from the scalp.
3. Depending on the barber-stylist's preference, use either hard rubber or metal combs.

4. Keep implements clean and sanitized.

5. Clean up the work area. Put everything back in its proper place.

6. For best results, the hair should be from two to three inches in length.

7. Shampoo the hair and leave it slightly damp.

8. If desired, apply a styling gel, lotion, or very warm water before, and sometimes during, the waving.

9. The hair must be thoroughly cooled before it is combed out. This may be accomplished by switching the dryer to cold and cooling the hair that has been dried.

10. Make sure that the blow-dryer is perfectly clean and free of dirt, grease, and hair, before using.

11. The air intake at the back of the dryer must be kept clear at all times.

REVIEW QUESTIONS

Air-Waving

1. What is air-waving?
2. By what other names is air-waving known?
3. List the equipment and implements used in air-waving.
4. Name two kinds of electrical styling dryers.
5. How does the barber-stylist control the air temperature of the styling dryer?
6. What three steps usually precede air-waving?
7. When towel drying the hair, in what condition is it to be left for air-waving?
8. In air-wave styling, what is generally used to make the hair more manageable?
9. In air-waving, what is used to control unruly hair?
10. In creating a ridge, to what area is the hot air directed?
11. In creating a ridge and wave that require more than one section, what should be their final appearance?
12. How is fullness created at the sides of the head?
13. When and why is hair spray used in air-waving?
14. For what type of hair is a conditioner recommended?
15. How is a styling dryer blowing hot air used?
16. When using a metal comb, why must it be kept away from the scalp?

Curling Iron Techniques

1. What is thermal waving and curling?
2. What are the two parts of the styling portion of the irons?
3. What degree of heat should be used on lightened, fine, or badly damaged hair?

4. How are the irons tested for desirable temperature?
5. In what position should the irons be held?
6. What type of combs must be used in iron curling?
7. What are volume iron curls used for?

Finger Waving Men's Hair

1. Define finger waving.
2. How is the client's clothing protected?
3. How should the hair be protected while being dried?
4. What type of hair is the easiest to finger wave?
5. Give two main points in judging a good finger-waved hairstyle.
6. Why are styling or waving lotions not harmful to the hair?
7. Prior to drying the hair, why are cotton, gauze, or paper protectors placed over the client's ears and forehead?

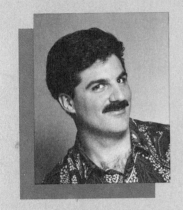

12

Mustache and Beard Design

Learning Objectives

After completing this chapter, you should be able to:

1. *Identify mustache and beard designs.*
2. *Design a mustache and beard for different facial features.*
3. *Determine the correct implements to use for certain mustache and beard designs.*
4. *Demonstrate a beard trim with shears, comb, and trimmer.*
5. *Demonstrate a beard trim with clippers, comb, and trimmer.*

Courtesy of: Hair: Sara Aiello. Photo: Jack Cutler. Grooming: Cheryl Esposito.

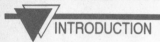

INTRODUCTION

In addition to cutting and styling hair, the barber-stylist should be able to offer clients a full range of services for grooming the hair and skin, including mustache and beard designing and trimming. These abilities give the barber-stylist the opportunity to exercise creativity and increase earnings. The client that wears a mustache and/or beard will frequent a shop that can provide complete service.

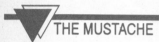

THE MUSTACHE

Mustaches have been worn by men of every social class throughout the world since prehistoric times. The mustache is worn primarily for personal adornment rather than utility, and the wearer usually is particular about how it is designed and maintained.

Care and artistry are required for this service, as well as sensitivity to the individual client's preference.

In addition to knowing how to trim and shape mustaches, the barber-stylist should be able to understand and apply the principles involved in mustache design. The following are some of the items that must be considered.

Suitable Mustache Designs

The client's facial features, hair growth, and personal taste must all be considered in designing a mustache. As in any hairstyling service, facial features are of primary importance in the selection process. The size of the mustache should correspond to the size of the features—a large design for heavy features, and a smaller design for fine, small, smooth facial features.

1. Large, coarse facial features—heavy mustache
2. Prominent nose—medium to large mustache
3. Long, narrow face—narrow to medium mustache
4. Extra-large mouth—pyramid-shaped mustache
5. Extra-small mouth—medium, short mustache
6. Smallish, regular features—small, triangular mustache
7. Wide mouth with prominent upper lip—heavy handlebar or large, divided mustache
8. Round face with regular features—semi-square mustache
9. Square face with prominent features—heavy, linear mustache with ends curving slightly downward
10. Important factors—length of mouth; size of nose; upper lip area; width of cheeks, jaw, and chin; density of hair growth

Procedure for Trimming a Mustache

1. Drape the client as for a haircut service.
2. Consult with the client regarding shape preferences.
3. Thin the mustache with comb and shears. (Fig. 12.1)
4. Trim the mustache to the desired length with shears. Check the length for evenness at the corners of the mouth. (Fig. 12.2)
5. Shape the mustache with a razor or trimmer. (Fig. 12.3)

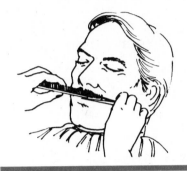 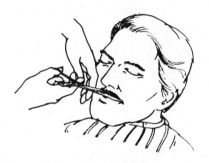 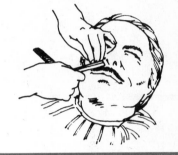

12.1 – Thinning the mustache	**12.2 – Trimming the mustache**	**12.3 – Shaping the mustache**

Additional Mustache Services

1. Waxing mustache ends
2. Penciling temporary color
3. Coloring for overall color evenness or compatibility

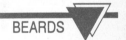

BEARDS

The purpose of a beard or goatee is to balance facial features and to correlate proportions of face, head, and body. Beard trimming usually is performed with scissors, comb, outliner (edger), and razor.

> **NOTE:** The following procedure is one way to perform beard designing and trimming. Other methods may be equally correct.

Beard Designing and Trimming

Preparation

1. Drape the client as for a haircut service.
2. Consult with the client as to the design of the beard. Determine any preferences regarding length, density, and shape.
3. Using a head rest, recline the client either slightly or totally

depending on your preference and the comfort of the client. This will allow the barber-stylist better visibility, dexterity, accessibility, positioning, and posture control.

Scissors, Comb, and Outliner Method

1. Trim excess hair with scissors and comb. (Fig. 12.4)
2. As an option, you may draw the desired beard design with an eyebrow pencil. (Fig. 12.5)
3. Starting in the middle (directly under the chin) outline the under part of the beard, working to the right side of the face up to the sideburn and ear area, then repeat for the left side. (Fig. 12.6)
4. Taper and blend the beard from the outlined areas up to just under the bottom lip, mustache, and cheek areas. (Fig. 12.7)

> **NOTE:** Remember to blend hair color as well as hair length. This is especially important for clients with gray or white hair in their beards. Color variations can make a design appear unbalanced if not blended correctly.

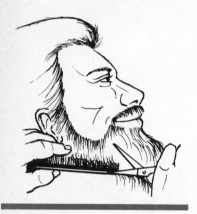

12.4 – Trimming excess hair

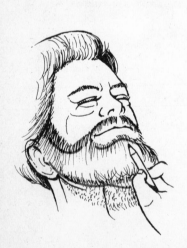

12.5 – Drawing beard design with eyebrow pencil

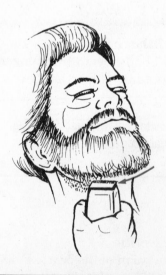

12.6 – Outlining the under part of the beard

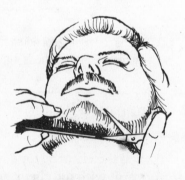

12.7 – Tapering and blending the beard

5. Return the client to a sitting position.
6. Outline the cheek and upper areas of the beard, blending with the sideburn area. (Fig. 12.8)
7. If a razor is used in Step 6, apply and massage lather into the area of the beard to be shaved. Shave the unwanted part of the beard. Remove the lather and penciled beard design. Apply after-shave lotion. (Fig. 12.9)
8. Trim and blend the mustache. (Fig. 12.10)
9. Check and retouch the beard with scissors and comb wherever necessary. Recomb or restyle the hair as needed for a finished look. (Fig. 12.11)

Clippers, Comb, and Outliner Method

Clippers may also be used for beard trimming, especially if one overall length is desired. Clipper cut beard trims are most successful on clients whose beards are of an even density and texture.

Most beard lengths will require the use of a clipper comb attachment. Follow steps 1 through 3 above, then proceed by choosing a comb attachment close to the length of the client's beard. If more than a light trim is required, select the next shortest length comb attachment. Repeat as required until desired beard length is achieved.

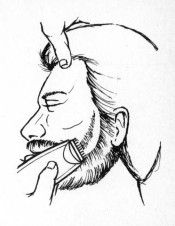

12.8 – Outlining the upper part of the beard

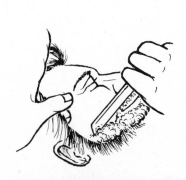

12.9 – Shaving unwanted part of the beard

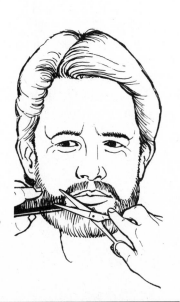

12.10 – Trimming mustache

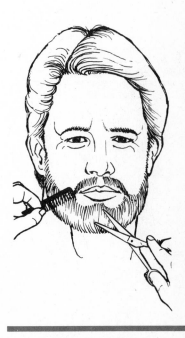

12.11 – Retouch work

NOTE: Many barber-stylists prefer to cut and style the client's hair prior to trimming the beard in order to maintain better precision when balancing the beard with the hairstyle.

CAUTION: Check with your state board regarding the use of razors for shaving cheek and neck areas during a beard trim. Today, many barber-stylists use outliners or edgers to achieve this part of the service.

There is tremendous versatility in the designs of beards. The fact that the beard, in some form or another, has survived from the age of the caveman to the present day is testimony of its acceptance by man as a permanent part of facial grooming.

REVIEW QUESTIONS

Mustaches and Beards

1. What is the primary reason for a man to wear a mustache?
2. How should a mustache be designed?
3. What is the basic consideration in determining the size of the mustache?
4. List five steps for trimming a mustache.
5. What are the primary implements used in beard trimming and designing?
6. List eight steps used in performing a beard trim with scissors, comb, and outliner.
7. What attachment may be necessary to perform clipper cut beard trims?
8. Why do some barber-stylists prefer to cut and style the hair before performing a beard trim service?

13

Permanent Waving

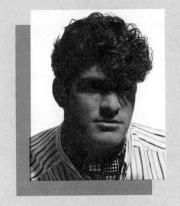

Learning Objectives

After completing this chapter, you should be able to:

1. *Identify the principal actions involved in permanent waving.*
2. *Discuss the chemical actions on the hair during permanent waving.*
3. *Describe the different types of permanent waving solutions.*
4. *Demonstrate a client consultation and hair analysis.*
5. *Demonstrate proper rodding and perming procedures.*
6. *Discuss safety precautions of permanent waving.*

Courtesy of: The Ice Cream Collection. NCA's S/S '92 Fashion Release.
Danny Ewert, Design Team Director. Jim Douglass, photographer.

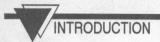

INTRODUCTION

Permanent waving is one of the most practical, versatile, and lucrative services a barber-stylist can offer because it provides clients with alternatives in hairstyling. Properly performed, perms can increase the fullness of fine, soft hair, redirect resistant growth patterns, restructure straight hair into waves or curls, and provide greater styling control. As with other chemical services, permanent waving requires maintenance and periodic re-application. The ability to develop creative perm styles will help to establish a loyal following of satisfied clients, repeat customers, and new referrals.

CHEMISTRY OF PERMANENT WAVING

Perm chemistry is being refined and improved constantly. Perms are available today using many different formulas designed for a wide variety of hair types. Waving lotions and neutralizers for both acid-balanced and alkaline perms are being developed with new conditioners, proteins, and natural ingredients that help to protect and condition the hair during and after perming.

Stop action processing is incorporated in many waving lotions to ensure optimum curl development. The curling takes place within a fixed time, without the risk of overprocessing or damaging the hair. Special pre-wrapping lotions have also been developed to compensate for hair with varying degrees of porosity.

Principal Actions in Permanent Waving

The process of permanent waving involves two principal actions on the hair.

1. Physical Action—the wrapping of hair around rods.
2. Chemical Action
   a) Waving lotion, which softens or breaks the internal structure of the hair.
   b) Neutralizer, which re-hardens or re-bonds the internal structure of the hair.

A clear understanding of the effects of physical and chemical actions during the permanent waving process will assist the barber-stylist in performing this valuable service correctly.

Chemical Actions

As **amino acids** form proteins, chemical reactions produce **peptide linkages.** The peptide linkages are held together by **cross-bonds** which consist of **sulphur** (SULL-fur) (also known as cystine [SISS-teen] or disulfide [die-SULL-fyde]), hydrogen, and salt bonds. When joined together with the peptide linkages, these cross-bonds help to build the **polypeptide** (polly-PEP-tyde) chains.

Hair develops and maintains its natural form by means of the physical (hydrogen or **H-bonds**) and the chemical (sulphur or **S-bonds**) cross-bonds in the cortical layer.

Processing

The physical bonds are the weaker of the two types and are easily broken by the processes of shampooing and rinsing.

The chemical action of the waving solution is required to break the chemical bonds and thus soften and expand the hair. During this process, the cystine is altered slightly to become **cysteine** (sis-TEE-in). Cystine is an amino acid component of many proteins especially keratin. Cysteine is an amino acid obtained by the reduction of cystine and important as a constituent of many proteins. The chemical action permits rearrangement of the inner structure of the hair so that it can assume the form and diameter of the rod. After the hair has assumed the desired shape, it must be neutralized chemically so that the hydrogen and sulphur cross-bonds in the cortical layer are permanently re-formed. Additionally, the cysteine is changed back to the cystine state. The action of oxidation and neutralization hardens the S-bonds of the hair into its newly constructed form. (Fig. 13.1 a-e)

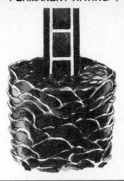

13.1a – Each hair strand is composed of many polypetide chains. This series of illustrations shows the behavior of one such chain.

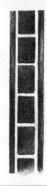

13.1b – Hair before processing—chemical bonds (links) give hair its strength and firmness.

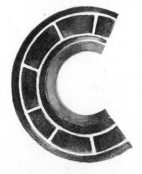

13.1c – Hair wound on rod—the hair bends to the curvature and size of the rod.

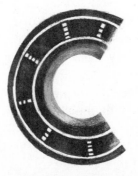

13.1d – During processing, waving lotion breaks the chemical cross-bonds, permitting the hair to adjust to the curvature of the rod while in this softened condition.

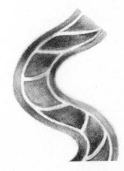

13.1e – The neutralizer re-forms the chemical bonds to conform with the wound position of the hair, and re-hardens the hair, thus creating the permanent wave.

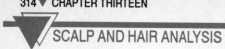

SCALP AND HAIR ANALYSIS

Before giving a permanent wave, it is very important to correctly and carefully analyze the client's scalp and hair condition. Learn all possible facts about the client's hair, including scalp condition, and the porosity, texture, elasticity, density, and length of hair.

Scalp Condition

The scalp should be examined very carefully. Abrasions on the scalp can make permanent waving dangerous to a client. An irritated scalp and badly damaged hair are both signs that a permanent wave should be postponed until the condition has been corrected.

Hair Porosity

Porosity is related very closely to the speed with which hair can accept any fluid. Speed of absorption determines the degree of hair porosity, and can be a measure for determining the required strength of waving solution. Unless pre-permanent analysis is closely observed, damaged hair may result.

The processing time for any permanent wave depends more on hair porosity than on any other factor. The more porous the hair, the less time processing takes, and the milder the waving solution required—regardless of texture. Before giving a permanent wave, determine the degree of porosity. (The various degrees of porosity are discussed in the chapter on hair.)

Porosity test. In order to test accurately for porosity, use three different areas: the front hairline, in front of the ears, and near the crown. Grasp a strand of dry hair. Hold the end firmly with the thumb and index finger of one hand, and slide the fingers of the other hand from the ends toward the scalp. If the fingers do not slide easily, or if the hair ruffles up as your fingers slide down the strand, the hair is porous. The more ruffles formed, the more porous is the hair, and the fewer ruffles formed, the less porous it is. If the fingers slide easily and no ruffles are formed, the cuticle layer lies close to the hair shaft. This type of hair is the least porous, most resistant, and will require a longer processing time. (Fig. 13.2 a-d)

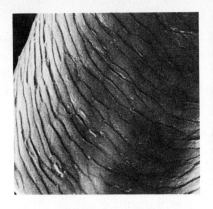

13.2a – Normal—moderate porosity

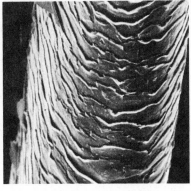

13.2b – Resistant—poor porosity

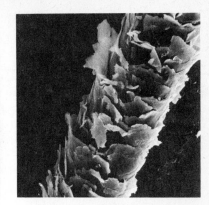

13.2c – Tinted—extreme porosity

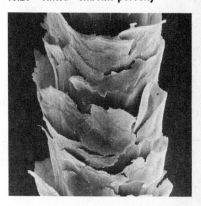

13.2d – Damaged—over-porous hair

Hair Texture

The texture and porosity of the hair are judged together in determining the processing time. Although porosity is the more important of the two, texture must also be considered. However, when coarse hair is very porous, it will process faster than fine hair that is not porous. (Fig. 13.3 a-c)

Hair texture should also be considered in deciding the size of the wave pattern and planning a hairstyle.

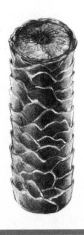

13.3a – Coarse

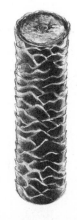

13.3b – Medium

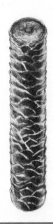

13.3c – Fine

Hair Elasticity

Hair elasticity is a very important factor to consider when giving a permanent wave. Without elasticity, there will be no curl in the hair. The greater the degree of elasticity, the longer the wave will remain in the hair because less relaxation of the hair occurs. Thus, the elastic qualities of hair will determine the success of a permanent wave.

1. Hair with very good elasticity will produce a resilient curl or firm wave.
2. Hair with good elasticity will produce a curl with average resilience.
3. Hair with fairly good elasticity will produce a slightly less resilient curl.
4. Hair with poor elasticity, also known as limp hair, will result in a very small amount of resilience in the curl.

A simple test for elastic qualities of the hair. Take a single dry hair and hold it between the thumb and forefinger of each hand. Slowly stretch it between them. The further it can be stretched without breaking, the more elastic is the hair. If the elasticity is good, the hair slowly contracts after stretching. Hair with poor elasticity will break quickly and easily when stretched.

Signs of poor elasticity include limpness, sponginess, and hair that tangles easily. Generally speaking, such hair will not develop a firm, strong wave. However, there are special waving solutions available that, if used in combination with smaller diameter rods, usually result in a satisfactory permanent wave.

Hair Density

Smaller blockings (sub-sections) and larger rods are often required for thickly growing hair. However, if the hair is thin per square inch, smaller (thinner) rods are required in order to form a good wave pattern close to the head. Avoid large blockings on a thin hair growth, as the strain may cause breakage.

Hair Length

Hair length is another important factor to consider. Waving hair of average length presents no real problem. However, if the client's hair length is six inches or more, a number of waving and wrapping problems may be created. The hair cannot be wrapped closely enough to develop a good, strong wave pattern near the scalp. In addition, the hair weight may pull the wave out of the hair very quickly. Therefore, in selecting a hairstyle it is important to carefully consider hair length, in addition to texture, elasticity, and density.

Choosing the Right Perming Technique

In order to decide which perming technique is right for a client, the hair must be evaluated and analyzed. Consult with the client to establish what the person expects a perm to accomplish—a tight, curly look or a loose, wavy look. This information helps in the selection of the correct perm product and technique.

Basic Manual Perming Skills

Successful perming requires manual dexterity. With practice, your skills in handling and manipulating hair will improve. Before actually applying a perm, you probably will spend considerable time practicing pre-perming skills such as blocking, sectioning, and wrapping.

Client Consultation

Every client has a different concept of how the perm should look. The only way to meet a client's expectations is to determine what they are. Talk to the client in a friendly but professional way. Take a few minutes to discuss:

1. The desired hairstyle and amount of curl. Photos or magazine pictures help to make this clear to both the client and the barber-stylist.
2. The client's lifestyle. Do they have leisure time, or a demanding schedule that requires a low-maintenance style?
3. How the hairstyle relates to overall personal image. Is the client concerned about current fashion trends?
4. Previous experience. Was the last perm satisfactory? If not, what were the problems?

The consultation with the client takes only a few minutes, but it is time well spent. It helps to establish your credibility as a professional, inspires the client's confidence, and makes the entire perming experience more satisfactory for both client and stylist.

Keep the information learned during the consultation as a written record, along with other important data, including the client's address and home and business phone numbers. An example of an organized format for maintaining client records is shown on page 318.

Release Statement

A release statement is used for any type of chemical treatment. It helps to protect the shop owner legally, in case of accidents or damages.

PERMANENT WAVE RECORD

Name _____ Tel._____

Address _____City _____

DESCRIPTION OF HAIR

Texture		Form	Length	Porosity	
coarse	soft	straight	short	very porous	less porous
medium	silky	wavy	medium	moderately porous	least porous
fine	wiry	curly	long	normal	resistant

Condition:
☐ virgin ☐ rewave ☐ dry ☐ oily ☐ very good ☐ good ☐ fair ☐ poor

If tinted or lightened, use: ☐ double end wrap ☐ water ☐ protein filler

previously waved with _____ system

TYPE OF PERMANENT WAVE

☐ alkaline ☐ acid ☐ body wave ☐ other _____ lotion _____ strength _____

Rod sizes: Top_____ sides_____ crown_____ nape_____

Results: ☐ good ☐ poor ☐ too tight ☐ too loose

Date	Stylist	Price		Date	Stylist	Price

RELEASE FORM

Client's Name _____ Address _____

Condition of Hair _____

Permanent Wave: Kind _____Given by _____

I fully understand that the permanent wave treatment which I have requested and am about to receive is ordinarily harmless to normal hair, but may damage my hair because of its present condition.
In view of this, I accept full responsibility for any possible damage that may result, directly or indirectly, to my hair.

Signature of Client _____

Witnessed By _____Date_____

Proper selection of perm rods is essential for successful permanent waving. The size of the rods controls the shape of the hair during the waving process.

Rods are made of plastic and vary in diameter, length, and design. They are available in various lengths: long, medium, and short ($3 \frac{1}{2}$ to $1 \frac{3}{4}$ inches in length). They also come in a variety of thicknesses, ranging from large to very thin—three quarters to one-eighth of an inch.

All rods must have some means of securing the hair and the rod into the desired position to prevent the curl from unwinding. (Fig. 13.4)

Types of Rods

There are two types of rods in general use: straight and concave.

The circumference and diameter of straight rods are the same for the rod's entire length. This type of rod creates a consistently sized wave.

Large, straight rods are usually used for a **body wave**. They permit the formation of a strong wave that is large enough to be dressed into any desired hairstyle. The body wave usually serves as a foundation for further styling.

Concave rods have a small diameter in the center, which gradually increases to a larger diameter at both ends. Concave rods are used when a definite wave pattern, close to the head, is desired.

When hair is wound on a concave rod, the outside hair of the winding forms a larger wave than the hair next to the rod. This creates a tighter wave at the hair ends, which gradually becomes slightly wider as it nears the scalp.

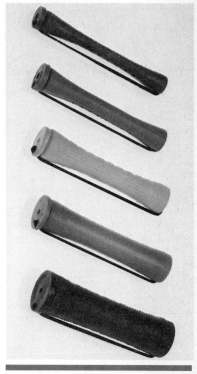

13.4 – Sizes of rods—top to bottom: extra small, small, medium, large, extra large

For success in permanent waving, it is absolutely essential that the proper waving lotion be selected. The chemical compounds in the waving lotion greatly influence the procedure to be followed in the waving process.

Pre-conditioning. Over-porous or damaged hair may require a pre-conditioning treatment before the application of waving lotion. Special fillers are now available that contain protein which conditions the hair and equalizes its porosity. Some fillers also contain lanolin and cholesterol, which may help to protect the hair against the harshness of the waving solution.

Conditioners. Alkaline permanent waving solutions tend to remove natural oils from the hair, causing it to dry out rapidly. Mineral oils, lanolin, or lanolin derivatives are added to the waving lotion, or may be used separately, to replace natural oils. The moisture content is preserved somewhat, and the feel and appearance of the hair improved, by permitting the conditioner to remain in the hair after the solution has been rinsed out.

Strengths of waving solutions. The strength of the waving solution can be adjusted either by increasing its pH or by increasing the amount of active ingredient, **ammonium thioglycolate** (a-**MOHN**-ee-um theye-oh-**GLEYE**-coh-layt). To adjust the pH of the solution, the ammonia content is either increased or decreased. However, it should not be increased to exceed pH 9.6, which is a strong solution.

Most manufacturers of permanent waving products market three or more strengths:

1. Weak or mild—for damaged, porous, or tinted hair
2. Average—for normal hair (having good porosity)
3. Stronger—for resistant hair (less porosity)

> **NOTE:** Manufacturers of permanent waving products are constantly improving their formulas. It is advisable to follow their directions explicitly.

Alkaline Perms

The main active ingredient or **reducing agent** in alkaline perms, ammonium thioglycolate, is a chemical compound made up of ammonia and thioglycolic acid. The pH of alkaline waving lotions generally falls within the range of 8.2 to 9.6, depending on the amount of ammonia. Because the lotion is more alkaline, the cuticle layers swell slightly and open, allowing the solution to penetrate more quickly than do acid-balanced lotions. Some alkaline perms are wrapped with waving lotion, others with water. Some require a plastic cap for processing, others do not. Therefore, it is extremely important to read the perm directions carefully before beginning.

The benefits of alkaline perms are:

- Strong curl patterns (perms that are lotion-wrapped usually produce stronger curls than water-wrapped perms).
- Fast processing time (varies from 5 to 20 minutes).
- Room temperature processing.

Generally, alkaline perms should be used when:

- Perming resistant hair.
- A strong/tight curl is desired.
- The client has a history of early curl relaxation.

Acid-Balanced Perms

The main active ingredient in acid-balanced waving lotions is **glyceryl monothioglycolate** (**GLIS**-ur-il mon-oh-theye-oh-**GLEYE**-cohlayt), which effectively reduces the pH. This lower pH is gentler on the hair and typically gives a softer curl than alkaline cold waves. Acid-balanced perms have a pH range of approximately 4.5 to 7.9 and usually penetrate the hair more slowly. Thus, they require a longer processing time and heat for curl development. Heat is used in one of two ways:

1. The perm is activated by heat created chemically with the product. This method is called **exothermic** (eck-so-**THUR**-mick).
2. The perm is activated by an outside heat source, usually a conventional hood-type hair dryer. This method is called **endothermic** (en-do-**THUR**-mick).

Recent advances in acid-balanced perm chemistry, however, have made it possible to process some acid-balanced perms at room temperature, without heat. These newer acid-balanced perms usually have a slightly higher pH, but still contain glyceryl monothioglycolate as the active ingredient.

All acid-balanced perms are water-wrapped, require a plastic cap, and may or may not require a pre-heated hood dryer for processing. Read the manufacturer's directions carefully before starting the perm.

The benefits of acid-balanced perms are:

- Softer curl patterns
- Slower, but more controllable processing time (usually 15 to 25 minutes)
- Gentler treatment for delicate hair types

Generally, acid-balanced perms should be used when:

- Perming delicate/fragile or color-treated hair.
- Soft, natural curl or wave pattern is desired.
- Style support, rather than strong curl, is required.

Neutralizers

Neutralizers for both acid-balanced and alkaline perms have the same important function: to establish permanently the new curl shape. Neutralizing is a very important step in the perming process. If the hair is not properly neutralized, the curl will relax or straighten within one to two shampooings. Generally, today's neutralizers are composed of a relatively small percentage of hydrogen peroxide, an oxidizing agent, at an acidic pH. As with waving lotions, there are slightly different procedures recommended for individual products. To achieve the best possible results, read the directions carefully.

Perm Selection

The type of perm chosen depends on the total hair evaluation and the client's wishes. The following is a general guide for choosing an alkaline or an acid-balanced perm.

Hair type	Perm Type
Coarse, resistant	Alkaline lotion wrap or alkaline water wrap
Fine, resistant	Alkaline lotion wrap or alkaline water wrap
Normal	Alkaline water wrap or acid-balanced
Normal, porous	Alkaline water wrap or acid-balanced
Normal, delicate	Acid-balanced
Tinted, non-porous	Alkaline water wrap or acid-balanced
Tinted, porous	Acid-balanced
Highlighted/frosted/ dimensionally colored	Acid-balanced
Highlighted, tinted	Acid-balanced
Bleached	Acid-balanced

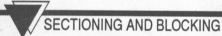

SECTIONING AND BLOCKING

Sectioning is dividing the head into uniform working panels.

Blocking (sub-sectioning) is the subdividing of panels into uniform, individual, rectangular rod sections. Uniform wave patterns depend on the following:

1. Uniformly arranged sections
2. Equally subdivided sections (blockings)
3. Clean and uniform partings (length and width)

In addition to the density and texture of the hair, the size of the blockings is determined by the diameter of the rods.

Depending on the pattern used in hair sectioning, the number of hair blockings may vary with each client. The average blocking for a standard wave generally should match the diameter of the rod being used. The length of the blocking can be a little shorter, but never longer than the length of the rod. If the rod is shorter than the length of the blocking, the hair will tend to slip off the ends of the rod during winding. (Figs. 13.5–13.7)

The size of the rods and blockings determines the size of the wave formation. Processing time has no bearing on the size of the wave pattern. Thicker hair with good elasticity gives a deeper wave formation. Thinner hair, usually fine in texture, gives a more shallow wave. The loss or increase of elasticity also affects the depth of the wave pattern.

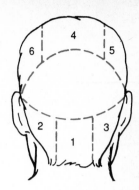

13.5 – Sectioning

Suggested Blockings and Rod Sizes

Although hair elasticity and texture both must be considered in the choice of rods, the texture should be the determining factor.

Coarse hair—good elasticity. Thickly growing hair requires smaller (narrower) blockings and larger rods, to permit better arrangement for a definite wave pattern.

Medium hair—average elasticity. Medium or average-textured hair requires smaller blockings and medium size rods.

Fine hair—poor elasticity. Thin hair requires smaller blockings and smaller (thinner) rods to prevent strain or breakage, and to form a good wave pattern close to the head.

Damaged hair—very poor elasticity. Use smaller hair sections and larger rods. If the damaged hair is fine in texture, use smaller hair blockings and medium rods.

Hair in nape area. Use smaller blockings and smaller rods.

Long hair. To permanently wave hair longer than six inches, wrap it smoothly and close to the scalp in smaller blockings, which permit the waving solution and neutralizer to penetrate more thoroughly.

The texture, elasticity, porosity, and condition of the client's hair all determine how the hair should be sectioned, blocked, which rods to use, and where the application of waving solution should begin. (Be guided by your instructor.)

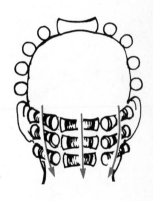

13.6 – Blocking (sub-sections)

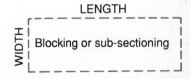

13.7 – Length denotes span of blocking. Width refers to the depth of the blocking. Small or large blockings usually refer to their width.

> **NOTE:** The size of the rods and blockings determines the size of the curl or wave pattern. Processing time has no bearing on the size of the wave pattern.

▼ WINDING OR WRAPPING THE HAIR

To form a uniform wave with a strong ridge, hair must be wrapped smoothly and neatly on each rod, without stretching. Hair is not stretched because the penetration of waving solutions causes the hair to expand. Tight wrapping or stretching interferes with this expansion and prevents penetration of the waving solution and neutralizer, which may cause hair breakage.

End Papers

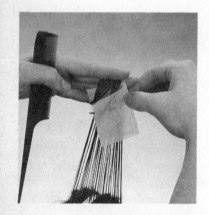

Porous end papers are very important aids in the proper wrapping or winding of the hair around curling rods. Properly used, end papers help in the formation of smooth and even waves. They also help to eliminate the possibility of **fish hooks** (flaws in the curling of hair which result in the tip of the hair bending in a direction opposite to that of the rest of the curl) and minimize the danger of broken hair ends. They are especially important in helping to smooth out the wrapping of uneven hair lengths.

There are three common methods of end paper application. Each method may be equally effective, if properly used.

1. The book end paper wrap (Fig. 13.8)
2. The single end paper wrap (Fig. 13.9)
3. The double end paper wrap (Figs. 13.10, 13.11)

13.8 – Book end wrap

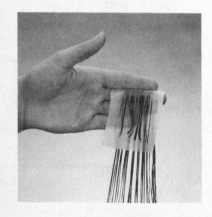

13.9 – Single end wrap

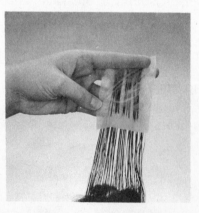

13.10 – Double end wrap

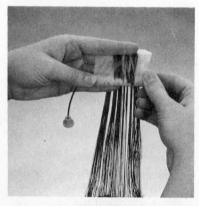

13.11 – Double end wrap rod position

Procedure

The step-by-step procedure for the book end paper wrap is illustrated by placing end papers, wrapping, and fastening curls as indicated. (Figs. 13.12–13.18)

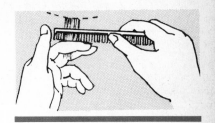

13.12 – Part and comb subsection up and out until all hair is evenly directed and distributed.

> **NOTE:** The blocking should not be longer than the rod. If it is, the hair will not wave evenly.

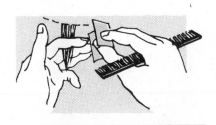

13.13 – Hold strand between the index and middle fingers. Fold and place the end paper over the strand, forming an envelope.

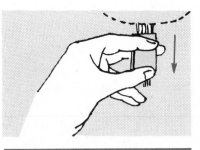

13.14 – Hold the strand smoothly and evenly. Slide the paper envelope a small fraction beyond the hair ends.

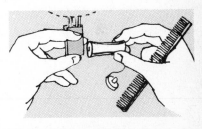

13.15 – With the right hand, pick up the rod.

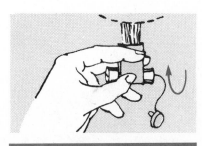

13.16 – Place the rod under the folded end paper, parallel with the partings. Draw end paper and rod toward hair ends until they are visible above the rod, and start winding end paper and hair under, toward the scalp.

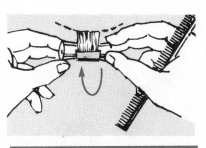

13.17 – Wind the hair smoothly, without tension, on the rod.

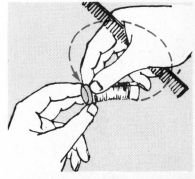

13.18 – Fasten the rod band evenly across the wound hair at the top of the rod.

CAUTION: When wrapping hair, always avoid bulkiness on the rod, which prevents the formation of a good curl since the hair cannot conform to the shape of the rod. The band should not cut into the hair or be twisted against the curl, to prevent breakage.

The preparation of the hair to receive the end wrap is the same for single, double, and book end wrapping techniques. (Figs. 13.19–13.24)

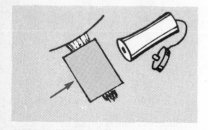

13.19 – Place the end paper on top of strand and hold it flat to prevent bunching.

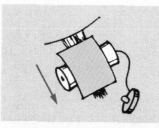

13.20 – Place rod under the strand, holding it parallel with the parting; then draw the end paper and rod downward until hair ends are covered.

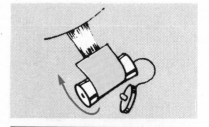

13.21 – Roll the end paper and strand under, using the thumb of each hand to keep the strand smooth. Wind strand on the rod to the scalp without tension. Fasten band at top of rod in the same manner as for book end paper wrap.

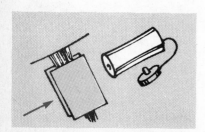

13.22 – Place one end paper beneath the hair strand and the other on top.

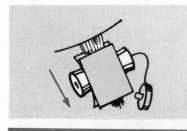

13.23 – Place rod under double end papers, parallel with hair part. Draw both toward hair ends.

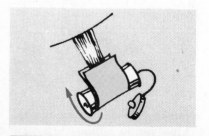

13.24 – Wind the strand smoothly on the rod to the scalp without tension. Then fasten band at top of rod as for book end paper wrap.

Placement of Curl in Blocking

Regardless of the type or size of rod used, it should be placed slightly off its base in order to give a close-to-the-head permanent, and to leave the hair easy to handle. Placing the rod slightly off its base helps to prevent the creation of excessive tension and hair breakage. (Fig. 13.25)

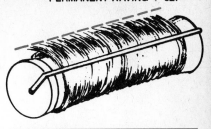

13.25 – Curl placed slightly off base

PRE-PERMANENT WAVE SHAMPOO

To help assure success, the hair should be shampooed prior to permanent waving. Even, longer-lasting waves can only be achieved with clean hair. In addition, clean hair allows the proper and even penetration of the waving solution and the neutralizer essential to successful permanent waving. If the solution penetrates the hair evenly, the curls and waves will be more uniform and manageable. Uneven or spottily curled hair is quite difficult to control.

Test Curls

Test curls help to determine how the client's hair will react to the permanent waving process. A test curl provides information on how to protect the client's hair and how to obtain the best possible results. They enable the barber-stylist to observe the following aspects of the hair:

1. Speed of wave formation
2. Overall picture of wave formation
3. Exact time when peak of wave formation is reached
4. Resistant areas

Procedure

1. Shampoo the hair and towel it dry.
2. Following the perm directions, wrap two or three rods in the most delicate areas of the hair.
3. Wrap a coil of cotton around the rod.
4. Apply waving lotion to the wrapped curls, being very careful not to allow the waving lotion to come in contact with unwrapped hair.
5. Set a timer and process the hair according to the perm directions.
6. Check the hair frequently.

To check a test curl, unfasten a rod and carefully (remember—hair is in a softened state) unwind the curl about one and one-half turns of the rod. Do not permit the hair to become loose or completely unwound. Hold the hair firmly by placing a thumb at each end of the rod. Move the rod gently toward the scalp so that the hair falls loosely into the wave pattern. Continue checking the rods until a firm and definite S is formed. The S reflects the size of the rod used. Be guided by the manufacturer's directions.

> **NOTE:** When judging test curls, different hair textures with varying degrees of elasticity will have slightly different S formations. Fine, thin hair is generally softer and has less bulk. The wave ridge might be less defined and more difficult to read. Coarse, thick hair has better elasticity and seems to reinforce itself, falling into the wave pattern more readily. The wave ridge will be stronger and better defined. Long hair may produce a wider scalp wave than short hair, because larger rods are used and the diameter of the wave widens toward the scalp.

When the optimum curl has been formed, rinse the curls with warm water; blot the curls thoroughly; apply, process, and rinse the neutralizer according to the perm directions; and gently dry these test curls. Evaluate the curl results. If the hair is over-processed, do not perm the rest of the hair until it is in better condition. If the test curl results are good, proceed with the perm, but do not re-perm these preliminary test curls.

> **NOTE:** Test curls also refer to checking for the S pattern during the permanent waving process.

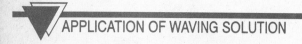

APPLICATION OF WAVING SOLUTION

Safety Measures

Always wear protective gloves. For the client's safety, apply protective cream or petroleum jelly around the hairline and neck, and cover the areas with strips of cotton. If the cotton strips become wet with solution, remove them, blot the areas with cool water, and replace the cotton with dry material. If the solution drips on the skin or scalp, absorb it with cotton pledgets saturated with cold water, followed by neutralizer. If the lotion is applied correctly there should be a minimum of dripping.

Protect client's eyes. If the waving solution gets into the client's eye, rinse immediately with cold water. Make sure the client obtains immediate medical attention.

Unless otherwise specified in the product instructions, apply waving solution liberally to the top and underside of each wound rod.

NOTE: Fine, thin hair may not require an application to the underside of the wound rod.

Start at the crown and progress systematically down each section. (Some stylists prefer to start at the top of head.) Be sure that the surface area of the wound hair is wet with lotion so penetration is even.

CAUTION: Be careful not to disturb the wrapping by dragging the nozzle over the curls. Do not leave the client alone while processing the hair. Do not interrupt the re-wet or saturation step. Complete it as quickly as possible.

Processing Time

The ability of the hair to absorb moisture may vary from time to time on the same individual, even while using the same solutions and procedures. Therefore, processing time may vary from one permanent wave to the next. A record of previous processing time is desirable to use as a guide. It is usually safe to anticipate the processing time to be less than that suggested by the manufacturer or a client's previous record card.

Factors affecting processing time include the strength of the solution; texture, porosity, length, and condition of the hair; atmospheric conditions; client's body heat; and the working speed of the stylist.

Re-saturation step during the processing time. Often, it is necessary to re-wet all the rods during the processing. This may be due to:

1. Evaporation of the solution or dryness of the hair.
2. Hair that has been saturated poorly.
3. Improper selection of the solution strength.
4. Failure to follow manufacturer's directions.

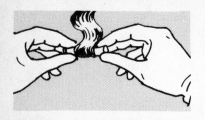

13.26 – Unwinding hair without pulling or stretching. Processed strand opens up into an *S* formation.

Reapplying the solution will hasten processing. Watch the wave development closely, since negligence may result in hair damage.

Wave Pattern Formation

As the hair is processing, the waves form a deep-ridged pattern. The wave has reached its peak when it forms a firm letter S. (Fig. 13.26)

The S pattern reaches a desirable peak only once. Shortly after the S is well formed, the hair may become frizzy unless processing is stopped. Frizziness indicates that the processing time has reached its absolute maximum. Beyond this point, the hair becomes over-processed and damaged.

Different conditions and hair textures will cause the quality of wave patterns to vary. Hair of good texture will show a firm, strong pattern, whereas hair that is weak or fine will not produce a firm pattern. (Fig. 13.27 a–e)

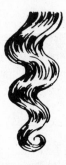

13.27a – A good permanent wave looks like this.

13.27b – Under-processed curl; result—little or no wave

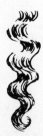

13.27c – Over-processed curl; result—narrow waves when wet, no waves when dry

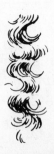

13.27d – Porous ends over-processed; result—frizzy ends

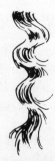

13.27e – Improper winding when hair ends are wound too tight; result—no wave or curl at hair ends

Over-Processing

Any solution that can process the hair properly can also over-process it. Solution left on the hair too long results in over-processing. Another cause of over-processing is that test curls were judged improperly. If neutralizer is used too sparingly the hair may continue to process, also causing over-processing.

Over-processed hair is easily detected. It is very curly when wet, completely frizzy when dry, and refuses to be combed into a suitable wave pattern. The elasticity of the hair has been damaged and the hair is unable to contract into the wave formation. The hair feels harsh after being dried. Reconditioning treatments should begin immediately.

Under-Processing

Under-processing results in a limp or weak wave formation. The ridges are not well defined and the hair retains little or no wave formation. Under-processing may be corrected by giving one or two reconditioning treatments. After these treatments, re-wrap the hair and apply a milder waving lotion, since the hair has already received some softening. Watch the wave formation closely.

NEUTRALIZATION OF THE HAIR

The waving solution produces the wave formation by rearranging the chemical bonds (links) in the cortex of the hair shaft. The rods hold the hair in this formation until it is re-hardened, or fixed, by neutralization. The neutralizer stops the action of the waving solution, re-forms the chemical bonds, and re-hardens the hair in its new curled position.

Rinsing and Preparation for Neutralization

Before applying the neutralizer, the waving solution must be thoroughly rinsed with warm water, followed by careful towel-blotting of each curl to remove excess moisture. To obtain the best results from towel-blotting, carefully press the towel with the fingers between each curl. (Fig. 13.28)

CAUTION: Do not rock or roll the rods while blotting. The hair is in a softened state and such movement may cause hair breakage.

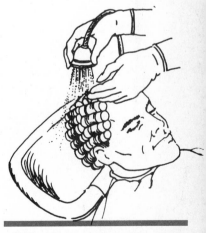

13.28 – Rinsing waving solution from hair

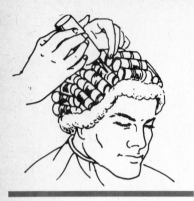

13.29 – Applying neutralizer with squeeze-applicator bottle

Methods of Neutralization

Neutralizers are packaged in the form of powders, liquids, or crystals and must be prepared immediately before their use, as directed by manufacturer.

There are two methods of neutralizer application in general use: the **direct** or **on-the-rod method** and the **conventional** or **splash-on method**.

Direct or on-the-rod method is also referred to as the **applicator** or **instant method**. Neutralizer comes in two forms: ready-for-use or to be mixed.

1. **Ready-for-use neutralizer:** snip off the tip of squeeze-applicator bottle, and apply. (Fig. 13.29)
2. **Neutralizer to be prepared:** mix it according to manufacturer's directions, pour it into the squeeze-applicator bottle, and apply.

Procedure. Apply the neutralizer directly to each curl in the same order as that followed in the application of the waving lotion. Start in the top center of the curl and apply it in either direction. Then apply it at the bottom of the curl, making sure that each curl is thoroughly saturated. Repeat if necessary.

> **NOTE:** A cotton pad saturated with neutralizer may be placed at the nape of the neck on the rim of the shampoo bowl, to assure that the neckline curls are in constant contact with the neutralizer.

Conventional or Splash-On Method. Mix the neutralizer with water, following the manufacturer's directions. Position the client at the shampoo bowl in the same manner as for a shampoo.

Procedure. Using a glass or plastic measuring cup, pour one-half of the neutralizer carefully over the curls, thoroughly saturating each curl. The neutralizer is caught in a plastic basin or pocket in the neutralizing bib attached to the client's neck.

Using large pads of cotton or sponge, reapply the neutralizer, thoroughly saturating each curl. Repeat two or three times.

> **NOTE:** The conventional method is rarely used today.

Removing Neutralizer

There are two methods for removing neutralizer from the hair, regardless of the method used to apply it.

Method 1. After the neutralizer is thoroughly applied, allow it to remain in the hair for five to eight minutes. Rinse the hair with tepid water and follow with a cool water rinse to re-harden the hair. Lightly towel-blot the hair. Remove the rods carefully and proceed to set and/or style the hair.

Method 2. After the neutralizer is thoroughly applied, allow it to set for five to eight minutes. Carefully remove the rods without stretching the hair and apply the balance of the neutralizer to the hair. Permit an additional minute of neutralizing time and then rinse with cool water. Proceed with setting and/or styling the hair.

CAUTION: Unless the hair is thoroughly and correctly neutralized, the permanent wave will not be successful and all the work done will be wasted. In addition, all the hair may be damaged.

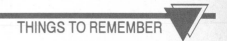

THINGS TO REMEMBER

Preparation

1. Select and arrange required materials.
2. Wash and sanitize the hands.
3. Seat the client comfortably at the shampoo bowl.
4. Adjust the towels and shampoo cape.
5. Carefully examine the condition of scalp and hair.

Drape Client

There are several ways in which a client may be draped for a permanent wave. Comfort and adequate protection are important during the entire procedure. One draping method is to place a small, folded towel around the neck, fasten the shampoo cape over it, and then place another towel over the cape. Fasten the towel securely.

Procedure

1. If hair is long, cut it before or after the shampoo. If hair is short, cut it after the permanent, if required.
2. Shampoo and thoroughly rinse the hair. Towel-dry and

moisten it with waving solution as recommended by the manufacturer.

3. Section and block (sub-section) the hair. Start wrapping in the nape area, or be guided by your instructor.

4. Apply protective cream and cotton strips around the client's hairline. The barber-stylist must wear gloves.

5. Apply the permanent waving solution as recommended by the manufacturer.

6. Test curl-wave formation immediately after saturating the hair with waving solution. Take frequent test curls on different areas of the head.

7. Process the hair for the required time. If re-wetting the curls is necessary, apply the solution in the same order followed originally. Protect the client with fresh protective cotton strips around the hairline and neck.

8. When the curls have processed sufficiently, rinse out the waving solution thoroughly. Use gentle water pressure and a tepid water temperature, unless the manufacturer's directions state otherwise.

9. Blot excess moisture from the hair wound on rods. Do not rock or roll the rods while blotting. The hair being in a softened state, any such movement may cause hair breakage.

10. Thoroughly apply neutralizer.

11. Unwind the rods and remove them carefully.

12. Apply the neutralizer again, if required.

13. Rinse the hair again, if required.

14. Towel-dry and set and/or style hair.

Important Reminders

A neutral or cream rinse, or hair cream, may be applied to protect the permanent and to facilitate the styling. If the manufacturer has included a special rinse with the product, its use will prevent excessive stretching while combing and will counteract any alkaline residue. Styling gel, if used, should be of a light consistency. Avoid excess tension in styling the hair.

Partial Perming

Perming only a section of a whole head of hair is called **partial perming**. Partial perming can be used on:

1. Clients who have long hair on the top and crown and very short, tapered sides and nape.
2. Clients who need volume and lift only in certain areas.
3. Designs that require curl support in the nape area but a smooth, sleek surface.
4. Previous perm has grown (and been trimmed off) sufficiently to re-perm top only. (Extends the life of original perm.)

Partial perming uses the same techniques and wrapping patterns already described. There are a few extra considerations, however.

1. When wrapping the hair, the area that will be left un-permed should be rolled on the next larger rod size so that the curl pattern of the permed hair will blend into the un-permed hair.
2. After wrapping the area to be permed, place a coil of cotton around the wrapped rods as well as around the entire hair-line.
3. Before applying the waving lotion, apply a heavy, creamy conditioner to the sections that will not be permed to protect this hair from the effects of the waving lotion (waving lotion softens and straightens unwrapped hair).

Many clients need the added texture and fullness that only a perm can give. A perm can also help overcome common hair problems. It can redirect a cowlick, help limp or unmanageable hair more easily maintain a style, and make sparse hair look fuller. (Figs. 13.30–13.32)

Perming techniques are basically the same for both men and women.

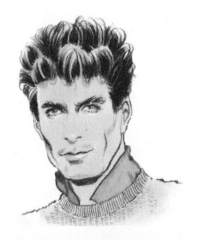

13.30 – Short curly style

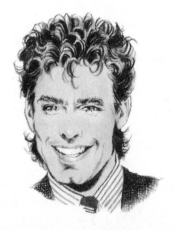

13.31 – Medium length style

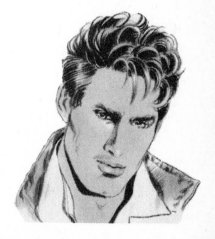

13.32 – Short wavy style

Reconditioning Treatments

Dry, brittle, damaged, or over-porous hair should be given reconditioning treatments. However, avoid any treatment requiring massage or heat just prior to a permanent wave. Such treatment could create a sensitive scalp.

Special Permanent Wave Fillers

Over-porous or damaged hair must be pre-conditioned before the application of waving solution. Special fillers that contain protein are now available that recondition the hair and equalize its porosity. Some fillers also contain lanolin and cholesterol, which may help to protect the hair against the harshness of the permanent waving solution.

After Care

Reconditioning treatments have a place in the after care of a permanent wave, and between permanent waves. The after care helps to keep the hair in the best possible condition. It includes regular hair care.

1. Shampoo the hair as needed with mild shampoo and rinse.
2. Use an appropriate hair conditioner as directed by the manufacturer.
3. Comb and brush the hair daily. Use the type of brush best suited to the hair. Avoid excessive brushing or combing in the opposite direction.
4. Suggest that the client have the hair trimmed and styled at regular intervals in order to make the hairstyle more serviceable.

To Tint or Wave

If a client requests both a permanent wave and a hair tint on the same day, advise against it for the following reasons.

1. If the tint is given first, the application of waving solution will lighten the hair and often cause an uneven color.

2. If the permanent wave is given first, the application of a tint will distort and weaken the wave pattern.
3. The combination of two chemical treatments on the same day may cause scalp irritation, hair breakage, and/or uneven color.

First give the permanent wave and postpone the tint treatment for at least a week to avoid distorting the wave pattern. Suggest a reconditioning treatment before the tint application.

Do not give a color rinse immediately after a permanent wave. It is also likely to disturb the wave pattern. If required, use a color rinse having a weak strength.

If the hair is to be lightened after the permanent wave, it should be reconditioned and the lightening treatment given at a later date.

NOTE: There is no exact rule of whether to perm or tint first. Each client's hair must be evaluated and then a determination made. However, porosity is probably the most important deciding factor.

Waving Tinted or Lightened Hair

Special precautions are recommended when waving tinted or lightened hair.

1. Shampoo the hair with a mild shampoo before waving.
2. Wrap the hair with a special conditioner, as required for damaged hair. Recommend a product designed for pre-perming only. The hair is already extra porous, therefore it will absorb too much of a regular conditioner, and interfere with penetration.
3. Use a special permanent waving solution according to the directions.
4. Give test curls, using a mild waving solution and a shorter processing time than is employed for normal hair.

Hair Tinted with Metallic Dye

Hair tinted with a metallic dye must first be treated with a dye remover to avoid hair discoloration or breakage. Do not wave the hair if the test curls break or discolor. This type of discoloration is very difficult to remove.

Curl Reduction

Sometimes a client is displeased after a permanent wave because the hair seems too curly. If the hair is fine, do not suggest curl reduction before shampooing two or three times. This type of hair relaxes to a greater extent than does normal or coarse hair. Usually, after the second shampoo, the hair has relaxed enough to be satisfactory.

If the hair has a normal or coarse texture, curl reduction may be done immediately following neutralization, or after a few days.

Permanent waving solution may be used to relax the curl, where required. Carefully comb it through the hair to widen and loosen the wave. When sufficiently relaxed, the hair is rinsed, towel-blotted, and neutralized.

If curl analysis and proper application have not been determined, hair could be damaged and breakage could occur.

> CAUTION: Do not attempt curl reduction in hair that has been over-processed. Such treatment will damage the hair further.

Permanent Waving Hair with a Partial Permanent

Previously permanently waved hair should be given reconditioning treatment. Leave the conditioning agent over the old permanent and cover this hair with two or three end papers. Then proceed with the usual permanent wave routine.

> NOTE: This is only one suggestion for permanent waving this type of hair. Your instructor's method is equally correct.

Items to Consider

Air conditioning. Because of its cooling effect, air conditioning may slow the action of the permanent waving solution. Additional time may be required.

Long hair. Because of its length, long hair may require smaller blockings or alternative rodding methods to assure thorough saturation of the waving lotion and neutralizer.

1. What is permanent waving?
2. The physical action involves the wrapping of the hair around _____.
3. The chemical action requires processing with a permanent waving solution, followed by _____.
4. Name two types of chemical solutions used in permanent waving.
5. What is the main action of a permanent waving solution?
6. What is the main action of the neutralizer?
7. What is the most important step before giving a permanent wave?
8. List six factors that a scalp and hair analysis should include.
9. What determines the choice of rods in permanent waving?
10. Why should hair be wrapped smoothly and without tension on each rod?
11. To achieve best results, what should guide the student?
12. What determines the size of the wave formation in permanent waving?
13. Why is it necessary to test curl-wave formation?
14. At what three points should curl-wave development be tested?
15. When does the wave pattern reach its peak?
16. What kind of hair texture will not form a firm wave pattern?
17. Why should safety rules be observed in permanent waving?
18. How is over-processed hair detected?
19. Why should a hair coloring treatment and a permanent wave not be given the same day?
20. Why should a color rinse not be given immediately following a permanent wave?
21. What determines the strength of waving solution used?
22. When may a permanent waving solution cause irritation to a healthy skin or scalp?
23. What must be done if the waving solution accidentally gets on the skin or scalp?
24. How may a permanent wave be relaxed, if it is too curly?
25. What strength waving solution is always recommended for tinted or lightened hair?
26. Why are special hair conditioners recommended for wrapping the hair?
27. In permanent waving, what determines the size of the blocking (sub-sectioning)?
28. What determines the length of rods used?
29. Which two hair factors determine the processing time during a permanent wave?
30. Why is hair elasticity so important in relation to permanent waving?

31. a. What are the benefits of alkaline perms? b. When should alkaline perms be used?
32. a. What are the benefits of acid-balanced perms? b. When should acid-balanced perms be used?
33. What is a partial perm?
34. How do you protect the hair that will not be permed during a partial perm process?

14

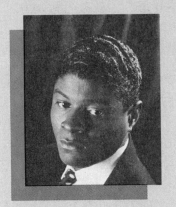

Chemical Hair Relaxing and Soft Curl Permanents

Learning Objectives

After completing this chapter, you should be able to:

1. *Define the purpose of chemical hair relaxing.*
2. *List the types of chemical hair relaxers.*
3. *Explain the difference between sodium hydroxide relaxer and thio relaxers.*
4. *List the basic products used in chemical hair relaxing.*
5. *Demonstrate the basic steps of chemical hair relaxing.*
6. *Define and perform a chemical blow-out.*
7. *Define a soft curl perm.*
8. *List the basic steps of a soft curl permanent procedure.*
9. *List safety precautions and procedures.*

Courtesy of: Hair: Sabrina Hill, North American Hairdresser Award winner in the Men's Makeover Category.

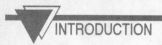

INTRODUCTION

Chemical hair relaxing is the process of rearranging the basic structure of overly curly hair into a straight form. When performed professionally, this service leaves the hair straight and able to be combed and styled into almost any manner desired. It is essential that the barber-stylist be able to perform this service.

Chemical hair processing or hair relaxing is not a difficult skill, but requires care and know-how. A thorough technical knowledge and expert manipulative skills are necessary to master the technique involved.

CHEMICAL HAIR RELAXING PRODUCTS

The basic products used in chemical hair relaxing are chemical hair relaxer, neutralizer, petroleum cream, shampoos designed specifically for hair relaxers, and conditioners.

Chemical Hair Relaxers

The two general types of hair relaxers are **sodium hydroxide** (SOH-dee-um heye-**DROK**-seyed), which does not require pre-shampooing, and **ammonium thioglycolate** (a-**MOH**-nee-um theye-oh-**GLEYE**-coh-layt), the use of which may require pre-shampooing.

Sodium hydroxide (a caustic type of hair relaxer, often called a hair straightener) both softens hair fibers and causes them to swell. As the solution penetrates the cortical layer, the cross-bonds are broken. The action of the comb, brush, or hands in smoothing the hair and distributing the chemical straightens the softened hair.

The strength of the sodium hydroxide solution may vary from 5 to 10 percent, and the pH factor from 10 to 14. In general, the more sodium hydroxide used and the higher the pH, the more quickly the chemical reaction will take place. The danger of hair damage will also increase.

Base and No Base Formulas

When using sodium hydroxide, there are two types of formulas—**base** and **no base**. The base formula is a petroleum cream that is designed to protect the client's skin and scalp during the chemical straightening process. This protective base is also important during a chemical straightening retouch. It is applied to protect hair that has been straightened previously, and to prevent over-processing and hair breakage.

Petroleum cream has a lighter consistency than petroleum jelly, and is formulated to melt at body temperature. The melting process ensures complete coverage of the scalp and other areas with a thin, oily protective coating. This helps to prevent burning and/or irritation of the scalp and skin. Previously treated hair should be protected with cream conditioner during the straightening process.

No base relaxers are also available. These relaxers have the same chemical reaction on the hair, although usually the reaction is milder. The procedure for the application of a no base relaxer is the same as for a regular relaxer, except that the base cream is not applied. It is advisable to use a protective cream around the hairline and over the ears.

> CAUTION: Because of the high alkaline content of sodium hydroxide, great care must be taken in its use.

Although ammonium thioglycolate (often called a **thio type relaxer**) is less drastic in its action than sodium hydroxide, it softens and relaxes overly curly hair by changing the hair's cystine linkage.

Neutralizer

A **neutralizer** also is known as a **stabilizer** or **fixative.** The neutralizer stops the action of any chemical relaxer that may remain in the hair after rinsing. The neutralizer for a thio type relaxer re-forms the cysteine cross-bonds in their new position and rehardens the hair.

Conditioners

Two types of conditioners are available:

1. Cream conditioners are applied to the scalp and hair, then carefully rinsed out. The hair is then towel dried. Setting lotion is applied and the hair is dried and set in the usual manner.
2. Protein (liquid) conditioners are applied to the scalp and hair prior to hairsetting and allowed to remain in the hair to serve as a setting lotion. Again, normal procedures are used for drying and styling.

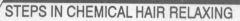

STEPS IN CHEMICAL HAIR RELAXING

All chemical hair relaxing involves three basic steps: processing, neutralizing, and conditioning.

Processing

When a chemical relaxer is applied, the hair begins to soften. As it does so, the chemical penetrates the hair to loosen and relax its natural curl.

Neutralizing

When the hair has been processed sufficiently, the chemical relaxer is rinsed out thoroughly with warm water, followed by either a built-in or a prescribed neutralizer.

Conditioning

Depending on the client's needs, the conditioner may be part of a series of hair treatments, or it may be applied to the hair before or after the relaxing treatment.

> CAUTION: Overly curly hair that has been damaged from heat appliances or other chemicals must be reconditioned before applying a relaxer. A chemical hair relaxer should not be used on hair treated with lighteners or metallic dyes since excessive damage or breakage could result.

Recommended Strength of Relaxer

The strength of relaxer used is determined by the strand test. The following guidelines help to determine which strength to use for the test.

1. Fine, tinted, or lightened hair—Use mild relaxer.
2. Normal, medium-textured virgin hair—Use regular relaxer.
3. Coarse virgin hair—Use strong or super relaxer.

It is important that the barber-stylist have a thorough understanding of the product being used and its action on the hair. The manufacturer's directions should be followed explicitly.

A working knowledge of human hair is particularly important in the case of over-curly hair. Before attempting to process over-curly hair, the barber-stylist must judge its texture, porosity, elasticity, and the extent, if any, of hair damage.

Client's Hair History

To help assure satisfactory results, as in the case of all chemical treatments, records should be kept of each hair relaxing treatment. These records should include the client's hair history and a release statement signed by the client, similar to that shown in the chapter on permanent waving.

RELAXER RECORD

Name _____ Tel. _____

Address _____ City _____ State _____ Zip _____

DESCRIPTION OF HAIR

Form	**Length**	**Texture**		**Porosity**	
☐ wavy	☐ short	☐ coarse	☐ soft	☐ very porous	☐ less porous
☐ curly	☐ medium	☐ medium	☐ silky	☐ moderately porous	☐ least porous
☐ extra-curly	☐ long	☐ fine	☐ wiry	☐ normal	☐ resistant

Condition

☐ virgin   ☐ retouched   ☐ dry   ☐ oily   ☐ lightened

Tinted with _____

Previsouly relaxed with (name of relaxer) _____

☐ Original sample of hair enclosed   ☐ not enclosed

TYPE OF RELAXER OR STRAIGHTENER

☐ whole head   ☐ retouch
☐ relaxer _____ strength_____   ☐ straightener _____ strength _____

Results

☐ good   ☐ poor   ☐ sample of relaxed hair enclosed   ☐ not enclosed

Date	Operator	Date	Operator

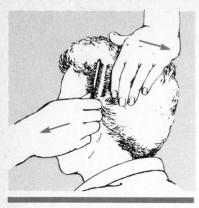

14.1 – Examining scalp

Before processing the hair, the barber-stylist must ascertain how the client's hair will react to the processor. Therefore a thorough scalp examination and a hair strand test are necessary.

Scalp Examination

Examine the scalp carefully for the presence or absence of eruptions, scratches, or abrasions in the same manner described in previous chapters. (Fig. 14.1)

> **NOTE:** Remember, no type of chemical hair relaxer should be applied if any blemishes or abrasions are found. Wait until the scalp is again healthy before treating the hair chemically.

Strand Test

The three strand tests that are employed include:
1. The finger test that determines the degree of hair porosity and is described in the chapter on permanent waving;
2. The pull test that determines the degree of elasticity and is also described in the permanent wave chapter; and
3. A relaxer test in which the relaxer is applied to a hair strand. The test strand's reaction to the chemical will indicate the ultimate results of the complete treatment. Take a small section of hair and thread it through a hole cut in a piece of waxed paper or aluminum foil. Apply relaxer to the hair. Do not use a base or cream. Allow it to remain on the hair for the required time and then remove it with a piece of dry cotton. If the test is satisfactory, proceed with the treatment.

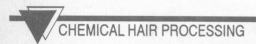

CHEMICAL HAIR PROCESSING

The following procedure is based primarily on products containing sodium hydroxide. As always, follow the manufacturer's directions and be guided by your instructor.

Implements and Supplies

Neutralizer or neutralizing shampoo	Chemical relaxer
Shampoo and cream rinse	Protective base
Conditioner-filler	Hair conditioner
Protective gloves	Towels
Comb and brush	Spatula
Timer	Absorbent cotton
Hair cloth or plastic cape	Neck strip
Record card	

Preparation

1. Select and arrange the required implements and supplies.
2. Wash and sanitize the hands.
3. Prepare and drape the client as for a shampoo.
4. Examine and evaluate the test results.
5. Do not shampoo.
6. Have client sign release card.
7. Hair ends may be trimmed after the chemical relaxer application.

Applying the Conditioner-Filler

In many cases a **conditioner-filler** is required before the chemical relaxer can be used. The conditioner-filler, usually a protein product, is applied to dry hair. It protects over-porous or slightly damaged hair from being over-processed. By evening out porosity, it permits uniform distribution and action of the chemical relaxer.

Gently rub the conditioner-filler onto the hair from the scalp to the hair ends, using either the hands or a comb. Towel-dry the hair or use a cool dryer (avoid the use of heat) to completely dry the hair.

Chemical Hair Relaxing (Processing)

The procedure for chemical hair relaxing is very similar to the technique followed in permanent waving. However, since the objective to be attained is exactly the reverse of permanent waving, some of the techniques must also be reversed.

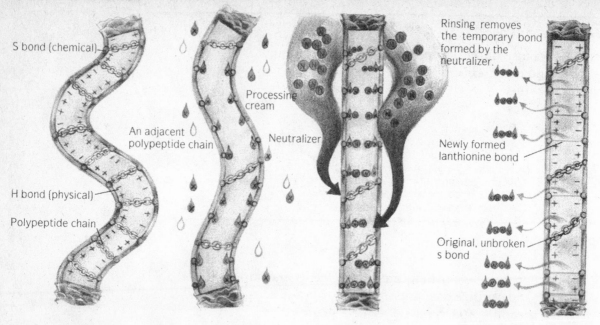

S bond (chemical)

An adjacent polypeptide chain

Processing cream

Neutralizer

Rinsing removes the temporary bond formed by the neutralizer.

Newly formed lanthionine bond

H bond (physical)

Polypeptide chain

Original, unbroken s bond

a. Both H and S bonds holding polypeptide chains in position

b. All H bonds broken and most S bonds broken—hand and comb manipulations starting to relax wave

c. Neutralizer fixes hair in a straight position after hair has been relaxed

d. Straightened hair after rinsing and proper drying; Lanthionine cross links now exist between polypeptide chains, keeping the hair in a permanently straight form. Drying re-forms the physical bonds.

14.2 – Chemical hair straightening process

As in permanent waving, the process requires the breaking down of the S-bonds and the H-bonds in the cortex. The relaxing process, however, requires that the hair be held or directed in a straight position. (Fig. 14.2)

Procedure for Sodium Hydroxide Relaxer

1. **Hair dried.** If moisture or perspiration is present, dry the client's hair and scalp.
2. **Application of protective base.** Most relaxers require the use of a petroleum base to protect the scalp from the active agents in the cream. The base is applied freely to the entire scalp with the fingers. The hairline around the forehead, nape of the neck, and over and around the ears must be completely covered. The base is actually *laid* on the scalp; it is not to be spread or rubbed on. Good coverage is important to protect the scalp and hairline from irritation. Any

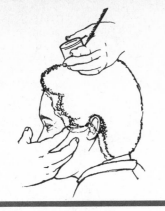

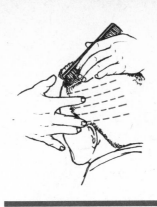

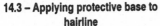

14.3 – Applying protective base to hairline

14.4 – Applying protective base to scalp

area that may come in contact with the relaxer must be protected. (Figs. 14.3, 14.4)

3. **Use of conditioner** (if recommended). In many cases it is necessary to apply a conditioner to the hair before applying the relaxer. Over-curly hair that has been damaged or weakened may break at the ends. The conditioner is used to strengthen the damaged and weakened hair and protect it against breakage.

4. **Applying the relaxer.** Use protective gloves. The relaxer must be applied with great caution. It must not be spread or rubbed on. The relaxer is laid on the hair shaft starting at the thickest part of the hair, for the action will take a little longer here. Extreme care must be taken not to let any relaxer touch the ears, the scalp, or the skin. The amount of cream used will vary, according to the thickness and length of the hair. The relaxer is applied to the entire scalp area and to the hair shaft, but not to the ends. The ends are the weakest part of the hair and therefore should receive the relaxer after the spreading-out procedure is completed.

5. **Spreading out the relaxer.** The spreading-out procedure follows the same pattern as that followed in applying the relaxer. There are three specific reasons for this procedure:

   a) To be sure the hair is completely covered, from the scalp.

   b) To be sure the hair is completely processed, from the scalp.

   c) To determine how fast the hair is being processed.

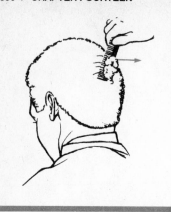

14.5 – Spreading out the relaxer with large-tooth comb

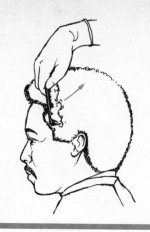

14.6 – Combing upward from the temples

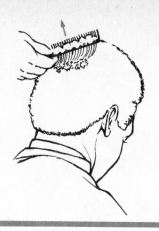

14.7 – Combing against the hair growth for total coverage

After spreading out the relaxer over the entire scalp area and hair shaft, it is laid on the ends and then applied to the front hairline.

6. **Use of a comb in spreading.** The relaxer may be spread over and through the hair by using a wide-tooth comb.
   a) Use the back of a comb to spread the relaxer over the entire head. (Fig. 14.5)
   b) Begin combing with wide-tooth comb.
   c) Comb in all directions.
   d) Comb first to one side, then to the other.
   e) Comb upward from the temples. (Fig. 14.6)
   f) By combing against the direction of hair growth, complete coverage will be obtained. (Fig. 14.7)
   g) The underneath hairs will be covered and straightened by combing away from the direction of natural growth.

7. **Testing.** In spreading the relaxer, the barber-stylist inspects the action by stretching the strands to see how fast the natural curl is being removed. If the action is too fast in any area, the relaxer should be washed from that particular section immediately. The spreading procedure can be continued over the rest of the head, and finally to the hair ends.

8. **Rinsing out the relaxer.** When the relaxer has reached its maximum action, it must be rinsed out rapidly and thoroughly. (Fig. 14.8)The water must be warm, but not hot. If the water is too hot, it may cause the processed hair to

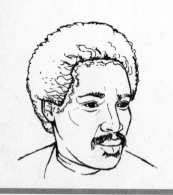

14.8 – Processor ready to be rinsed

revert. If the water is too cold, it will not remove the relaxer sufficiently. Unless the relaxer is completely removed, the chemical action continues on the hair.

CAUTION: Do not get any relaxer or rinse water into the client's eyes or on the skin. If this should happen, rinse the area thoroughly with warm water. In the rinsing process the stream of water must be directed out from the scalp rather than toward the scalp.

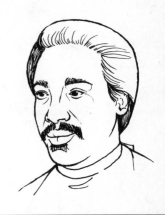

14.9 – After the hair has been shampooed and combed

9. **Shampooing the hair.** The shampoo (cream shampoo is recommended) is worked gently into the hair. The hair is very fragile at this point and tangled ends can be broken easily. Use tepid water and avoid firm manipulations, rubbing, or tangling the hair. Most processed hair requires at least three shampooings. (Fig. 14.9)

10. **Applying stabilizer.** After the hair has been shampooed, a stabilizer helps to keep the hair in a processed state. The hair is completely saturated with the stabilizer and is then combed through with a wide-tooth comb. The comb is used to:
   a) keep the hair straight;
   b) completely saturate the hair with the fixative; and
   c) remove any tangles without too much pulling.

11. **Applying color rinse.** To remove any reddish cast caused by the relaxer a color rinse may be applied, following the application of a stabilizer or a shampoo. Towel-dry the hair and apply a color rinse.

NOTE: If the reddish cast is not evident until the hair has been dried, the color rinse may be applied to the dried hair.

12. **Applying conditioner.** Some manufacturers recommend the use of a conditioner to the scalp and hair to restore some of the natural oils that have been removed by the

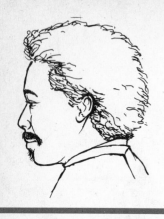

14.10 – Before: unruly hair

chemical hair relaxer. Before applying the conditioner, the hair and scalp is usually towel-dried.

13. Style the hair as desired.
14. If necessary, adjust a hair net (trainer) and thoroughly dry the hair with warm, not hot, air.
15. Carefully remove the hair net and re-comb the hair into a natural looking hairstyle. (Figs. 14.10, 14.11)

Final Clean-Up

1. Discard all used supplies.
2. Cleanse and sanitize all implements and equipment.
3. Wash and sanitize the hands.
4. Complete the hair processing record card.

> **NOTE:** Different products used for processing the hair require different methods of handling the hair during the processing and stabilizing period. Always follow the manufacturer's directions and be guided by your instructor.

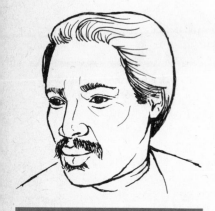

14.11 – After: hair processed and styled

Retouching

Follow all steps for a regular chemical hair relaxing treatment, with the exception that the relaxer is applied only to the new growth.

> **NOTE:** Before proceeding with any chemical relaxing treatment, it is essential that strand tests be taken to determine the ability of the client's hair to withstand the chemicals.

AMMONIUM THIOGLYCOLATE RELAXER (Thio Relaxer)

The procedure is somewhat different when using an ammonium thioglycolate product, commonly known as a thio relaxer.

Procedure for Thio Relaxer

1. Preparation of the client is the same as previously described.
2. Shampoo the hair with a neutral shampoo. Be careful not to irritate the scalp.

3. Towel-dry the hair, leaving it slightly damp.
4. If necessary, or if recommended by manufacturer, apply a hair conditioner as previously described.
5. Prepare the stabilizer before applying the relaxer.
6. Use protective gloves or cream on the hands. Apply the relaxer as previously described.
7. The spreading-out and testing procedure is the same as that followed for sodium hydroxide products.
8. When the hair has been sufficiently processed, the relaxer is rinsed out in a three-step process.
   a) Rinse about 50 percent of the relaxer from the hair with warm water.
   b) Comb the hair smooth and straight for about five minutes with the remaining relaxer left in the hair, to change the cystine linkages into a straight position.
   c) Rinse the remaining relaxer thoroughly from the hair with warm water, keeping the hair smooth and straight while rinsing.
9. After the relaxer is completely rinsed from the hair, apply a stabilizer as previously described, and proceed in the same manner as outlined for sodium hydroxide treatment.

Completion. Final clean-up is the same as previously described.

Retouching

Follow all steps for a regular chemical hair relaxing treatment, with the exception that the relaxer is applied only to the new growth.

THE CHEMICAL BLOW-OUT

Overly curly hair has unique characteristics that require rather special styling techniques.

A **chemical blow-out** or texturizer is a combination of chemical hair straightening and hairstyling which creates a well-groomed style. The procedure may be performed with either a thio hair relaxer or a sodium hydroxide straightener. The primary consideration with either method is not to over-relax the hair to the point where the blow-out process becomes impossible to perform.

Since the chemical used in a thio treatment is not extremely strong and will not straighten overly curly hair completely, it may be used for almost its entire recommended application time.

Sodium hydroxide, however, is an extremely potent chemical and may process the hair very quickly to the point where a blow-out cannot be performed. When using sodium hydroxide, timing becomes very important. Extreme care must be taken to control the amount of processing, and the chemical should not be kept on the hair for more than 40 percent of the recommended processing time.

The procedures for both the thio and the sodium hydroxide method have been explained thoroughly in this chapter. After all chemicals have been rinsed out of the hair, the stabilizer (neutralizer) applied to stop the chemical process, and then rinsed out, a good conditioner must be applied to the hair. Failure to condition this weakened hair thoroughly, prior to the blow-out procedure, could result in hair breakage. The conditioner will help to minimize possible damage or breakage and enable the hair to withstand the necessary combing.

Using a wide-tooth comb, hair lifter, or pick, comb the hair upward and slightly forward. The hair closest to the scalp gives direction to the hair; therefore it must be picked upward and outward. Start at the crown and continue until all of the hair has been combed out from the scalp and distributed evenly around the head. By combing in a circular pattern, splits are usually avoided.

The client is now placed under the dryer and the hair allowed to dry. The time permitted for drying depends on the length and thickness of the hair.

The dried hair is ready for shaping. Evenness is very important at this point. The hair length is checked to make sure that the shortest hair is used as the guide for the balance of the head. The barber-stylist must visualize the style and the length of hair planned for the blow-out.

Cutting should be started at the sides. The hair is evened out around the head with an electric clippers or scissors, while the picking of the hair outward from the scalp continues at the same time. The hair should be cut in the direction in which it is to be combed. The object is to achieve a smooth, even cut that is properly contoured. The final cutting should be done only with scissors, to even out loose or ragged ends.

Outline the hairstyle at the sides, around the ears, and in the nape area, using either scissors or an outliner. After the hair is cut to the desired style the finishing touches are applied. Fluff the hair slightly with the lifter, where required, and spray lightly. The lifter or pick is used to improve the smoothness of the style.

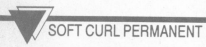

SOFT CURL PERMANENT

Soft curl permanent waving is a method of permanently waving overly curly hair. The following procedure can be used for both men and women.

CAUTION: The product used contains ammonium thioglycolate.
1. Do not use it on bleached, tinted, or damaged hair, or on hair that has been colored with metallic dye or compound henna.
2. Do not use it on hair that has been relaxed with sodium hydroxide.
3. If permanent waving lotion or neutralizer accidentally gets into the client's eye, flush the eye immediately with water and refer the client to a doctor.

To achieve a soft curl permanent, it is important to follow the manufacturer's or your instructor's directions explicitly. Doing otherwise may give poor results and may damage the client's hair and skin.

Procedure

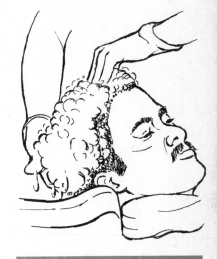

14.12 – Shampoo the hair.

1. Examine the client's scalp. Do not use permanent waving gel or cream if the scalp shows any signs of abrasions or lesions, or if the client has experienced an allergic reaction to a previous perm.
2. Shampoo and rinse the hair thoroughly. Towel it dry, leaving it damp. (Fig. 14.12)
3. Remove any tangles with a large-tooth comb. (Fig. 14.13)
4. Part hair into 4–5 sections, as recommended by your instructor. (Figs. 14.14,14.15)

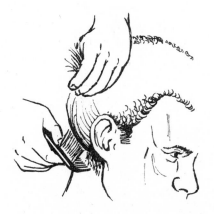

14.13 – Remove tangles from hair.

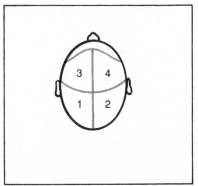

14.14 – Four sections—part hair down center from forehead to nape. Part across, starting behind the ear. Extend part from ear to ear.

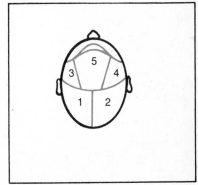

14.15 – Five sections—part across, starting behind the ear. Extend part from ear to ear. Divide front area into sections. Divide back area into two sections.

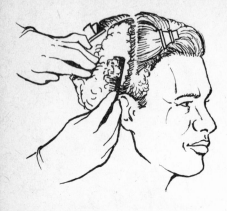

14.16 – Part hair into sections and coat with thio gel.

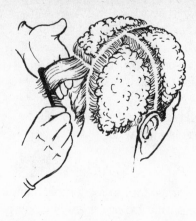

14.17 – Comb thio gel through hair.

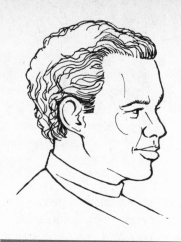

14.18 – Rinse hair.

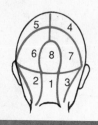

14.19 – Divide hair into eight sections.

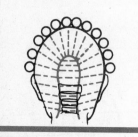

14.20 – Sub-section as you wrap.

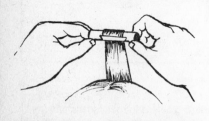

14.21 – Wrap hair on rods.

> **NOTE:** If manufacturer requires it, put a protective cream on the entire scalp, including around the hairline.

5. Put on protective gloves.
6. Apply thio gel or cream to one section at a time, using a hair-coloring brush, fingers, or the back of a comb. Use the rat tail of the comb or brush to part the hair and begin the application of thio gel or cream to the hair nearest the scalp, preferably starting at the nape area. Work the gel or cream to the ends of the hair. (Fig. 14.16)
7. Comb the gel or cream through the entire head, first with a wide-tooth comb, then with a smaller-toothed comb. (Fig. 14.17)
8. When the hair becomes supple and flexible rinse it with tepid water and towel dry. Do not tangle the hair. (Fig. 14.18)
9. Section the hair into nine sections. (Fig. 14.19) Sub-section as you wrap the hair. (Fig. 14.20)
10. Wrap the hair on desired size of curling rods. (Fig. 14.21) Use small (thin) curling rods for tighter curls and larger ones for looser curls. If the hair is short, use short rods since they make it easier to wrap and control short, curly hair.

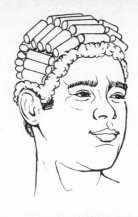

14.22 – Protect client's skin with cotton around hairline.

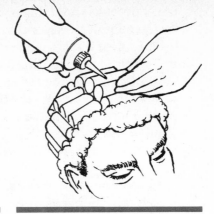

14.23 – Apply thio gel to curls.

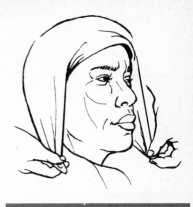

14.24 – Cover hair with plastic cap.

11. After wrapping is complete, protect the client's skin by placing cotton around the hairline and neck. (Fig. 14.22)
12. Apply thio gel or cream to all the curls until they are thoroughly saturated. (Fig. 14.23)
13. Cover the client's head with a plastic cap. (Fig. 14.24)
14. Seat the client under a preheated dryer for 15 to 25 minutes, or as recommended by the manufacturer. (Fig. 14.25)
15. Take a test curl, and if the desired curl pattern has not developed, keep the client under the dryer for another ten minutes or until a curl pattern develops. (Fig. 14.26)
16. When the desired curl pattern has been reached, rinse the hair thoroughly with warm (not hot) water. (Fig. 14.27) Blot each curl with a towel.

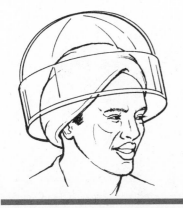

14.25 – Process under preheated dryer.

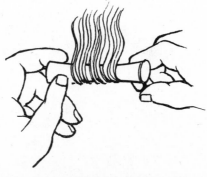

14.26 – Test a curl.

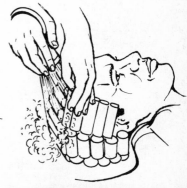

14.27 – Rinse the hair.

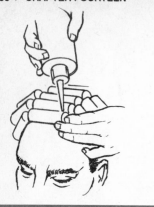

14.28 – Apply neutralizer.

17. Use a prepared neutralizer, or mix neutralizer as directed by the manufacturer, and saturate each curl twice. (Fig. 14.28) Allow the neutralizer to remain on the curls for five to ten minutes, or as directed by the manufacturer.

18. Carefully remove the rods and apply the balance of the neutralizer to the hair. Work it through with the fingers for thorough distribution, and allow it to remain on the hair for another five minutes. (Fig. 14.29)

19. Rinse the hair thoroughly with cool water and towel-blot. (Fig. 14.30)

20. Trim any uneven hair ends. (Fig. 14.31)

21. Apply conditioner as directed by the manufacturer.

22. Air-dry the hair or style as desired. (Fig. 14.32)

Figures 14.33 and 14.34 illustrate a hairstyle before and after a soft curl permanent, respectively.

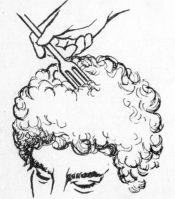

14.29 – Work neutralizer through hair.

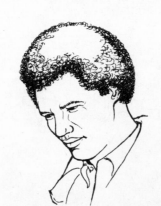

14.30 – Rinse hair.

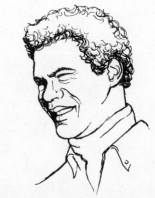

14.31 – Trim hair ends.

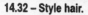

14.32 – Style hair.

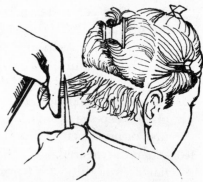

14.33 – Before soft curl permanent

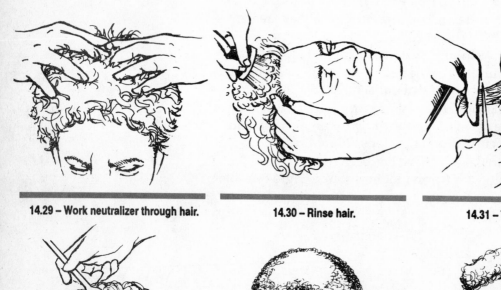

14.34 – After soft curl permanent

Alternate Method

Steps 1 through 7 are the same

Step 8: When the hair has become supple and flexible (do not rinse), section and wrap in the usual manner (steps 9 and 10).

NOTE: Use small curling rods for tighter curls and larger ones for looser curls.

To protect the client's skin, place cotton around the head and neck (step 11).

Apply a thio permanent wave lotion to each curl as directed by the manufacturer. Steps 13 through 21 are the same.

After Care

1. Do not comb or brush the curls when wet; use a lifting pick instead.
2. Shampoo about once a week using a mild shampoo.
3. Conditioner or curl activator should be used daily to maintain flexibility, sheen, and proper moisture balance of the hair.

SAFETY PRECAUTIONS AND REMINDERS

1. Know the texture of the hair to be treated.
2. Check the elasticity of the hair for its ability to stretch and return to its normal length without breaking.
3. Check the porosity of the hair and its ability to absorb moisture.
4. Do not relax damaged hair. Suggest a series of reconditioning treatments.
5. Always read and follow the manufacturer's instructions before giving a relaxing treatment.
6. Have all implements and materials ready before you start the treatment.
7. Never give a chemical hair relaxing treatment to hair that has recently been straightened by a hot pressing comb.
8. Do not use a hot comb after a relaxing treatment. To do so will damage the hair.

9.   Avoid rubbing the relaxer on the hair. Lay it on the hair shaft.

10. Do not give a relaxing treatment if the client suffers from nausea or if redness and irritation appear within or around the skin test area.

11. Strand test to be sure the relaxing treatment can be given safely.

12. Examine the scalp for abrasions; if any are present, do not give a relaxing treatment.

13. Apply a petroleum base to protect the scalp from the active agents in the relaxer (if required by the manufacturer).

14. If a base is used, after the application check carefully to see that the scalp has been covered completely and thoroughly. Failure to cover the scalp carefully can result in a burning or irritation by the chemicals being used.

15. Always use great care and caution when applying the relaxer.

16. Never leave the client alone while the relaxer is on the hair.

17. Wear protective gloves when giving a relaxing treatment.

18. Use extreme care when applying the relaxer to avoid spilling it on the ears, scalp, or skin.

19. When rinsing the relaxer from the hair, be very careful that the water is not too hot. If hot water is used, the hair will revert to its natural curly shape.

20. Be sure to shampoo and rinse the relaxer from the hair thoroughly. Failure to do so will cause the relaxer to continue to act, resulting in hair damage.

21. When rinsing the shampoo from the hair, always work the fingers from the scalp to the ends, following the water stream to prevent tangling the hair.

22. The application of a stabilizer to the hair following the shampoo is important to keep the hair relaxed or straight.

23. Use a wide-tooth comb and avoid pulling when combing the hair.

24. To help restore some of the natural oils removed by the chemicals, apply a conditioner after the hair and scalp are towel-dried, and before combing.

25. When retouching the new growth, do not allow the relaxer to touch the already relaxed hair.

26. Avoid scratching the scalp with the comb or fingernails.

27. Avoid leaving the chemical relaxer on the hair any longer than is necessary to straighten it.

28. Avoid harsh or rough handling of the scalp and the hair.

29. To avoid hair damage, do not use hot irons on processed hair.
30. Avoid getting chemicals or rinse water into the eyes.
31. Do not give a vigorous shampoo.
32. Do not use a strong relaxer on fine hair.
33. If hair ends are damaged, trim the hair before a relaxing treatment is given.
34. Test the action of the relaxing agent frequently to determine how fast the natural curl can be removed.
35. When drying the hair, extreme heat from the dryer should be avoided to prevent hair damage and scalp irritation.
36. To remove a reddish cast caused by the relaxer, apply a color rinse to the hair.
37. Always fill out a record card at the completion of each treatment.

REVIEW QUESTIONS

Chemical Hair Relaxing
and Soft Curl Permanents

1. What is the action of a chemical hair relaxer?
2. What is the purpose of analyzing the client's hair prior to applying a chemical relaxer?
3. List four hair conditions to consider in a hair analysis.
4. What chemical compound is required in addition to the chemical relaxing agent? By what other term is it known?
5. What test should be given before a client receives a chemical relaxing treatment?
6. If a client's hair has been receiving hot comb treatments, when can a chemical relaxing treatment be given?
7. What are three purposes of strand testing in the chemical relaxing procedure?
8. Why is a scalp examination especially important prior to a chemical hair relaxing treatment?
9. What is the purpose of the client's record card?
10. Why is it necessary to have the client sign a release?
11. What hair condition should prevent treatment with a chemical hair relaxer?
12. What is the purpose of the base that is applied to the entire scalp and surrounding areas?
13. Why are protective gloves used when applying the chemical relaxer?
14. After the hair has been treated with sodium hydroxide relaxer, why

should the hair be rinsed thoroughly prior to the application of a shampoo?

15. Why should the hair be combed carefully without touching the scalp before applying the relaxer?

16. Why is a cream shampoo preferred for chemically relaxed hair?

17. Why is it important to keep chemically relaxed hair from tangling during a shampoo?

18. Why should the hair have at least three shampoo applications after being treated with a sodium hydroxide hair relaxer?

19. What is the action of the stabilizer in chemical hair relaxing?

20. When should the hair be combed after chemical relaxing?

21. How is a chemical relaxing retouch given?

22. When should the hair be shampooed in giving a thio relaxing treatment?

23. How is thio cream removed from the hair?

24. How are the underneath hairs covered in comb spreading?

25. What are some of the advantages of using a comb in spreading the relaxer?

26. What type of combs are used in spreading the relaxer?

27. After a relaxing treatment, why is it recommended that a conditioner be applied to the scalp and hair?

28. What may be used if the hair develops a reddish cast after a relaxing treatment?

29. Why are hot irons not to be used on the hair after a relaxing treatment?

30. Why must a relaxing treatment not be given to hair that has received a hot comb treatment?

31. Define a soft curl permanent.

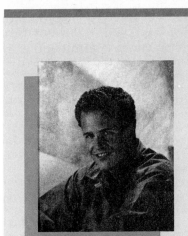

Hair Coloring

Learning Objectives

After completing this chapter, you should be able to:

1. *Discuss the principles of color theory and relate their importance to hair coloring.*
2. *Identify hair color classifications, explain their action on the hair, and give examples of their use.*
3. *Demonstrate the correct preparation for coloring hair.*
4. *Demonstrate the correct procedures for applying tints and lighteners.*
5. *List safety precautions to follow during hair coloring procedures.*

Courtesy of: Matrix Essentials, Inc.

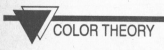

INTRODUCTION

Hair coloring (tinting) is the science and art of changing the color of the hair. **Hair bleaching** (lightening) is the partial or total removal of natural pigment or artificial color from the hair. Skill in both hair coloring and lightening requires thorough practice, determination, and study.

(The terms *tinting* and *coloring* are used interchangeably in this text. Most barber-stylists prefer to use the term *lighten* instead of *bleach*.)

There are many reasons for coloring or lightening the hair. Some of these include:

1. To restore gray hair to its original color.
2. To change the natural color of hair to a more attractive shade.
3. To restore hair to its natural color.
4. To create decorative effects.
5. To enhance or create highlights.

Typical clients are:

1. Those who enjoy fashion changes.
2. Those with prematurely gray hair.
3. Those who wish to maintain a youthful appearance.

A successful barber-stylist should understand the correct process for selecting and applying coloring and lightening products. Also necessary is knowledge of the chemical reactions of tints and lighteners on hair.

Hair coloring includes processes of adding artificial pigment to either natural or previously colored hair; adding artificial pigment to pre-lightened hair; and diffusing natural pigment and adding artificial pigment in one step.

COLOR THEORY

The theory of color pigment must be understood before you begin applying hair coloring products to clients' hair. It is only through this knowledge that correct color formulation can be chosen for each client.

Color is created by the movement of light rays either as they are absorbed or reflected by artificial pigment added to the hair in the tinting process, or by natural hair pigment.

Natural hair color is created by the reflection or absorption of light rays by melanin. The size, amount, and distribution of melanin determines hair color. Greater numbers of large melanin molecules distributed throughout the cortex create dark colors. Fewer, smaller melanin molecules create light colors. The various combinations in the size, amount, and distribution of melanin create all natural hair colors.

The Laws of Color

The laws of color regulate the mixing of dyes and pigment to make other colors. They are based in science and adapted to art. The laws of color serve as guidelines for harmonious color mixing.

Primary Colors

Primary colors are basic or true colors that are not created by combining other colors. The three primary colors are yellow, red, and blue. All other colors are created by some combination of red, yellow, or blue.

Secondary Colors

Secondary colors are created by mixing equal amounts of two primary colors. Mixed in equal parts, yellow and blue create green, blue and red create violet, and red and yellow create orange.

Tertiary Colors

Tertiary colors are created by mixing equal amounts of one primary color with one of its adjacent secondary colors. The tertiary colors are red-violet, blue-violet, blue-green, yellow-green, yellow-orange, and red-orange.

Quaternary Colors

Quaternary colors are all other combinations that create any color that has not been previously described.

Complementary Colors

Complementary colors are any two colors situated directly across from each other on the color wheel. When mixed together their action is to neutralize each other. For example, when mixed in equal amounts, red and green neutralize each other, creating brown. Orange and blue neutralize each other, and yellow and violet neutralize each other. Complementary colors are always composed of a primary and a secondary color, and complementary pairs always consist of all three primary colors. For example, if you look at the color wheel, you see that the complement of red (a primary color) is green (a secondary color). Green is made up of blue and yellow (both primary colors)—so all three primaries are represented in this complementary pair.

Tone

Tone refers to whether a color is warm or cool. The **warm colors**—also known as highlighting colors—are red, orange, and yellow. The **cool colors**—also known as ash or drab—are blue, green, and violet.

Level

Level indicates the degree of lightness or darkness of a color. Every color can be made either lighter or darker, thus changing the level, by the addition of white or black. Hair colors, both natural and color-treated, are classified by level on a scale of one to ten, one indicating black and ten indicating the lightest blond. The **level system** is crucial to formulating, matching, and correcting colors.

THE LEVEL SYSTEM

Level 10 — Lightest blond
Level 9 — Very light blond
Level 8 — Light blond
Level 7 — Medium blond
Level 6 — Dark blond
Level 5 — Lightest brown
Level 4 — Light brown
Level 3 — Medium brown
Level 2 — Dark brown
Level 1 — Black

Saturation

Saturation refers to the degree of concentration or amount of pigment in the color. For example, a saturated red is very vivid. Any color can be more or less saturated. A more saturated product creates a dramatic change in hair color.

▼ CLASSIFICATIONS OF HAIR COLOR

Hair color is divided into three classifications: temporary, semi-permanent, and permanent. These classifications indicate **color fastness**, or its ability to remain on the hair, and are determined by the chemical composition and molecular weight of the pigments and dyes within the products. (Fig. 15.1)

Temporary colors utilize pigment and dye molecules of the greatest molecular weight, making these molecules the largest in the three classifications of hair color. The large size of the color molecule prevents penetration of the cuticle layer of the hair shaft and allows only a coating action on the outside of the strand.

THREE CLASSIFICATIONS OF COLOR

	Temporary	Semipermanent	Permanent
Molecular weight of dye molecule	Large	Medium	Small
pH	Acid	Slightly alkaline	Alkaline
Reaction or change	Physical	Chemical & physical	Chemical & physical
Color fastness	Removed with shampooing	Fades gradually	Permanent
Color changes	Deposits	Deposits	Lightens & deposits

15.1 – Three classifications of color

The chemical composition of a temporary color is acid in reaction and makes only a physical change rather than a chemical change in the shaft. This creates a color that is designed to be removed completely with the next shampoo.

Semi-permanent pigment and dye molecules are of a lesser molecular weight than those of temporary colors. These smaller molecules have the physical capability to partially penetrate the hair shaft. The chemical composition of semi-permanent colors is mildly alkaline in reaction, thus causing the cortex to swell and the cuticle to raise to allow some penetration. This mild alkaline solution, combined with a mild oxidizer, creates a classification of color that becomes self-penetrating.

The semi-permanent colors make a mild chemical change as well as a physical change. These changes create a color designed to be removed gradually through shampooing, leaving behind a slight diffusion of color that often goes unnoticed.

Permanent pigment and dye molecules have the lowest molecular weight, making them the smallest used in the three classifications of hair color. These molecules are small enough to enter through the cuticle and penetrate deep into the cortex, creating a color as permanent as current technology allows.

Permanent tints are alkaline in reaction. This creates the same chemical process as with semi-permanent colors, in that the cortex swells, the cuticle raises and separates, and small pigment and dye molecules can enter the shaft. After the addition of a full strength oxidizer, the product is able to diffuse melanin as the artificial color molecules swell and become a part of the structure of the cortex. As the color is shampooed and dried, it begins to return to its normal pH. This causes the cortex to shrink and the cuticle to close. The color molecules become trapped beneath the cuticle. Even though the color fades eventually, the cortex undergoes permanent chemical and structural changes.

Temporary Hair Coloring

As explained previously, temporary hair coloring products are designed to remain on the hair until it is shampooed. The color coats the hair shaft rather than penetrating it. Thus it can only deposit pigment; it cannot lighten. (Fig. 15.2) A patch test is usually unnecessary for this type of hair color. However, it is wise to always consult the manufacturer's directions.

Types of Temporary Hair Coloring

1. **Color rinses** are used to highlight the color or add color to the hair. These rinses contain certified colors and remain on the hair until the next shampoo.

   Two types of color rinses are available: instant and concentrated. Instant rinses are applied straight from the bottle and remain in the hair. Concentrated rinses are mixed with hot water before application, processed for 5 to 10 minutes, and then rinsed. Both types of rinses may leave traces of the darker shades on combs, brushes, and clothing.
2. **Highlighting color shampoos** combine the action of a color rinse with that of a shampoo. These shampoos generally contain certified colors, give highlights, and impart color tones to the hair.
3. **Crayons** are sticks of coloring in all shades, compounded with soaps or synthetic waxes, sometimes used to color gray or white hair between hair tint retouches. Crayons are often used by men as a temporary coloring for mustaches.

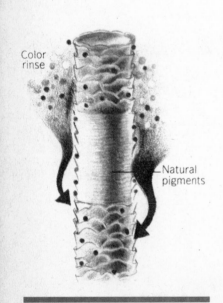

Color rinse

Natural pigments

15.2 – Action of temporary hair color

They come in several colors: blond; light, medium, and dark brown; black; and auburn.

4. **Hair color sprays** are applied to dry hair from aerosol containers. Color sprays are usually available in vibrant colors and are generally used for special or party effects.

5. **Hair color mousses** and gels are now available that combine highlighting and styling effects in one product.

Semi-Permanent Hair Coloring

Semi-permanent hair colorings are formulated to last three to four weeks (depending on frequency of shampooing, type of shampoo, and general porosity of the hair) and gradually are rinsed from the hair by shampooing. These tints are considered **deposition colors** as color is deposited in the cortical layer of the hair, as well as coating the shaft. Semi-permanent tints are considered self-penetrating because basic and direct dyes are utilized, rather than pigments that must be mixed with hydrogen peroxide for color development, and a mild oxidizer in the formulation opens the cuticle and allows some penetration. Because semi-permanent tints do not change the basic structure of the hair, they cannot lighten natural hair color.

Semi-permanent colors are used:

1. To cover or blend partially gray hair without affecting its natural color. Most semi-permanent colors are designed to cover hair that is no more than 25 percent gray.
2. To enhance or blend partially gray hair without affecting its natural color. This can be done successfully on almost any percentage of gray, depending upon the desired color.
3. To highlight and enhance the color tones of the hair. Semi-permanent colors can be used to add golden or red highlights, and to deepen the color of the hair. This type of color is especially effective on ethnic clients and clients whose natural hair color is too light or too drab to set off their complexions.
4. To serve as a non-peroxide toner for pre-lightened hair. Pre-lightened hair is porous and the toner will penetrate.

The illustration (Fig. 15.3) indicates how this type of hair coloring works on the hair shaft.

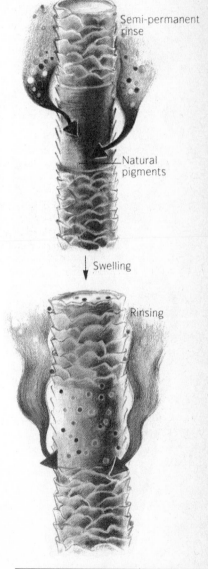

15.3 – Action of semi-permanent hair color

Permanent Hair Coloring

Permanent hair colorings are designed to penetrate the cuticle and deposit molecules into the cortex. Due to the penetration and the addition of peroxide, these colors can both **lift** and **deposit**. (Fig. 15.4)

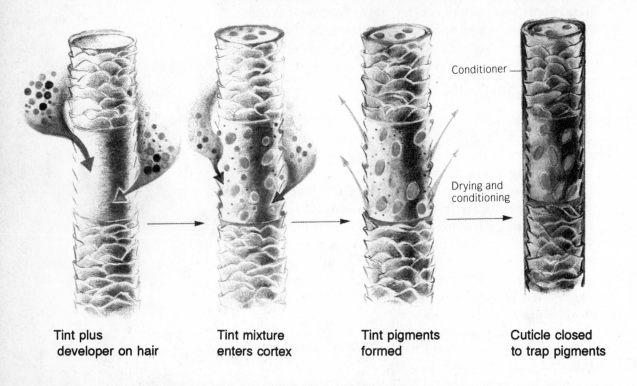

Conditioner —

Drying and conditioning

| Tint plus developer on hair | Tint mixture enters cortex | Tint pigments formed | Cuticle closed to trap pigments |

15.4 – Action of permanent hair color

Permanent hair colors fall into four classifications: oxidation tints, vegetable tints, metallic dyes, and compound dyes.

1. Professional permanent hair dyes are based almost entirely on the use of **oxidation tints**. Oxidation tints are also known as **aniline derivative tints, penetrating tints, synthetic-organic tints,** and **amino tints.** Tints can lighten and deposit color in a single process and are available in a wide variety of colors. **Toners** also fall into the category of permanent color. Toners are aniline derivative products of pale, delicate shades designed for use on pre-lightened hair.

   Most oxidation tints contain aniline derivatives and require a **predisposition test** before the service is performed.

As long as the hair is of normal strength and kept in good condition, oxidation tints are compatible with other professional chemical services.

Oxidation tints are sold in bottles, canisters, and tubes, in either a semi-liquid or cream form. These products must be mixed with hydrogen peroxide, which activates the chemical reaction known as **oxidation**. This reaction begins as soon as the two compounds are combined, so the mixed tint must be used immediately. Any leftover tint must be discarded since it deteriorates quickly.

NOTE: Check MSDS (Material Safety Data Sheets) for the proper disposal of leftover tints and containers.

Timing the application of the tint depends upon the product and the volume of peroxide selected. Consult the manufacturer's directions and your instructor for assistance. A strand test should always be taken to ensure satisfactory results.

2. **Vegetable tints** are hair coloring products made from various plants, such as herbs and flowers. In the past, indigo, camomile, sage, Egyptian henna, and other plants were used to color the hair. Henna is still used as a professional hair coloring product, but it should be used with some caution. Henna has a coating action that, if over-used, can build up on the hair and prevent penetration of other chemicals. Henna also penetrates the cortex and attaches to the salt bonds. Both of these actions may leave the hair unfit for other professional treatments.

3. **Metallic** or **mineral dyes** are advertised as *color restorers* or *progressive colors*. The metallic ingredients, such as lead acetate or silver nitrate, react with the keratin in the hair, turning it brown. This reaction creates a colored film coating which creates a dull metallic appearance. Repeated treatments damage the hair and can react adversely with many professional chemical services. Metallic dyes are not professional coloring products.

4. **Compound dyes** are metallic or mineral dyes combined with a vegetable tint. The metallic salts are added to give the product more staying power and to create different colors. Like metallic dyes, compound dyes are not used professionally.

Test for Allergy

Allergy to aniline derivative tints is unpredictable. Some clients may be sensitive, and others may suddenly develop a sensitivity after years of use. To identify an allergic client, the U.S. Federal Food, Drug, and Cosmetic Act prescribes that a patch or predisposition test be given 24 to 48 hours prior to each application of an aniline derivative tint or toner.

CAUTION: Aniline derivative tints must never be used on the eyelashes or eyebrows. To do so may cause blindness.

▼ LIGHTENERS

Lighteners diffuse hair color by use of a bleach formula, hydrogen peroxide, and the chemical heat produced by the combination of ingredients. (Fig. 15.5)

The hair pigment goes through different stages of color as it lightens. The amount of change depends on how much pigment the hair has, and the length of time the lightening agent is processed. Hair goes through seven stages of lightening from the darkest to the lightest: a natural head of black hair will go from black to brown, to red, to red-gold, to yellow, and finally to pale yellow (almost white). (Fig. 15.6)

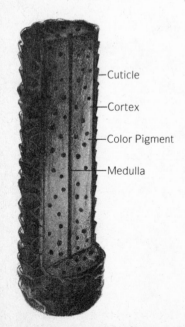
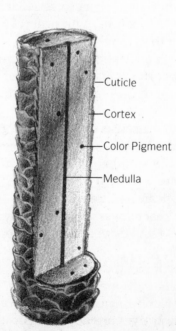
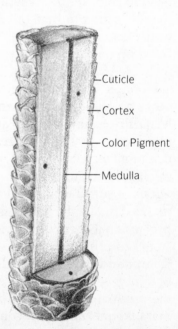

Cuticle
Cortex
Color Pigment
Medulla

Cuticle
Cortex
Color Pigment
Medulla

Cuticle
Cortex
Color Pigment
Medulla

15.5 – Hair lighteners are used to diffuse pigment.

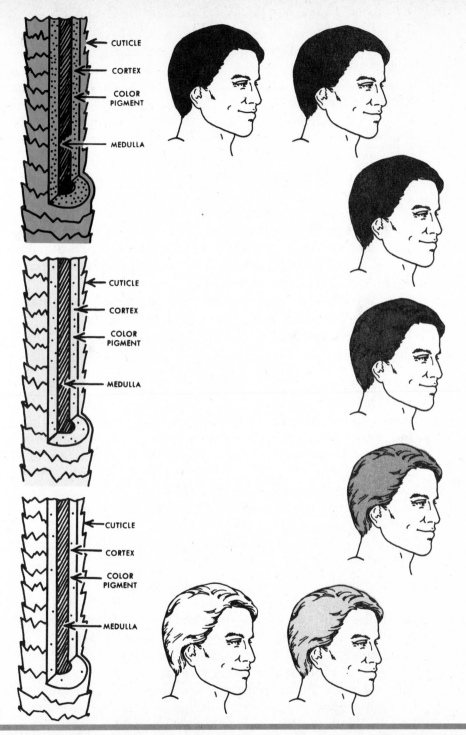

15.6 – Seven stages in lightening from dark hair to pale yellow (almost white). A virgin head of dark hair passes through seven stages before it arrives at the almost white stage. The change in the color depends upon the type of lightener chosen and the length of time that it remains on the hair.

CAUTION: Clients with dark hair may not be able to be lightened to a very pale blond color without extreme damage to their hair.

Action of Lighteners

Lighteners may be used for two purposes:

1. As a color treatment, to lighten hair to the final shade.
2. As a preliminary treatment, to prepare the hair for the application of a toner or tint (double-process application).
   a) Toner—A lightener is always necessary before applying delicate toner shades.
   b) Tint—If the client desires a shade much lighter than the natural shade, a lightener can be used to remove some color before the tint is applied.

Toners

Toners are aniline derivative tints, require a 24 to 48 hour patch test, and consist of pale and delicate colors. Toners usually have a very different color appearance than the final shade such as purple, blue, orange, pink—colors uncommon to natural hair color. As toner color oxidizes it goes through several visual color changes. A strand test should be done to determine the processing time required for a desired shade.

Toners require a double-process application. The first process is the lightener, the second is the toner.

Pre-Lightening to Create a Foundation for Toners

After the hair goes through the seven stages of lightening, the color left in the hair is known as its **foundation**. Achieving the correct foundation is necessary for proper toner development.

Manufacturers of toners provide literature that recommends the proper foundation to achieve a desired color. As a general rule, the paler the desired color, the lighter the foundation must be. It is important to follow the guide closely. Over-lightened hair will grab the base color of the toner, while under-lightened hair will appear to have more red, yellow, or orange than the intended color.

Many clients buy and use hair coloring products at home. Therefore, it is important to be able to recognize and understand their effects. Such coloring agents must be removed and the hair reconditioned prior to any other chemical service.

Hair treated with a metallic or other coating dye looks dry and dull. It is generally harsh and brittle to the touch. These colorings usually fade to unnatural tones. Silver dyes have a greenish cast, lead dyes leave a purple color, and those containing copper turn red.

Test for Metallic Salts and Coating Dyes

1. In a glass container, mix one ounce (30 ml) of 20 volume (6 percent) peroxide and 20 drops of 28 percent ammonia water.
2. Cut a strand of the client's hair, bind it with tape, and immerse it in the solution for 30 minutes.
3. Remove, towel dry, and observe the strand.

Hair dyed with lead will lighten immediately. Hair treated with silver will show no reaction at all. This indicates that other chemicals will not be successful because they will not be able to penetrate the coating.

Hair treated with copper will start to boil, and will pull apart easily. This hair would be severely damaged or destroyed if other chemicals such as those found in permanent colors or perm solutions were applied to it.

Hair treated with a coating dye either will not change color or will lighten in spots. This hair will not receive chemical services easily, and the length of time necessary for penetration may very well damage the hair.

Removing Coatings from the Hair

Removal of metallic dyes from the hair shaft may be attempted, but is not always effective. Performing a strand test will indicate whether the metallic deposits have been removed. If not, the entire application must be repeated until the hair shaft is sufficiently free of metal salts to perform other chemical services.

Materials Needed

- 70 percent alcohol
- Concentrated shampoo for oily hair

- Mineral, castor, vegetable, or commercially prepared color-removing oil

Procedure

1. Apply 70 percent alcohol to dry hair.
2. Allow alcohol to stand for five minutes.
3. Apply the heavy oil thoroughly to the hair.
4. Cover the hair completely with a plastic bag.
5. Place under a hot dryer for 30 minutes.
6. To remove, saturate with concentrated shampoo.
7. Work the shampoo into the oil for three minutes, then rinse with warm water.
8. Repeat the shampoo steps until the oil is removed completely.

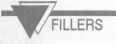

FILLERS

A **filler** is a dual-purpose hair coloring product that is able both to create a color base and to equalize excessive porosity. The two general classifications of fillers are protein and non-protein, both of which are manufactured in gel, cream, and liquid forms. Fillers are available in clear, neutral, and a variety of colors.

A clear filler is designed to correct porosity without affecting color. A neutral filler (a balance of all three primary colors) has minimal saturation and color correction abilities but has full power to equalize porosity. The colored fillers are pre-oxidized color that remain true during application and which will be subdued by the tint.

PREPARATION FOR HAIR COLORING

Before beginning any hair coloring application, a clear understanding is needed of the importance of a consultation and safety procedures, for both the well-being of the client and the successful outcome of the service.

Consultation

Always consult with the client regarding color preference before applying a tint or toner to the hair. Consultations should be held in a well-lighted room, providing either a strong natural light or incandescent lighting. Fluorescent lighting is not suitable for judging hair colors.

Consider that skin tones change with age. The natural color of the client's hair, which harmonized with the skin coloring at the age of 20 or 30, may seem harsh and unbecoming at the age of 40 or 50. For clients in this age group, keep to the lighter shades of color.

HAIR COLOR RECORD

Name _____ Tel. _____

Address _____ City _____

Patch Test: Negative ☐   Positive ☐   Date _____

DESCRIPTION OF HAIR

Form   **Length**   **Texture**   **Porosity**

☐ straight   ☐ short   ☐ coarse   ☐ very porous   ☐ resistant
☐ wavy   ☐ medium   ☐ medium   ☐ porous   ☐ very resistant
☐ curly   ☐ long   ☐ fine   ☐ normal   ☐ perm. waved

Natural hair color _____

Condition

☐ normal   ☐ dry   ☐ oily   ☐ faded   ☐ streaked   _____ % gray

Previously lightened with _____ for _____ (time)

Previously tinted with _____ for _____ (time)

☐ original sample enclosed   ☐ not enclosed

Desired hair color _____

CORRECTIVE TREATMENTS

Color filler used _____   Corrective treatments with_____

HAIR TINTING PROCESS

whole head_____   retouch _____   inches (cm)   shade desired _____

Formula: color _____   lightener _____

Results:

☐ good   ☐ poor   ☐ too light   ☐ too dark   ☐ streaked

Date	Operator	Price	Date	Operator	Price

Examining Scalp and Hair

The scalp and hair are examined carefully to determine if it is safe to use an aniline derivative tint and whether any special hair tinting problems exist.

An aniline derivative tint should not be used if any of the following conditions are present:

1. Signs of a positive skin test, such as redness, swelling, itching, and/or blisters.
2. Scalp sores or eruptions.
3. Contagious scalp or hair disease.
4. Presence of metallic or compound dyes.

If the scalp and hair are healthy, carefully observe and record the following data on a record card.

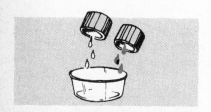

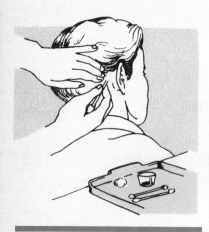

1. **Type of hair**—degree of porosity: either very receptive, moderately receptive, very resistant, or moderately resistant.
2. **Texture of hair**—coarse, medium, fine, or wiry.
3. **Color of hair**—natural or colored and the percentage of gray hair.

15.7 – For permanent tints, mix a capful of tint with a capful of hydrogen peroxide.

15.8 – First wash patch test area behind ear. Then apply tint mixture.

Patch Test

The patch test must be given 24 hours before each aniline derivative tinting or toner treatment. The tint used for the skin test must be of the same shade and mixture as the tint to be used.

Procedure

1. Select the test area, either behind the ear extending partly into the hairline, or on the inner fold of the elbow.
2. Wash an area about the size of a quarter with mild soap and water.
3. Dry the test area by patting with absorbent cotton or a clean towel.
4. Prepare the test solution by mixing one capful of tint and one capful of 20–volume peroxide, or as directed by the manufacturer. (Fig. 15.7)
5. Apply enough test solution with a cotton-tipped applicator to cover the area previously cleansed. (Figs. 15.8, 15.9)
6. Allow the test area to dry. Leave it uncovered and undisturbed for 24 hours.
7. Examine the test area for either negative or positive reactions.

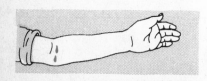

15.9 – A patch test may also be given at the inner bend of the elbow.

Patch Test for Semi-Permanent Tints

In giving a client a patch test for a semi-permanent tint, the test solution is applied in the same manner as for a permanent tint, except that the semi-permanent tint is not mixed with hydrogen peroxide. (Fig. 15.10) Apply the tint full strength to the test area with a cotton-tipped applicator.

A **negative skin test** will show no signs of inflammation; hence, an aniline derivative or semi-permanent tint may be applied.

A **positive skin test** is recognized by the presence of redness, swelling, burning, itching, blisters, or eruptions. The client may also suffer from a headache and vomiting. A client showing such symptoms is allergic to aniline derivative tint, and under no circumstances should this particular kind of tint be used. The client must get immediate medical attention; otherwise, complications may ensue.

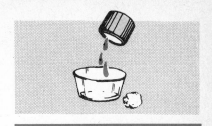

15.10 – Measure one capful of full strength tint.

How to Give Strand Tests

A strand test is given prior to any complete color application to determine the actual color and the condition of the hair.

Strand Test for Semi-Permanent Tints

Semi-permanent tints do not require the addition of hydrogen peroxide to the coloring material. Give the strand test in the following manner:

1. Gently shake the tint container.
2. Pour a small quantity of tint (about one teaspoon) into a glass or plastic bowl.
3. Apply the tint with a brush to the full length of a hair strand. Retain it on the hair until the desired shade has developed.
4. Remove any excess color with a piece of wet towel or cotton, and dry and examine the hair strand. If the results are satisfactory, proceed with the tint application.

Should the color produced in the strand test be different from the color desired, select another shade and perform the strand test again. (Fig. 15.11)

Strand Test for Permanent Tints

Single-application tints, double-action tints, and toners require the addition of 20–volume hydrogen peroxide to the coloring material.

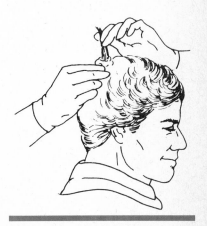

15.11 – Strand testing

For these tints, mix one-half teaspoon or one bottle cap of the selected color with equal amount of 20–volume hydrogen peroxide. (Use a plastic spoon.) Then follow the same instructions as for the strand test for semi-permanent tints.

> CAUTION: If strand testing for semi-permanent and permanent tints show discoloration that might indicate the presence of a metallic dye, corrective steps must be taken before tint application.

How to Remove Tint Stains from Skin

As a rule, soap and water will remove most tint stains. However, use one of the following methods for a difficult stain removal.

1. Wet a piece of cotton with the left-over tint. With a rotary movement cover the stain areas; follow with a damp towel. Apply a small amount of face cream and wipe clean.
2. Use a prepared tint stain remover.

Hair Coloring Applications

Hair coloring applications fall into two main classifications: **single-process coloring** and **double-process coloring.**

Single-process coloring achieves the desired result with a single application. The application itself may incorporate several steps, but one application creates the desired color. It is also known as single-application coloring, one-step coloring, one-step tinting, and single-application tinting.

Examples of single-process coloring include:

- Virgin tint applications
- Tint retouch applications
- Semi-permanent rinse applications
- Temporary color applications

Double-process coloring requires two separate and distinct applications to achieve the desired color. It is also known as double-application coloring, two-step coloring, two-step tinting, and double-application tinting.

Examples of double-process coloring include:

- Bleach and toner applications
- Pre-softening and tinting applications
- Filler and tint applications

TEMPORARY COLOR RINSES

Clients may be hesitant about a permanent hair color change. Temporary color rinses may be used to give a preview of how a color change will look.

Temporary color rinses also are satisfactory for clients who want to highlight the color of their hair or add slight color to gray hair. These rinses wash out with soap and water, but as a rule remain color-true from shampoo to shampoo. They come in various color shades: blond, brown, black, red, silver, and slate. These rinses are applied easily and quickly and are valuable as an introduction to semi-permanent or permanent hair coloring.

They can be used as follows:

1. To bring out highlights in hair of any shade.
2. To temporarily restore faded hair to its natural shade.
3. To neutralize the yellowish tinge of white or gray hair.
4. To tone down over-lightened hair.

Testing for Color Selection

Before applying a color rinse to the hair give a preliminary strand test, which will indicate whether the proper color selection was made and the correct length of time to leave the color rinse on the hair.

How to Give a Strand Test with a Temporary Rinse

1. Drape the client for a wet hair service.
2. Mix a small amount of the selected color rinse with warm water.
3. Apply the mixture to a full hair strand. Retain it on the hair as directed by the manufacturer.

4. Rinse, dry, and examine the hair strand. If the results are satisfactory, proceed with the color rinse treatment.

Should the color produced on the test strand be different from the color desired, select another and perform the strand test again.

Implements and Materials

Glass or plastic bowls
Timer
Shampoo
Neck strip
Protective gloves
Record card

Applicators — (Fig. 15.12)
  Swab stick
  Brush
  Plastic bottle
Comb
Plastic cape and towels
Cotton
Color rinse
Temporary rinse

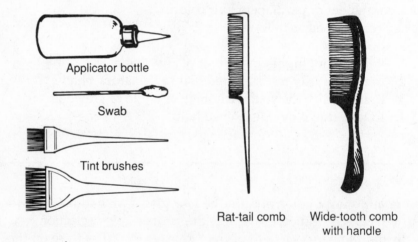

Applicator bottle

Swab

Tint brushes

Rat-tail comb   Wide-tooth comb with handle

15.12 – Applicators and combs used for hair coloring

NOTE: The procedures that follow represent two methods of applying a color rinse to the client's hair. Your instructor may have developed other techniques that are equally correct.

Preparation

The client is usually given a haircut prior to a color rinse application.

1. Assemble all necessary supplies.
2. Prepare the client. Protect the clothing with a plastic cape and a towel.
3. Examine the client's scalp and hair.
4. Select the desired shade of color rinse.
5. Prepare the color rinse.
6. Give a color strand test.

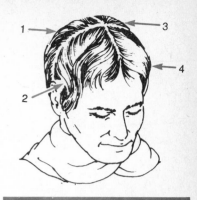

15.13 – Section hair properly.

Procedure for Color Rinse Applications

1. Shampoo, rinse, and towel-blot the hair. (Excess moisture must be removed to prevent diluting the color.)
2. Prepare the color rinse.
3. A plastic applicator bottle, or a glass, plastic, or porcelain bowl may be used to hold the mixture.
4. The rinse may be applied by using any one of the following methods:

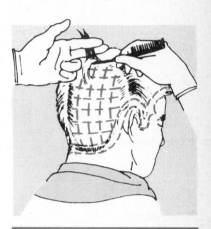

15.14 – Part each strand with applicator brush.

Brush-on Method

1. With an applicator brush apply the mixture around the front hairline. Manipulate the brush in short, rotary movements over the temple areas to lock in the color. This area is usually resistant.
2. Continue the application, working from the side areas toward the front.
3. Apply around the nape line and work upward to the crown area.
4. Brush the color rinse throughout the hair.
5. Check for complete coverage.
6. Leave the rinse on for the desired length of time.
7. Follow the manufacturer's directions for either rinsing or towel-blotting.
8. Style the hair.
9. Fill out a record card.
10. Clean up the work area. Discard all used material and return any unused material and supplies to their proper places. (Figs. 15.13—15.15)

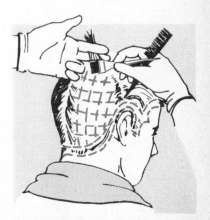

15.15 – Apply tint to each strand, first on the top side and then on the under side.

NOTE: There are many kinds of temporary color rinses. For easy application they are usually prepared in a liquid form. To prepare a correct mixture the manufacturer's directions must be followed.

Applicator Method

The applicator method is very similar to the brush-on method. The only difference is that the tint mixture is applied with the applicator bottle and worked in with the cushion tips of the fingers. (Figs. 15.16, 15.17)

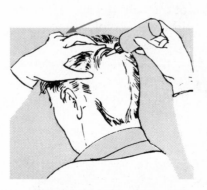 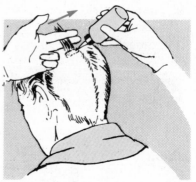

15.16 – Use nozzle of plastic bottle to subdivide section into one-quarter inch strands.

15.17 – Apply tint along strand near the scalp.

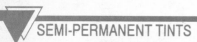

SEMI-PERMANENT TINTS

Semi-permanent tints offer a form of hair coloring suitable for the client who may have been reluctant previously.

A semi-permanent tint fills the gap between a temporary color rinse and a permanent hair color tint, without replacing either of them. Such tints may improve the tone of drab or dull natural hair color without bleaching the hair.

Semi-permanent tints depend on the original color and texture of the hair, the shade used, and length of development time for successful results.

A wide range of colors are available. The results obtained will depend mainly on the original color, as well as the texture of the client's hair. The various shades may be blended to create individual color tones.

There are specifically designed blue-gray or silver-gray shades for hair ranging from 10 percent to 100 percent gray.

Characteristics of Semi-Permanent Tints

1. Semi-permanent tints do not require the addition of hydrogen peroxide.
2. The color is self-penetrating.
3. The color is applied the same way each time.
4. Retouching is eliminated.
5. Color does not rub off, because it has penetrated the hair shaft slightly.
6. Hair will return to its natural color in four to six weeks, provided a mild, non-stripping shampoo is used.
7. Semi-permanent tints require a 24–hour patch test.
8. Some semi-permanent hair colorings require pre-shampooing, others do not.

NOTE: Be guided by your instructor and manufacturer's directions.

Types of Semi-Permanent Tints

Semi-permanent tints are available that cover gray completely but do not affect the remaining pigmented hair. There are also tints that make gray hair more beautifully gray without changing the natural pigment, as well as those that add color and highlights to hair with no gray.

Selecting Color Shades for Semi-Permanent Tints

If the client's hair is slightly sprinkled with gray select a shade that matches the natural hair color. If the hair is 50 percent or more gray select one shade darker.

Implements and Materials

Timer	Cotton
Comb	Color chart
Glass or plastic bowls	Clips
Towels	Tint cape
Applicators:	Protective gloves
Tint brushes	Mild shampoo
Swab sticks	Selected semi-permanent tint
Plastic bottles	Acid or normalizing rinse
Record card	Talcum powder

Preliminary Steps

1. Examine the client's scalp for irritation or abrasion.
2. Give a preliminary patch test 24 hours before tinting.
3. If the patch test is negative, proceed with the tinting after performing a strand test.

Preparation

1. Assemble all necessary supplies.
2. Prepare the client. Protect the clothing with a towel and tint cape.
3. Re-examine the client's scalp.
4. If required, give a mild shampoo.
5. Towel-dry the hair.
6. Put on protective gloves.
7. Give a color strand test.

> **NOTE:** The procedure herein described is one way to apply a semi-permanent hair coloring. However, your instructor may have developed a particular technique that is equally correct.

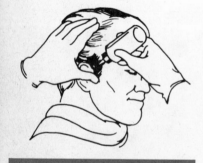

15.18 – Applying tint to sideburn

Procedure

The semi-permanent tint is applied with an applicator bottle to sectioned hair, or applied at the shampoo bowl with a brush or applicator bottle.

1. Apply tint to the temples and sideburn areas. (Fig. 15.18)
2. Apply tint to the hair throughout the scalp area.

3. With the fingers, gently work the color through the hair until it is thoroughly saturated. (Do not massage into the scalp.)
4. If the hair is long, pile it loosely on the top of the head.
5. During color development, be guided by your instructor or the manufacturer's directions as to whether to use a plastic cap covering. (Fig. 15.19)
6. Perform a strand test for color.
7. When the color has developed, wet the hair with warm water, and work up a lather. (Fig. 15.20)
8. Rinse the hair with warm water until the water runs clear.
9. Give an acid or normalizing rinse.
10. Remove stains if necessary
11. Complete the service in the usual manner.
12. Fill out a record card.
13. Clean up. Discard all used material and return any unused material and supplies to their proper places.

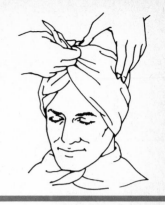

15.19 – Use plastic cap covering, if recommended.

CAUTION: Client should be seated in a reclining position to avoid getting tint in the eyes. If an inclined position is used, the client must hold a towel over the forehead and eyes to protect the eyes from the tint.

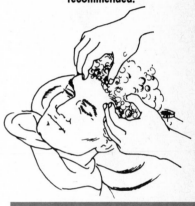

15.20 – Rinse with warm water and work up a lather.

Special Problems

Some semi-permanent hair colorings have a tendency to build up color on the hair shaft with repeated applications. If this should occur follow this procedure for coloring the new growth.

1. Apply the color only to the new growth.
2. Retain until the desired color shade develops.
3. When the color has developed, wet the hair with warm water and blend the color through the hair with a large-toothed comb.

HIGHLIGHTING SHAMPOO TINTS ▽

Highlighting shampoo tints are preparations containing aniline derivative tints combined with hydrogen peroxide and a neutral shampoo base. They are used when a very slight change in hair shade is desired. A 24-hour patch test is required. These tints serve to cleanse the hair and highlight its natural color in a single operation.

Method of Application

The hair is cut before the mixture is evenly distributed over the entire head at the shampoo bowl. Retain from 8 to 15 minutes. Rinse thoroughly.

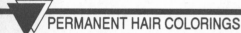

PERMANENT HAIR COLORINGS

Practically all professional permanent hair coloring is done with the use of oxidizing-penetrating tints containing an aniline derivative (a coal tar product).

Penetrating tints may be either single-application or double-application tints.

Single-application tints (cream or liquid) perform two activities: they lighten and add color to the hair in a single application.

Double-application tints (cream or liquid) perform only one activity at a time. For a complete color change or when a toner is desired, they require two separate and distinct applications to the hair:

1. The application of a lightener (bleach) or softener.
2. The application of a tint or toner.

Both tints penetrate the cuticle of the hair to the cortical layer. Here they are oxidized, by the peroxide that has been added, into color pigments that are distributed throughout the hair in much the same manner as the natural pigment.

When the developer (hydrogen peroxide) is mixed with the tint, oxidation begins. For this reason, the tint mixture must be applied immediately to the hair. After the mixture is applied to the hair, the oxidation continues until the color has developed to the desired shade. Timing the development of the applied tint requires a thorough study of the product being used.

Single-Application Tints

Single-application tints provide a simplified method of hair coloring. In one application, the hair can be colored permanently without requiring pre-shampooing, pre-softening, or pre-bleaching. In most instances, single-application tints contain a lightening agent and a shampoo with an oil base, combined with an aniline derivative tint. When ready for use, 20–volume hydrogen peroxide is added in fixed proportions, according to the manufacturer's directions.

A single-application tint is applied on dry hair only. If the hair is extremely soiled and a shampoo is necessary, the hair must be dried thoroughly before applying the tint. The choice of shades varies from deepest black to lightest blond.

Single-application tints:

1. save time by eliminating pre-shampooing or pre-lightening.
2. leave no line of demarcation.
3. color the hair lighter or darker than the client's natural color.
4. blend in gray or white hair to match the client's natural hair shade.
5. tone down streaks, off-shades, discoloration, and faded hair ends.
6. are available as creams, liquids, or gels.

Color Selection
Some general rules for single-application color selection are:

1. To match the natural color of hair and to cover gray, select the color closest to the natural shade.
2. To brighten or lighten hair color and to cover gray, select a shade lighter than the natural color. The selected tint must contain enough color to produce the desired shade on gray hair.
3. To darken the hair and cover gray, select a color darker than the natural hair color.
4. Study the manufacturer's color chart for correct color selections.

CAUTION: The color chart used for a color selection must be from the same manufacturer as the tint product. Each manufacturer's color charts conform to a particular manufacturer's tint products.

Single Application for Virgin Hair

Preliminary

1. Give a patch test 24 hours before tinting.
2. If the patch test is negative and the scalp is normal, without irritation or abrasions, proceed with the color application after giving a strand test.

Materials and Supplies

Materials and supplies are the same as listed previously for semi-permanent tints with the following exception: include permanent tint and 20–volume hydrogen peroxide.

> **NOTE:** Whether a haircut is given before or after a permanent hair coloring application depends mainly on the length of the hair and the preference of the barber-stylist. If the hair is quite long, give the haircut first. However, if the hair is short, cut the hair after the tint application.

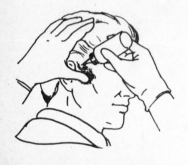

15.21 – Applying tint to sideburns and temples; spread it with thumb. Do not rub.

Preparation

1. Assemble all necessary supplies.
2. Prepare the client. Protect the clothing with a towel and tint cape, since tint can stain clothing permanently.
3. Re-examine the client's scalp.
4. Select the desired shade of color.
5. Give a color strand test.
6. Prepare the formula.
7. Put on protective gloves.

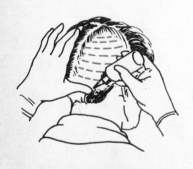

15.22 – Applying tint to nape area; spread it with thumb. Do not rub.

Procedure

1. If the hair is long enough, it may be sectioned into the four standard partings for a tint application. If the hair is short, it may be parted by lifting the hair with the nozzle of the applicator bottle, or with the comb.
2. Apply tint to the grayest areas first, such as temples, sideburns, and the nape area, since these areas usually are more resistant to color. (Figs. 15.21, 15.22)
3. Apply the tint to the scalp area by making one-quarter inch partings. The hair may be lifted with the nozzle tip of the

applicator bottle. Except when tinting longer hair, the tint is applied about one-half inch from the scalp to the ends. After the head has been completely covered, additional tint is applied to the scalp area. Since the scalp area receives the benefit of body heat, the tint in this area processes more quickly. (Fig. 15.23)

4. After the scalp area is completely covered, gently comb or work the tint through the hair shaft until it is thoroughly saturated. Do not massage. (Fig. 15.24)
5. Check for complete coverage. Apply additional tint to areas, if needed.
6. Strand test for color. (Fig. 15.25)
7. Retain the tint on the hair for the required time as indicated by the strand test.
8. When the desired color has developed, rinse with warm water.
9. Give a mild shampoo. (Fig. 15.26)
10. Rinse thoroughly with lukewarm water to remove excess color and shampoo.
11. Remove color stains, if necessary.
12. Dry and comb or style hair as desired.
13. Fill out a record card.
14. Clean up. Discard all used material and return any unused material and supplies to their proper places.

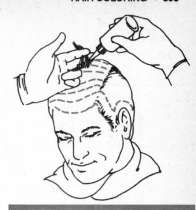

15.23 – Applying tint to the top area and to the sides and back of the head

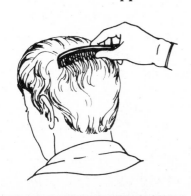

15.24 – Using comb, gently blend tint throughout hair for evenness.

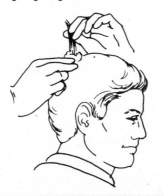

15.25 – Strand testing

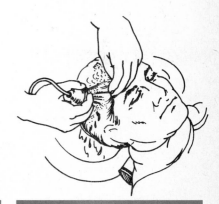

15.26 – Giving a mild shampoo

Single-Application Tint Retouch

For a satisfactory retouch, the barber-stylist must possess a high degree of skill and a uniform method of application. If the retouch

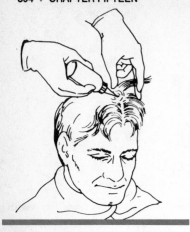

15.27 – Applying tint to new growth

is performed incorrectly, light and dark streaks may appear over the entire head.

Procedure

To retouch the new growth, follow the same preparation as for coloring virgin hair. Refer to the record card for correct color selection and other data.

1. Apply the tint first to new growth at sideburns, temples, and nape area.
2. Rest of head. Apply the tint to new growth in one-quarter inch strands. Do not overlap. Check frequently for color development. (Fig. 15.27)
3. When color has almost developed, dilute the remaining tint by adding a mild shampoo or warm water. Apply and gently work the mixture through the hair with the fingertips. Then comb-blend from the scalp to the hair ends for even distribution.
4. Process for the required time. Rinse with warm water to remove excess color.
5. Give a mild (non-strip) shampoo and rinse thoroughly.
6. Dry and comb, or style hair as desired.
7. Remove color stains, if necessary.
8. Fill out a record card.
9. Clean up in the usual manner.

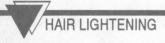

HAIR LIGHTENING

Lightening the hair is usually a preparatory process for the application of a single-action, penetrating tint or toner. A lightening product is used to lighten the hair to the desired shade.

Do not promise a client that dark hair can be lightened to a very pale blond shade if red pigment predominates.

Whatever the reason for lightening, it is important to select the right lightener and the best mixture for the degree of color change desired. To make an intelligent choice, follow the manufacturer's literature and color charts.

Types of Lighteners

Lighteners are classified as oil lighteners, cream lighteners, and powder or paste lighteners.

1. **Oil lighteners** are usually mixtures of hydrogen peroxide with a sulfonated oil.

   a) **Colored oil lighteners** add temporary color and high-light the hair as they lighten. The colors contained are certified and may be used without a patch test. They remove pigment and add color tones at the same time. Basically, they are classified according to their action on the hair, namely:

      1. **Gold**—lightens and adds red highlights.
      2. **Silver**—lightens and adds silvery highlights to gray or white hair and minimizes red and gold tones on other shades.
      3. **Red**—lightens and adds red highlights.
      4. **Drab**—lightens and adds ash highlights. Tones down or reduces red and gold tones.

   b) **Neutral oil lightener** removes pigment without add-ing color tone. It may be used to pre-soften hair for tint application.

2. **Cream lighteners** are the most popular types of lighteners. They are easy to apply and will not run, drip, or dry out. They are easy to control and contain conditioning agents, bluing, and thickener, which provide the following benefits:

   a) The conditioning agents give some protection to the hair.
   b) The bluing agent helps to drab undesirable red and gold tones.
   c) The thickener gives control when applying.

3. **Powder or paste lighteners**, also called quick lighteners, contain an oxygen-releasing booster and inert substances for quicker and stronger action.

   a) Paste lighteners will hold and not run, but will dry out quickly.
   b) Cream lighteners can be controlled to prevent overlap-ping.
   c) Powder lighteners do not contain conditioning agents and may dry the hair and irritate the scalp.

If the scalp shows any sensitivity or abrasions, lighteners are not recommended.

Action of Hair Lighteners

Hair lighteners, depending on the manufacturer's directions, can be used as follows:

1. To lighten the entire head of hair.
2. To lighten the hair to a particular shade.
3. To brighten and lighten the existing shade.
4. To tip, streak, or frost certain parts of the hair.
5. To lighten hair that has already been tinted.
6. To remove undesirable casts and off-shades.
7. To correct dark streaks or spots in hair that has already been lightened or tinted.

Lightening creates a desired color foundation. This new color foundation may be the finished result or it may be the first step of a double-process application. Before beginning the lightening process, it is important to understand that achieving the desired shade requires that you consider not only the virgin hair color, how long the product should be left on to achieve the desired stage of lightening, and the resulting porosity of the hair shaft, but also selection of the appropriate product to achieve the desired color foundation.

CAUTION: A patch test is required only if followed with a toner or tint application.

Choice of Hair Lighteners

Together with manufacturer's directions, be guided by the following general rules:

1. Choose a cream lightener (blue base) when pre-lightening for pastel toners, such as blond, silver, platinum, or beige.
2. Choose a neutral oil lightener for the purpose of lightening the hair without adding color.
3. Choose an oil lightener (drab series) to avoid red and gold highlights in the natural color of the hair.

Hydrogen Peroxide Review

The lightening agent for removing pigment from the hair shaft is hydrogen peroxide. The active ingredient in hydrogen peroxide is oxygen gas, and to speed the liberation of the oxygen gas, a small quantity of 28 percent ammonia water is added. Commercial lightening products now contain substances that modify or prevent a straw-like appearance or reddish or brassy tones in the hair.

Hydrogen peroxide, when properly used, can lighten, soften, and oxidize the hair. For the purpose of hair lightening, it is used as a 6 percent solution, capable of producing 20 volumes of oxygen gas. A weaker strength of peroxide is not suitable for lightening and tinting. The use of a higher strength, even though it may speed up the lightening action, may be harmful to the hair.

Hydrogen peroxide is available in the form of a liquid, cream, powder, or tablet. The liquid peroxide should be purchased in pint sizes, kept closed when not in use and stored in a cool, dark, dry place. Do not permit peroxide to come in contact with metal. When liquid peroxide is kept too long, exposed to air, or stored in a warm place, it will weaken in strength. When using the tablets, powder, or cream, follow the manufacturer's directions.

Uses of Hydrogen Peroxide

As a lightening agent, hydrogen peroxide solution softens the cuticle of the hair shaft, and lightens the shade of the coloring matter in the hair.

Lightening makes the hair porous and lighter in color. The final shade can range from light to golden brown, to gold and pale gold, depending upon the basic color of the hair or the formula of the lightener. Continued use of lighteners will make some hair over-dry and brittle.

As a softening agent, hydrogen peroxide solution softens the cuticle of the hair and makes it more receptive to the penetrating action of an aniline derivative tint. Care must be taken to control the softening process so that the hair is not lightened. It is also used to pre-soften gray hair before applying a toner.

As an oxidizing agent, hydrogen peroxide solution is used in all aniline derivative hair tints. It acts as a developer to liberate oxygen gas which changes para-phenylenediamine into a dark-colored compound capable of tinting the hair.

Preliminary Lightening Strand Test

A preliminary strand test is necessary to judge the length of time to leave any lightening mixture on the hair, and to discover the condition of the hair.

Patch Test for Toners

A patch test must be made 24 hours before a toner is applied. To save the client's time, the strand test for lightening should be done the day of the patch test.

Lightening Virgin Hair

Implements and Materials for Hair Lightening

The procedure of lightening hair may require the use of the following:

Towels	Plastic cape
Shampoo and rinse	Cotton
Comb	Record card
Talcum powder	Peroxide (20 volume)
Lightening agent	Protective gloves
Glass or plastic bowls	Measuring glass or cup
Timer	Applicator bottle (plastic, with measurements listed)

If a paste lightener is to be used, a brush applicator or swab will be needed also.

Procedure for Short Hair

The following instructions for applying lightening products are general guidelines. Always follow the manufacturer's directions.

1. Prepare the client. Adjust a tint cape and towel to cover and protect the client's clothing.
2. Examine the scalp and hair. Do not give a lightening treatment to a client with eruptions or abrasions on the scalp. Do not brush or shampoo hair.
3. Section the hair into four quarters.
4. Put on protective gloves.
5. Prepare lightener and use immediately to prevent deterioration. Carefully follow the manufacturer's directions.

NOTE: The order of applying the lightener around the head is important. If the hair seems resistant or especially dark around the crown, it is advisable to start at the back of the head to allow extra time of contact in this region.

6. Apply lightener in partings of one-eighth of an inch, from the scalp to the hair ends on both the top and underside of the hair strand. Continue to do this until the entire head is completed. For even distribution, gently comb-blend the lightener through the hair. Be sure to keep the hair moist with the lightener during the bleaching process. (Figs. 15.28, 15.29)

7. Test for color. Make the first strand test about 15 minutes before the completion of the time required as indicated by the preliminary strand test. Remove the lightening mixture from the strand with a wet towel or cotton. Dry the strand. If the shade is not light enough, reapply the mixture and continue testing frequently until the desired shade is almost developed.

8. Remove the lightener. When the desired shade is reached, rinse the hair and scalp with cool water and shampoo the hair lightly with a mild shampoo.

9. Dry the hair with a towel or under a cool dryer.

10. Again examine the scalp for abrasions and the hair for breakage. If the scalp and hair are normal, toner may be applied. (Consult the section on toners in this chapter.)

11. Fill out a record card.

12. Clean the shampoo bowl, sanitize all implements, discard any used supplies, and put the work bench in order.

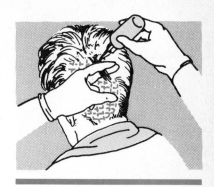

15.28 – Applying lightener to the hair

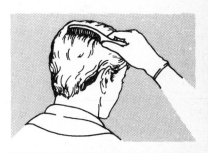

15.29 – Comb-blending lightener through the hair

Procedure for Longer Hair

The procedure for applying a lightener to longer hair is the same as for short hair, with the following variations.

Steps 1 through 5 are the same as for short hair.

6. Apply the lightener in one-eighth inch partings starting about one-half inch from the scalp and extending the lightener to a point where the hair shaft shows signs of damage. Apply lightener to both the top and underside of the hair strand. Continue until the entire head is completed. Work the mixture into the hair with the fingers. Because the lightener makes the hair fragile, do not comb it through the hair. Keep the hair moist with lightener.

7. Test for color. Make the first strand test about 15 minutes before the completion of the time required as indicated by the preliminary test. Remove the mixture from the strand with a wet towel or cotton. Dry the strand. If the shade is not

light enough, reapply the mixture and continue testing frequently until the desired shade is almost developed.

Towel-blot any excess lightener from the hair. If necessary, prepare a fresh mixture of lightener. Using one-eighth inch partings, apply lightener over the entire scalp area, on previously lightened hair, and through the hair ends. Work the lightener through the hair ends with the fingertips. Do not massage the scalp. Retain the lightener on the hair for the required length of time.

Follow steps 8 through 12 of the procedure for short hair.

Lightener Retouch

A lightener retouch is the term commonly used when a lightener is applied only to the new growth of hair from the scalp to match the rest of the lightened hair. Black or dark brown hair requires retouch applications more frequently than all lighter shades. In retouching, the lightener is applied to the new growth only, with the following exceptions:

1. If another color is desired.
2. If a lighter shade is desired.
3. If the color has become heavy or dull from several applications.

For any of these conditions, wait until the new growth is almost light enough or has developed fully. Then bring the remainder of the lightener through the hair shaft. One to five minutes is ample time to correct any of the above conditions.

Retouch Procedure

The client's record card should be consulted as a guide to the lightener used previously and the time required for the shade to develop.

Cream lightener generally is used for a lightener retouch because it prevents the overlapping of the previously lightened hair.

The procedure for a lightener retouch is the same as that for lightening a virgin head, except that the mixture is applied only to the new growth of hair. (Fig. 15.30)

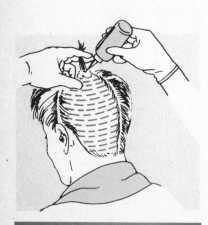

15.30 – Applying lightener to new growth—spread with thumb.

CAUTION: Be careful not to overlap the lightener with the previously lightened or tinted hair. To do so may cause breakage and/or streaks.

Double-Application Tints

Double-application tints (two-process tints) can be used advantageously to achieve a complete color change. These tints require the use of two basic products, each one having a distinct action on the hair. First, a product is used to lighten the hair. Then aniline derivative tint is applied, which colors the hair. A patch test is required. Careful judgment is important in selecting the first shade.

Pre-Lighten or Pre-Soften

When using a double-application tint there is no lightening action. When a color is added to color, the result is a darker shade. Use the following suggestions as a guide to pre-soften or pre-lighten the hair:

1. If the client desires a complete color change to a lighter color, pre-lighten the hair before applying the tint.
2. Pre-soften resistant gray hair before color application.
3. Pre-soften gray hair before a toner application.
4. Pre-lighten the hair to gold or pale yellow before a toner application.

Color Selection for Double-Application Tints

1. If the client's hair is completely gray, select the exact color desired.
2. If the hair is about 50 percent gray, select a color that is one shade lighter.
3. If the hair is about 25 percent gray, select a color that is two to three shades lighter.

Double-Application Tint for Virgin Hair

Preliminary

1. Give a patch test 24 hours before tinting.
2. If the patch test is negative and the scalp is normal, proceed with the color treatment.

Preparation

1. Arrange all necessary supplies.
2. Prepare the client.

3. If the hair is pre-softened, dry it under a cool dryer. If the hair is pre-lightened, shampoo it lightly, rinse it, and dry it thoroughly.
4. Select the desired color.
5. Perform a color strand test.
6. Put on protective gloves.
7. Prepare the formula.

NOTE: For damaged hair or hair ends, first apply filler to these areas to equalize hair porosity.

Procedure

1. Section the hair according to its length. If it is long enough, section it into four quarters.
2. Apply tint to the areas where gray hair is most prevalent. Use a plastic bottle with a nozzle or brush to apply the tint. Hold a strand of one-quarter inch, spread between the index and middle fingers in an upward direction, away from the scalp. Apply tint evenly to both sides of the strand, going from the scalp to the hair ends if the hair is short, and from the scalp to within one-half to one inch of the hair ends, if the hair is longer. When all sections have been treated, check for complete coverage and apply more tint where needed. Allow the tint to remain on the hair for the required length of time, which can be judged by frequent strand tests.
3. When performing a strand test, wet a small piece of cotton with soap and water or shampoo. Wring out some of the moisture. Select a section of hair where the tint was applied first or where gray hair was most evident. Remove the tint with wet cotton. If the desired shade has not been reached, re-moisten this strand of hair with the tint, and leave it on for another five to ten minutes. Then test again for color.

NOTE: It is impossible to give definite instructions as to the length of time required for color development, since this will vary depending on the product used and the porosity of the hair.

---

4. Apply tint to the hair ends. After the developing time has almost elapsed, distribute the tint through the hair ends using a large-tooth comb or fingers. For damaged hair ends, apply color filler before the tint application or mix the filler with the remaining tint and apply it to the hair ends.
5. Rinse the hair. Spray it thoroughly with water using a strong force. This serves to set the color and remove all excess tint from the hair.
6. Remove any stains with commercial tint remover or cream.
7. Shampoo the hair with a mild shampoo and rinse it thoroughly.
8. Give a neutral rinse.
9. Set, dry, and style the hair.
10. Fill out the record card.
11. Clean up in the usual manner.

Double-Application Tint Retouch

To match the color for a retouch application, consult the client's record card. The preparation is the same as for tinting virgin hair.

Procedure

1. Section the hair into four quarters.
2. Outline the partings with tint and then apply tint to the section where the softener or lightener was last applied.
3. Subdivide one section at a time into one-quarter inch strands. Hold the hair upward and away from the scalp and apply color along the part.
4. Distribute the color evenly along the part, out to the previously tinted hair, being careful not to overlap the previously tinted hair.
5. Take frequent strand tests.
6. When the desired color has developed, be guided by your instructor as to diluting the remainder of tint with warm water, to be applied to the hair shaft.
7. After the color has been distributed through the hair ends, check the development frequently until the new growth and hair shaft are the same color.
8. Rinse thoroughly, to remove all excess color.
9. Remove any stains from the hairline, ears, and neck.
10. Shampoo the hair with mild shampoo and rinse it thoroughly.

11. Complete the service in the usual manner.
12. Fill out the record card.
13. Clean up in the usual manner.

Keep Up To Date

Manufacturers are constantly improving and developing new hair coloring products. Be sure to attend seminars and trade shows as often as possible to keep abreast of such changes.

Toners

Double-Application Method

Toners are aniline derivative tints. They consist primarily of pale, delicate colors.

Toners are applied in the same manner as double-application tints. Most of them require a patch test.

Pre-Lightening for Toners

Pre-lightening is required for color effect. Hair should be pre-lightened to gold or pale yellow, depending on the color to be used. Toners penetrate and deposit color in the same manner as other tints. They are dependent upon the preliminary lightening, which must leave the hair both light and porous. Some toners, especially the extreme pale shades, require more pre-lightening than others. In addition, the lightener must be kept on long enough to achieve the desired porosity. Coarse, resistant, or dark hair requires a longer lightening time than naturally blond hair.

Although naturally blond hair may reach the pale yellow stage very quickly, it may not be porous enough to retain a toner.

White or gray hair requires a certain amount of pre-lightening to increase porosity. Since white or gray hair is almost colorless, it needs pre-lightening before the application of a blond, silver, or pastel shade toner. When gray hair is a mixture of light and dark strands, pre-lightening is especially important, although lengthy lightening will not be necessary.

Choosing Toner Shades

Pastel colors, such as silver, ash, platinum, and beige, are usually considered to be in good taste. For the client who wants extremely light hair, blond colors are a good choice. For gray hair and skin tone changes that accompany advancing years, the lighter silver tones are becoming. For extremely pale toner shades such as very light silver, platinum, or beige, the hair must be pre-bleached to pale yellow or almost white.

Age and complexion should be considered when choosing the color tone to be used.

Toning of Men's Hair

Pre-lighten the hair before applying the toner. After the client has been properly prepared, proceed as follows:

1. Apply a suitable toner shade.
2. When the hair is completely covered, distribute the toner with the fingertips. Do not comb it through the hair.
3. Leave the toner on the hair for the length of time indicated by the strand test.
4. Rinse with cool water.
5. Cleanse the hair lightly with a non-strip shampoo.
6. Apply a cool water rinse again to the hair.
7. Style the client's hair as desired.

Toner Retouch

A toner retouch must be given the same careful consideration as you would give a two-color tint retouch application. The new growth must be pre-lightened to the same degree of lightness as was given in the first toner application. The lightener is applied to the new growth only. To overlap the lightener on previously lightened hair will damage it.

After the lightening process has been completed, the toner is applied to the entire length of the hair in the usual manner.

Suggestions and Reminders

Toners are completely dependent upon the proper preliminary lightening treatment, which must leave the hair light and porous enough to receive the pale toner shades. A strand test should be made first, and a complete explanation as to the possible outcome given the client.

It is always possible that the hair cannot be decolorized sufficiently for the color choice without serious damage resulting. If red or gold pigment is not eliminated during lightening, the use of toner color can result in a greenish cast, or the color may not take at all. When this happens, the shade of toner used must be deeper.

During the application and development period, toner colors are quite different from the final shade. For instance, ash blond will appear somewhat brown; silver blond will have a bluish cast; and platinum will appear violet.

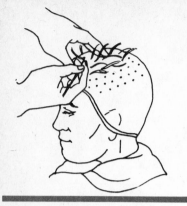

15.31 – Drawing strands with crochet hook

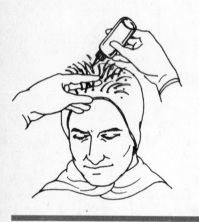

15.32 – Applying lightener

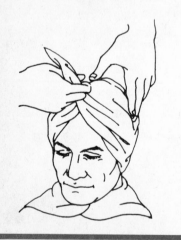

15.33 – Covering head with aluminum foil or plastic cap to hasten the process

Frosting, Tipping, and Streaking

For partial lightening, such as frosting, tipping, and streaking, quick lighteners are often advisable.

1. **Frosting.** Strands of hair are lightened over various parts of the head, using a perforated cap in order to protect the scalp. Strands of hair are pulled through the holes in the cap. The effect achieved will depend on where and how many strands of hair are treated.
2. **Tipping** is similar to frosting. Wisps of hair are lightened in various areas, usually across the front of the head. This produces a contrast with the darker shade of hair. The strands of hair are drawn through the holes in a perforated cap.
3. **Streaking.** This is a lightened strand, usually at the front hairline. The width and placement of the lightened strand depend on the feather effect to be achieved.

Cap Technique for Frosting or Tipping

1. Shampoo and dry the hair.
2. Comb the hair gently.
3. Adjust a perforated cap over the head.
4. Draw strands of hair through the holes with crochet hook. (Fig. 15.31)
5. Apply the lightener. (Fig. 15.32)
6. To hasten the process, cover the head with aluminum foil or a plastic cap. (Fig. 15.33)
7. When the hair is sufficiently lightened, remove the aluminum foil or plastic cap.
8. With the perforated cap still on, shampoo or rinse off the lightener. Towel dry.
9. Apply toner in the usual manner.
10. Style the hair as desired.

Foil Technique

Another method of adding color highlights to hair is a foil technique. This involves weaving out (taking alternating strands from a subsection) small strands of hair from a subsection. The selected strands are then placed over foil or plastic wrap, and the appropriate lightener or high-lift tint is applied. The foil is folded to prevent lifting any unwoven hair and processed as desired. With this technique, the colorist can strategically place highlights.

> **NOTE:** A lamp or dryer may be used to speed up and even out the lightening process, whenever an off-the-scalp procedure is used.

Special Problems in Hair Tinting and Lightening

Fillers

Fillers are preparations that are available in liquid or cream form. They are employed to revitalize, recondition, and correct abused, lightened, tinted, or damaged hair. There are two general classifications of fillers: conditioner fillers, which are colorless; and color fillers, which range in shades from pale blue to deep brown.

When to Use a Color Filler

If the hair is damaged, and if there is any doubt that the finished color will be an even shade, a color filler is recommended. A filler is applied after the hair has been pre-lightened and before the application of a toner or tint. A filler is also used for clients who have tinted or lightened hair and desire to return it to the natural color. Color fillers have the ability to:

1. deposit color to faded hair shafts and ends;
2. help hair to hold color;
3. help to ensure a uniform color from the scalp to the hair ends;
4. prevent color streaking;
5. prevent off-color results;
6. prevent dullness;
7. give more uniform color in a tint back to the natural shade.

How to Use Color Fillers

Color fillers may be used directly from the containers to damaged hair prior to tinting, or they may be added to the remainder of the tint and applied to damaged hair ends. To obtain satisfactory results, select the color filler to match the same basic shade as the toner or tint to be used.

Reconditioning Damaged Hair

The frequent use of compound henna and metallic dyes coats and damages the hair. Hair in this state must be reconditioned before it can successfully be tinted or lightened. Careless application by the barber-stylist of tinting or lightening agents to the hair may result in breakage or a dry, brittle condition. The use of highly alkaline shampoos or soapless oil shampoos, the improper use of water temperature and hair dryers, or extreme exposure to the elements also may cause hair to become damaged.

Hair may need reconditioning for reasons other than damage resulting from the use of harmful products. Sometimes hair is naturally brittle, thin, and lifeless. Both neglect and the client's physical condition may contribute to these conditions.

Hair is considered damaged when it:

1. is over-porous.
2. is brittle and dry.
3. breaks easily.
4. has lost its elasticity.
5. is rough and harsh to the touch.
6. is spongy and mats easily when wetted.
7. rejects color or absorbs too much color during a tinting process.

Any of these hair conditions may create trouble during a tinting or lightening treatment. Therefore, damaged hair should receive reconditioning treatments prior to and after the application of these chemical agents.

Reconditioning Treatment

To restore damaged hair to a more normal condition, commercial products containing lanolin or protein substances should be used. The reconditioning agent is applied to the hair. If heat is applied, use a heating cap, a steamer, or a heating lamp according to the manufacturer's directions. As to the frequency and length of time for each treatment, be guided by your instructor.

Tint Back to Natural Color

Each tint back to natural color must be handled as an individual situation. The determining factors in the selection of the tint shade are the present condition and color of the hair, the final result desired, and the original color. Check the natural shade of the hair next to the scalp.

Select an appropriate shade of filler to correspond with the tint to be used. Without the use of an appropriate filler, it will be difficult to obtain a uniform color from the scalp to hair ends, since hair porosity will vary in degree and area.

Such hair coloring problems require two or more strand tests.

Lightening Streaked Hair

Streaks of discoloration may appear on the hair caused by unsuccessful or unskilled lightener applications.

To correct streaked hair:

1. Prepare the lightening formula as for virgin hair.
2. Apply the mixture only to the darker streaks.
3. Work one strand at a time.
4. Allow the mixture to remain until all the streaks are removed.
5. Shampoo the hair.

COLORING MUSTACHES AND BEARDS

Mustaches

An aniline derivative tint should never be used for coloring mustaches; to do so may cause serious irritation or damage to the delicate membrane in the nostrils and the lips. Harmless commercial products are available to color mustaches.

> **NOTE:** The procedure given here is one way to apply hair coloring to mustaches and beards. Your instructor may use a different technique that is equally correct.

Harmless Commercial Products

1. **Crayons** are sticks that come in several colors: blond, medium and dark brown, black, and auburn. The end of the stick, used like a pencil, is applied by rubbing it directly on the mustache until the desired shade is reached.

CAUTION: To avoid staining the skin, a fine-toothed comb may be inserted in the mustache, close to the skin. Then the end of the stick is rubbed on the mustache.

2. **Pomade in tubes**, consisting of harmless ingredients, is formulated specifically for coloring mustaches. It comes in the following shades: black, brown, blond, chatain (chestnut), and white (neutral). The pomade is applied to the mustache with a small brush and is stroked from the nostrils downward until full coverage is achieved.

    Waxing. The pomade also contains a wax ingredient. When the outer ends of the mustache are rolled or twisted, they will remain in that position until the pomade is removed.

3. **Two-bottle set solutions** also are available for coloring mustaches. The choice of colors is limited to brown and black.

CAUTION: Never shave around the mustache immediately before or after the color application. To do so may cause the product to irritate shaved areas.

Implements and Supplies

Petroleum jelly

Stain remover

Cotton

Coloring solutions (No. 1 and No. 2)

Towels

Applicator sticks

Procedure

1. Place the client in a comfortable position.
2. Place a clean towel across the chest.
3. Wash the mustache with warm, soapy water.
4. Apply petroleum jelly around the mustache and on the edge of the upper lip.
5. Apply solution No. 1. Remove the cap and moisten a cotton-tipped applicator in the solution. Touch the tip of the applicator to a towel to remove excess moisture. Apply the solution to the mustache, moistening it completely. Replace

the cap on bottle No. 1. Discard the applicator immediately. Moisten a fresh cotton-tipped applicator with stain remover and place it on the edge of a towel for future use. Replace the cap on the stain remover bottle.

6. Apply solution No. 2 to the mustache in the same manner as solution No. 1. If the skin becomes stained, use stain remover immediately. Replace the cap on bottle No. 2.
7. Wash the mustache with soap and cool water.
8. Remove any stains with stain remover. Replace the bottle cap.
9. Style the mustache as desired.
10. Clean up in the usual manner.

Beards

The same products that are used for coloring mustaches may be used to color beards.

1. **Crayons.** For even distribution and to avoid staining the skin, crayon should be applied to the beard while holding the hair with a fine-toothed comb.
2. **Pomade.** The pomade is applied with a small brush to particular areas of the beard held with a fine-toothed comb. Combing the hair with the comb will distribute the pomade evenly and avoid staining the skin.
3. **Liquid.** The liquid form may also be used to color beards. The procedure is the same as for coloring mustaches.

SAFETY MEASURES IN HAIR COLORING

Hair Tinting

1. Make a 24–hour patch test before the application of a tint or toner.
2. Examine the scalp before applying a tint.
3. Do not apply tint if abrasions are present on the scalp.
4. Use only sanitized swabs, brushes, applicator bottles, combs, and linens.
5. Always wash your hands before and after serving a client.
6. Do not brush the hair prior to a tint.
7. Do not apply a tint without reading the manufacturer's directions.

8. Make a strand test for color, breakage, and/or hair discoloration.
9. Choose a shade of tint that harmonizes with the general complexion.
10. Use an applicator bottle or bowl (plastic or glass) for mixing the tint.
11. Do not mix tint before ready for use; discard leftover tint.
12. If required, use the correct shade of color filler.
13. Make frequent strand tests until the desired shade is reached.
14. Suggest a reconditioning treatment for tinted hair.
15. Do not apply tint if metallic or compound dye is present.
16. Do not apply tint if a patch test is positive.
17. Give a strand test for the correct color shade before applying tint.
18. Do not use an alkaline or harsh shampoo for tint removal.
19. Do not use water that is too hot for removing tint.
20. Protect the client's clothing by proper draping.
21. Do not permit tint to come in contact with the client's eyes.
22. Do not overlap during a tint retouch.
23. Do not neglect to fill out a tint record card.
24. Do not apply hydrogen peroxide or any material containing hydrogen peroxide directly over dyes known or believed to contain a metallic salt. Breakage or complete disintegration of the hair may result.
25. Wear protective gloves.

Hair Lightening

1. Analyze the condition of the hair and suggest reconditioning treatments, if required.
2. When working with a cream or paste lightener, it must be the thickness of whipped cream to avoid dripping or running, causing overlapping.
3. Apply lightener to resistant areas first. Pick up one-eighth inch sections when applying lightener. This will ensure complete coverage.
4. Make frequent strand tests until the desired shade is reached.
5. After completing the lightener application, check the skin and remove any lightener from these areas.
6. Check the towel around the client's neck. Lightener on the

towel that is allowed to come in contact with the skin will cause irritation.

7. Lightened hair is fragile and requires special care. Use only a very mild shampoo, and cool water for rinsing.
8. If a preliminary shampoo is necessary, comb the hair carefully. Avoid irritating the scalp during the shampoo or when combing the hair.
9. Work as rapidly as possible when applying the lightener to produce a uniform shade without streaking.
10. Never allow lightener to stand; use it immediately.
11. Cap all bottles to avoid loss of strength.
12. Keep a completed record card of all lightening treatments.

HAIR COLORING GLOSSARY

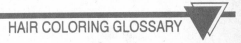

accelerator: (See *activator*)

accent color: A concentrated color product that can be added to permanent, semi-permanent, or temporary hair color to intensify or tone down the color. Another word for concentrate.

acid: An aqueous (water-based) solution having a pH less than 7.0 on the pH scale.

activator: An additive used to quicken the action or progress of a chemical. Another word for booster, accelerator, protenator, or catalyst.

alkaline: An aqueous (water-based) solution having a pH greater than 7.0 on the pH scale. The opposite of acid.

allergy: A reaction due to extreme sensitivity to certain foods or chemicals.

allergy test: A test to determine the possibility or degree of sensitivity, also known as a patch test, predisposition test, or skin test.

amino acids: The group of molecules that the body uses to synthesize protein. There are some 22 different amino acids found in living protein that serve as units of structure in protein.

ammonia: A colorless pungent gas composed of hydrogen and nitrogen; in water solution it is called ammonia water. Used in hair color to swell the cuticle. When mixed with hydrogen peroxide, activates the oxidation process on melanin and allows the melanin to decolorize.

ammonium hydroxide: An alkaline solution of ammonia in water, commonly used in the manufacture of permanent hair color, lightener preparations, and hair relaxers.

analysis (hair): An examination of the hair to determine its condition and natural color. (See *consultation; condition*)

aqueous: Descriptive term for water solution or any medium that is largely composed of water.

ash: A tone or shade dominated by greens, blues, violets, or grays. May be used to counteract unwanted warm tones.

base (alkali): (See *pH alkaline*)

base color: (See *color base*)

bleeding: Seepage of tint/lightener from foil or cap due to improper application.

blending: A merging of one tint or tone with another.

blonding: A term applied to lightening the hair.

bonds: The means by which atoms are joined together to make molecules.

booster: (See *activator*)

brassy tone: Red, orange, or gold tones in the hair.

breakage: A condition in which hair splits and breaks off.

build-up: Repeated coatings on the hair shaft.

catalyst: A substance used to alter the speed of a chemical reaction.

caustic: Strongly alkaline materials. At very high pH levels, can burn or destroy protein or tissue by chemical action.

certified color: A color that meets certain standards for purity and is certified by the FDA.

cetyl alcohol: Fatty alcohol used as an emollient. It is also used as a stabilizer for emulsion systems and in hair color and cream developer as a thickener.

chelating stabilizer: A molecule that binds metal ions and renders them inactive.

chemical change: Alteration in the chemical composition of a substance.

citric acid: Organic acid derived from citrus fruits and used for pH adjustment. Primarily used to adjust the acid-alkali balance. Has some antioxidant and preservative qualities. Used medicinally as a mild astringent.

coating: Residue left on the outside of the hair shaft.

color: Visual sensation caused by light.

color additive: (See *accent color*)

color base: The combination of dyes that make up the tonal foundation of a specific hair color.

color lift: The amount of change natural or artificial pigment undergoes when lightened by a substance.

color mixing: Combining two or more shades together for a custom color.

color refresher: 1. Color applied to mid-shaft and ends to give a more uniform color appearance to the hair. 2. Color applied by a shampoo-in method to enhance the natural color. Also called *color wash, color enhancer.*

color remover: A product designed to remove artificial pigment from the hair.

color test: The process of removing product from a hair strand to monitor the progress of color development during tinting or lightening.

color wheel: The arrangement of primary, secondary, and tertiary colors in the order of their relationships to each other. A tool for formulating.

complementary colors: A primary and secondary color positioned opposite each other on the color wheel. When these two colors are combined, they create a neutral color. Combinations are as follows: blue/orange, red/green, yellow/violet.

concentrate: (See *accent color*)

condition: The existing state of the hair: elasticity, strength, texture, porosity, and evidence of previous treatments.

consultation: Verbal communication with a client to determine desired result. [See *analysis (hair)*]

contributing pigment: The current level and tone of the hair; refers to both natural contributing pigment and decolorized (or lightened) contributing pigment. (See *undertone*)

cool tones: (See *ash*)

corrective coloring: The process of correcting an undesirable color.

cortex: The second layer of hair. A fibrous protein core of the hair fiber containing melanin pigment.

coverage: Reference to the ability of a color product to cover gray, white, or other colors of hair.

cuticle: The translucent protein outer layer of the hair fiber.

cysteic acid: A chemical substance in the hair fiber, produced by the interaction of hydrogen peroxide on the disulfide bond (cystine).

cysteine: The disulfide amino acid that joins protein chains together.

D & C colors: Colors selected from a certified list approved by the U.S. Food and Drug Administration for use in drug and cosmetic products.

decolorize: A chemical process involving the lightening of the natural color pigment or artificial color from the hair.

degree: Term used to describe various units of measurement.

dense: Thick, compact, or crowded.

deposit: Describes the color product in terms of its ability to add color pigment to the hair. Color added equals deposit.

deposit-only color: A category of color products between permanent and semi-permanent colors. Formulated to only deposit color, not lift. They contain oxidation dyes and utilize low-volume developer.

depth: The lightness or darkness of a specific hair color. (See *value; level*)

developer: An oxidizing agent, usually hydrogen peroxide, that reacts chemically with coloring material to develop color molecules and create a change in natural hair color.

development time (oxidation period): The time required for a permanent color or lightener to completely develop.

diffused: Broken down, scattered; not limited to one spot.

direct dye: A pre-formed color that dyes the fiber directly without the need for oxidation.

discoloration: The development of undesired shades through chemical reaction.

double process: A technique requiring two separate procedures in which the hair is decolorized or pre-lightened with a lightener before the depositing color is applied.

drab: Term used to describe hair color shades containing no red or gold. (See *ash; dull*)

drabber: Concentrated color, used to reduce red or gold highlights.

dull: A word used to describe hair or hair color without sheen.

dye: Artificial pigment.

dye intermediate: A material that develops into color only after reaction with developer (hydrogen peroxide). Also known as oxidation dyes.

dye solvents or **dye remover:** (See *color remover*)

dye stock: (See *color base*)

elasticity: The ability of the hair to stretch and return to normal.

enzyme: A protein molecule found in living cells that initiates a chemical process.

fade: To lose color through exposure to the elements or other factors.

fillers: 1. Color product used as a color refresher or to fill damaged hair in preparation for hair coloring. 2. Any liquid-like substance to help fill a void. (See *color refresher*)

formulas: Mixtures of two or more ingredients.

formulate: The art of mixing to create a blend or balance of two or more ingredients.

gray hair: Hair with decreasing amounts of natural pigment. Hair with no natural pigment is actually white. White hairs look gray when mingled with the still pigmented hair.

hair: A slender, thread-like outgrowth of the skin of the head and body.

hair root: That part of the hair contained within the follicle, below the surface of the scalp.

hair shaft: Visible part of each strand of hair. It is made up of an outer layer called the cuticle, an innermost layer called the medulla, and an in-between layer called the cortex. The cortex layer is where color changes are made.

hard water: Water that contains minerals and metallic salts as impurities.

henna: A plant-extracted coloring that produces bright shades of red. The active ingredient is lawsone. Henna permanently colors the hair by coating and penetrating the hair shaft. (See *progressive dye*)

high lift tinting: A single-process color treatment with a higher degree of lightening action and a minimal amount of color deposit.

highlighting: The introduction of a lighter color in small, selected sections to increase lightness of hair. Generally not strongly contrasting from the natural color.

hydrogen peroxide: An oxidizing chemical made up of two parts hydrogen, two parts oxygen (H_2O_2), used to aid the processing of permanent hair color and lighteners. Also referred to as a developer, available in liquid or cream.

level: A unit of measurement, used to evaluate the lightness or darkness of a color, excluding tone.

level system: In hair coloring, a system colorists use to analyze the lightness or darkness of a hair color.

lift: The lightening action of a hair color or lightening product on the hair's natural pigment.

lightener: The chemical compound that lightens the hair by dispersing, dissolving, and decolorizing the natural hair pigment. (See *pre-lighten*)

lightening: (See *decolorize*)

line of demarcation: An obvious difference between two colors on the hair shaft.

litmus paper: A chemically treated paper used to test the acidity or alkalinity of products.

medulla: The center structure of the hair shaft. Very little is known about its actual function.

melanin: The tiny grains of pigment in the hair cortex that create natural hair color.

melanocytes: Cells in the hair bulb that manufacture melanin.

melanoprotein: The protein coating of a melanosome.

melanosome: Protein-coated granule containing melanin.

metallic dyes: Soluble metal salts such as lead, silver, and bismuth that produce colors on the hair fiber by progressive build-up and exposure to air.

modifier: A chemical found as an ingredient in permanent hair colors. Its function is to alter the dye intermediates.

molecule: Two or more atoms chemically joined together; the smallest part of a compound.

neutral: 1. A color balanced between warm and cool, which does not reflect a highlight of any primary or secondary color. 2. Also refers to a pH of seven.

neutralization: The process that counterbalances or cancels the action of an agent or color.

neutralize: Render neutral; counterbalance of action or influence. (See *neutral*)

new growth: The part of the hair shaft that is between previously chemically treated hair and the scalp.

nonalkaline: (See *acid*)

off the scalp lightener: A liquid, cream, or gel form of lightener that can be used directly on the scalp.

opaque: Allowing no light to shine through.

outgrowth: (See *new growth*)

overlap: Occurs when the application of color or lightener goes beyond the line of demarcation.

over-porosity: The condition where hair reaches an undesirable stage of porosity requiring correction.

oxidation: 1. The reaction of dye intermediates with hydrogen peroxide found in hair coloring developers. 2. The interaction of hydrogen peroxide on the natural pigment.

oxidative hair color: A product containing oxidation dyes that require hydrogen peroxide to develop the permanent color.

para tint: A tint made from oxidation dyes.

para-phenylenediamine: An oxidation dye used in most permanent hair colors, often abbreviated as P.P.D.

patch test: A test required by the Food and Drug Act. Made by applying a small amount of the hair coloring preparation to the skin of the arm or behind the ear to determine possible allergies (hypersensitivity). Also called predisposition or skin test.

penetrating color: Color that enters or penetrates the cortex or second layer of the hair shaft.

permanent color: 1. Hair color products that do not wash out by shampooing. 2. A category of hair color products mixed with developer that create a lasting color change.

peroxide: (See *hydrogen peroxide*)

peroxide residue: Traces of peroxide left in the hair after treatment with lightener or tint.

persulfate: In hair coloring, a chemical ingredient commonly used in activators. It increases the speed of the decolorization process. (See *activator*)

pH: The quantity that expresses the acid/alkali balance. A pH of seven is the neutral value for pure water. Any pH below seven is acidic; any pH above seven is alkaline. The skin is mildly acidic and generally in the pH 4.5 to 5.5 range.

pH scale: A numerical scale from zero (very acid) to 14 (very alkaline); used to describe the degree of acidity or alkalinity.

pigment: Any substance or matter used as coloring; natural or artificial color.

porosity: Ability of the hair to absorb water or other liquids.

powder lightener: (See *off the scalp lightener*)

pre-bleaching: (See *pre-lighten*)

predisposition test: (See *patch test*)

pre-lighten: Generally the first step of double-process hair coloring, used to lift or lighten the natural pigment. (See *decolorize*)

pre-soften: The process of treating gray or very resistant hair to allow for better penetration of color.

primary colors: Pigments or colors that are fundamental and cannot be made by mixing colors together. Red, yellow, and blue are the primary colors.

prism: A transparent glass or crystal solid that breaks up white light into its component colors of the spectrum.

processing time: The time required for the chemical treatment to react on the hair.

progressive dyes or **progressive dye system:** 1. A coloring system that produces increased absorption with each application. 2. Color products that deepen or increase absorption over a period of time during processing.

regrowth: (See *new growth*)

resistant hair: Hair that is difficult to penetrate with moisture or chemical solutions.

retouch: Application of color or lightening mixture to new growth of hair.

salt and pepper: The descriptive term for a mixture of dark and gray or white hair.

secondary color: Colors made by combining two primary colors in equal proportion; green, orange, and violet are secondary colors.

semi-permanent hair coloring: Hair coloring that lasts through several shampoos. It penetrates the hair shaft and stains the cuticle layer, slowly diffusing out with each shampoo.

sensitivity: A skin highly reactive to the presence of a specific chemical. Skin reddens or becomes irritated shortly after application of the chemical. On removal of the chemical, the reaction subsides.

shade: 1. A term used to describe a specific color. 2. The visible difference between two colors.

sheen: The ability of the hair to shine, gleam, or reflect light.

single-process color: Refers to an oxidative tint solution that lifts or lightens while also depositing color in one application. (See *oxidative hair color*)

soap cap: The application of a tint diluted with a shampoo and worked through the hair like shampoo.

softening agent: A mild alkaline product applied prior to the color treatment, to increase porosity, swell the cuticle layer of the hair, and increase color absorption. Tint that has not been mixed with developer is frequently used. (See *pre-soften*)

solution: A blended mixture of solid, liquid, or gaseous substances in a liquid medium.

solvent: Carrier liquid in which other components may be dissolved.

specialist: One who concentrates on only one part or branch of a subject or profession.

spectrum: The series of colored bands refracted and arranged in the order of their wave lengths by the passage of white light through a prism. Shading continuously from red (produced by the longest wave visible) to violet (produced by the shortest): red, orange, yellow, green, blue, indigo, and violet.

spot lightening: Color correcting using a lightening mixture to lighten darker areas.

spot tinting: Application of a tint to areas insufficiently colored in order to produce even results throughout.

stabilizer: General name for ingredient that prolongs lifetime, appearance, and performance of a product.

stage: A term used to describe a visible color change that natural hair color goes through while being lightened.

stain remover: Chemical used to remove tint stains from skin.

strand test: Test given before treatment to determine development time, color result, and the ability of the hair to withstand the effects of chemicals.

stripping: (See *color remover*)

surfactant: A short way of saying surface active agent. A molecule that is composed of an oil-loving (oleophilic) part and a water-loving (hydrophilic) part. They act as a bridge to allow oil and water to mix. Wetting agents, emulsifiers, cleansers, solubilizers, dispersing aids, and thickeners are usually surfactants.

tablespoon: One-half of an ounce, three teaspoons, 15 milliliters.

teaspoon: One-sixth of an ounce, one-third of a tablespoon, five milliliters.

temporary coloring or **temporary rinses:** Color made from pre-formed dyes that are applied to the hair, but are readily removed with shampoo.

terminology: The special words or terms used in science, art, or business.

tertiary colors: The mixture of a primary and an adjacent secondary color on the color wheel. Red-orange, yellow-orange, yellow-green, blue-green, blue-violet, red-violet. Also referred to as inter-mediary colors.

texture, hair: The diameter of an individual hair strand. Termed: coarse, medium, or fine.

tint: Permanent oxidizing hair color product having the ability to lift and deposit color in the same process.

tint back: To return hair back to its original or natural color.

tone: A term used to describe the warmth or coolness in color.

toner: A pastel color to be used after pre-lightening.

toning: Adding color to modify the end result.

touch-up: (See *retouch*)

translucent: The property of letting diffused light pass through.

tyrosinase: The enzyme (tyrosinase) that reacts together with the amino acid (tyrosine) to form the hair's natural melanin.

tyrosine: The amino acid (tyrosine) that reacts together with the enzyme (tyrosinase) to form the hair's natural melanin.

undertone: The underlying color that emerges during the lifting process of melanin, which contributes to the end result. When lightening hair, a residual warmth in tone always occurs.

urea peroxide: A peroxide compound occasionally used in hair color. When added to an alkaline color mixture, it releases oxygen.

value: (See *level; depth*)

vegetable color: A color derived from plant sources.

virgin hair: Natural hair that has not undergone any chemical or physical abuse.

viscosity: A term referring to the thickness of the solution.

volume: The concentration of hydrogen peroxide in water solution. Expressed as volumes of oxygen liberated per volume of solution, 20 volume peroxide would thus liberate 20 pints (9.4 liters) of oxygen gas for each pint (liter) of solution.

warm: Containing red, orange, yellow, or gold tones.

REVIEW QUESTIONS

Hair Coloring

1. Define hair tinting.
2. Give three reasons why a client may wish to have the hair tinted.
3. What three points should a barber-stylist know in order to be successful in the technique of hair coloring?
4. Define a virgin head of hair.
5. What are the three main groups of hair coloring?
6. List three temporary hair colorings.
7. For how long are semi-permanent hair tints designed?
8. List four types of permanent hair colorings.
9. What are aniline derivative tints?
10. State two reasons why aniline derivative tints require a 24–hour patch test.
11. Briefly describe the action of aniline derivative tints.
12. How is a skin test given for permanent tints?
13. In giving a patch test for a semi-permanent tint, how does the procedure differ from that given for a permanent tint?
14. How is a positive skin reaction recognized?
15. What are two very important factors to consider when selecting a color shade?
16. Why should a preliminary strand test be given before the application of a tint?
17. List four conditions that would prohibit the application of an aniline derivative tint.
18. Why should an accurate record of each hair coloring treatment be kept?
19. What can be used to lighten and deposit color in the hair in one tint application?
20. List three advantages of single-application tints.
21. List three important points to remember when using a double-application penetrating tint.
22. What are two purposes of highlighting shampoo tints?
23. When is pre-lightening required?
24. When is pre-softening required?

25. Why is the hair not massaged vigorously prior to a tinting treatment?
26. What type of dyes are never used professionally?
27. List four characteristics of semi-permanent tints.
28. List two reasons for using a temporary color rinse.
29. How are tint stains removed from the skin and scalp?
30. In a retouch, to which part of the hair is a permanent tint applied?

Hair Lightening

1. Define hair lightening.
2. List three types of commercial lighteners.
3. What agent is used for lightening pigment in the hair shaft?
4. What strength hydrogen peroxide is commonly used?
5. Why do lightening products contain small quantities of 28 percent ammonia water?
6. When used as a softening agent, what reaction does hydrogen peroxide have on the hair?
7. List the two important reasons for a preliminary strand test prior to lightening the hair.
8. Why is a patch test required prior to a toner application?
9. What are three causes for over-lightened hair?
10. To which part of the hair is a lightener retouch applied?
11. Why should cool water be used during the shampoo following hair lightening?
12. What effects do lightening products have on the hair?
13. Define the word *toners*.
14. How are toners applied?
15. Why does white or gray hair require some pre-lightening prior to application of a toner?
16. On what parts of the hair shaft are frosting, tipping, and streaking usually applied?

Miscellaneous

1. Why should lightened hair receive corrective treatment?
2. What purposes are served by conditioner fillers?
3. Name two types of fillers.
4. List two reasons for using a color filler.
5. What kind of hair treatment may be used to prevent porous areas of the hair shaft from absorbing too much tint?
6. List two methods by which tint may be removed from the hair.
7. Each color removing treatment must be handled as an _____problem.
8. Why must the tint remover be rinsed thoroughly from the hair?
9. List three precautionary measures to follow when tinting hair back to its natural shade.

Coloring Mustaches and Beards

10. Briefly define the following terms: a) color filler; b) coating; c) dye removal; d) oxidation.

1. What kind of tint should never be used to color mustaches? Give reason.
2. List three harmless products that may be used to color mustaches and beards.

16

Men's Hairpieces

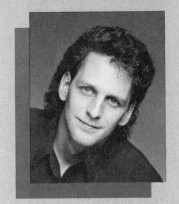

Learning Objectives:

After completing this chapter, you should be able to:

1. *Discuss reasons why men purchase hairpieces.*
2. *Identify the types of hair used in the manufacture of hairpieces.*
3. *List the different types of hairpiece bases that are available.*
4. *Demonstrate how to measure a client for a hairpiece.*
5. *Demonstrate fitting and cutting-in of hairpieces.*
6. *Demonstrate correct cleaning methods for hairpieces.*
7. *Discuss alternative hair replacement methods.*
8. *Discuss selling of hairpieces in the barber-styling shop.*

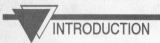

INTRODUCTION

The care and fitting of men's hairpieces is a rapidly growing service in the barber-styling field. The professional barber-stylist who can design, fit, and cut-in a hairpiece into a natural style opens the door to an increased clientele.

Men wear hairpieces for a variety of personal reasons that usually originate from the desire or need to cover thinning or balding areas of the head.

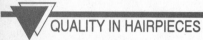

QUALITY IN HAIRPIECES

The quality of a hairpiece varies with the kind of hair it contains, the way it is constructed, and how it is fitted.

Types of Hair

Human hair is the most desirable choice for a quality hairpiece. The hairpieces most commonly available are made of Caucasian and Oriental hair. First quality human hair is usually in virgin condition, thereby assuring minimal oxidation. Oriental hair has many good qualities. However, the usual straight, coarse texture and dark color often require waving and/or coloring in order to match the client's hair. This processing diminishes the strength of the hair and oxidation occurs when exposed to sunlight and natural elements.

Animal hair usually originates from angora or yak, the angora being finer and the yak coarser. Angora used at the front hairline will create a softer, more natural look.

Synthetic hair is used primarily in the production of full wigs, rather than in toupees. It is difficult to match the texture of synthetic hair with human hair, which makes blending difficult. Synthetic fibers also possess a high gloss, which make them more noticeable. The positive factors of synthetics are that the fibers will not oxidize or lose the style. The continuing research of synthetic fibers may eventually result in the production of a hairpiece fiber equal in quality to that of human hair.

Hairpieces constructed of synthetic hair or a blend of human and synthetic or animal hair have the following disadvantages:

1. They are difficult to handle, tending to mat and tangle easily.
2. They are stiff and have a glassy surface shine.
3. Human hair shades cannot be duplicated readily.

Since most of the hair used in hairpieces is imported, it must be prepared for use. The usual process includes:

1. chemically cleaning the hair with an acid solution;
2. sorting the hair by color and length;
3. aligning or root-turning the hair, meaning that all the hair is turned in the same direction as it would grow on the head; and
4. giving the hair a permatizing bath.

Bases and Construction

Hairpieces are available with hard, soft, net, plastic, or combination bases.

The types of construction include:

1. Wefted—machine made
2. Handmade—usually ventilated
3. Ventilated—with lace front
4. Hard base

Stock and Custom Hairpieces

Hairpieces are available from manufacturers and distributors in stock sizes and colors. The barber-stylist can maintain an inventory of these products. Custom hairpieces are designed and measured by the barber-stylist before ordering them from the supplier.

A pattern or contour analysis should be done prior to selling any hairpiece. The contour analysis will help to determine whether a client has the option of purchasing a stock hairpiece.

Implements and Supplies Used for Men's Hairpieces

Most of the implements and supplies required for men's hairpiece services are available in the barber-styling shop. The remainder can be obtained easily from a supply company. (Fig. 16.1)

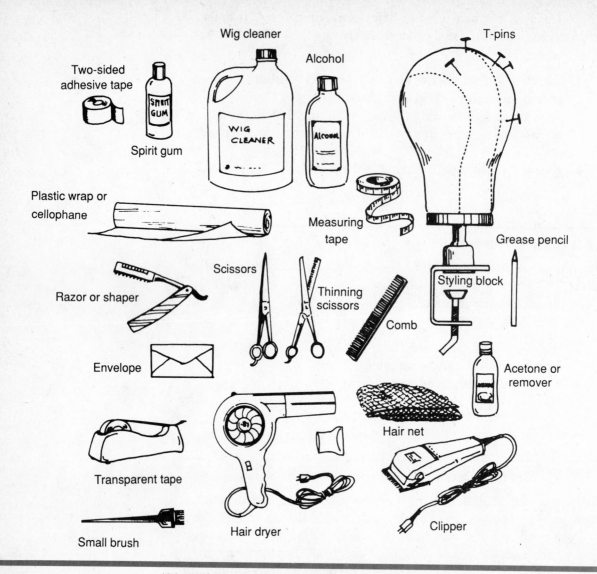

Two-sided adhesive tape

Spirit gum

Wig cleaner

Alcohol

T-pins

Plastic wrap or cellophane

Measuring tape

Grease pencil

Styling block

Razor or shaper

Scissors

Thinning scissors

Comb

Envelope

Acetone or remover

Hair net

Transparent tape

Hair dryer

Clipper

Small brush

16.1 – Implements and supplies used for men's hairpieces

MEASURING THE CLIENT FOR A HAIRPIECE

Preliminary Haircut

To achieve a natural look, the client's hair should be allowed to grow fairly long, thus making it much easier to blend it with that of the hairpiece. When cutting the client's hair, trim it very lightly. Leave a low neckline and keep the hair close to the ears at the sides. (Figs. 16.2 and 16.3)

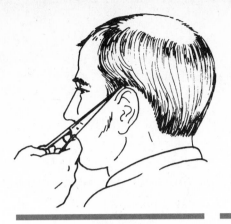

16.2 – Trim hair around ears.

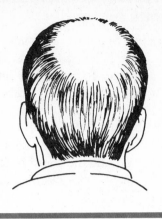

16.3 – Leave a low neckline.

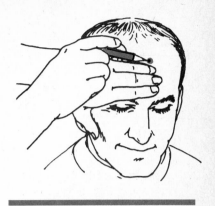

16.4 – Indicate where the hairpiece will begin.

When finished with the haircut, gather the longest of the cuttings and put it in an envelope for possible use as a color guide.

Tape Measurement

For a front hairline to look natural, it should not be too low on the forehead. You should try to follow the original natural hairline as closely as possible. Place three fingers above the eyebrow, directly in line with the center of the nose. Make a dot with grease pencil on the forehead to indicate where the hairpiece is to begin. (Fig. 16.4)

Place a tape measure on the dot. Measure the length to where the back hair begins and mark the tape measure. Be sure to measure back to where substantial growth begins—disregard sparse hair between the forehead and crown bald areas. (Fig. 16.5)

The next measurement is across the top, directly over the side-burn (normally about one and one-half inches behind the forehead dot). This is the place where the front hairline of the hairpiece blends in with the client's own hair at the sides of the head. Measure across the crown area if it is noticeably different from the front width. (Fig. 16.6)

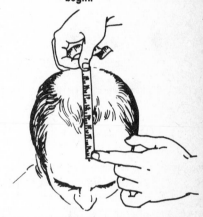

16.5 – Measure from front to where the back hair begins.

Manufacturer's Code

The sizes of men's hairpieces are commonly referred to by these measurements. For example: a six-by-four inch piece would be six inches long from front to back, and four inches wide. The larger number refers to the length unless otherwise indicated.

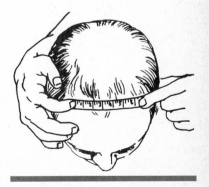

16.6 – Measure across the top.

Pattern Measurements

Tape measurements alone can be used by experienced designers in most cases. For beginners and for odd-shaped areas, a pattern may be preferable. To assemble, prepare plastic wrap, 12 strips of three-quarter-inch transparent tape (preferably the dull-finish type for easy writing), and a grease pencil. (Fig. 16.7)

Take two feet of plastic wrap (Fig. 16.8) and place it on top of the client's head. Twist the sides until they conform to the contour of the head. While the client holds the plastic wrap, place each pre-cut strip of tape across the bald area to stiffen the pattern and hold its shape. (Fig. 16.9)

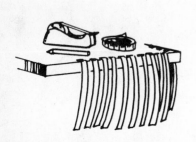

16.7 – **Assemble materials needed for pattern measurements.**

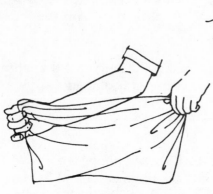

16.8 – **Use two feet of plastic wrap.**

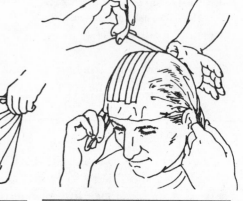

16.9 – **Place plastic wrap on client's head and shape.**

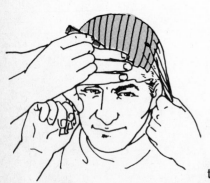

16.10 – **Indicate new hairline on pattern.**

NOTE: The instructions contained in this chapter represent the best available information on the fitting and servicing of hairpieces. However, your instructor may have developed different, equally correct techniques.

Next, place three fingers above the eyebrows and make a dot on the pattern to indicate the new hairline. (Fig. 16.10) Place additional dots as follows:

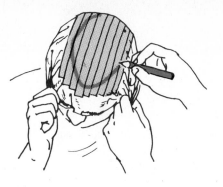

16.11 – Outline balding area on pattern.

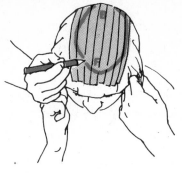

16.12 – Mark the front and back parts of the pattern.

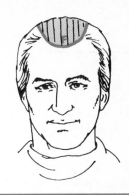

16.13 – Replace cut pattern over balding area.

1. two dots on each side where the front hairline is to meet the client's own hairline;
2. two dots in back of the head on each side of the balding spot;
3. one dot at the center back edge of the bald spot to determine the length of the area to be covered.

Connect the dots with a pencil to outline the balding area. Ignore minor irregularities and sparse areas. (Fig. 16.11)

Mark the front part of the pattern **F** and back **B** as in Fig. 16.12. Then remove and cut around the edge with scissors. After cutting the outline, replace the pattern over the balding area (Fig. 16.13). Make sure the bald area is covered exactly. It is better to have a foundation that is slightly smaller than one that is too large. However, accuracy is very important.

NOTE: Another method for taking a pattern is with a plaster-cast type material. Some hairpiece manufacturers prefer this method. It gives a true-to-shape form of the bald area. This is the same material used in setting broken bones. Check with manufacturers for the method they prefer and the availability of supplies.

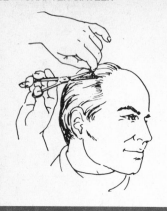

16.14 – Take swatch of hair from side with thinning shears.

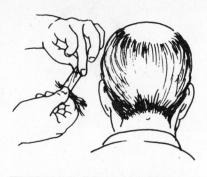

16.15 – Tape swatch and mark it with an S.

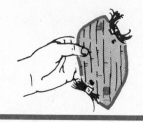

16.16 – Attach swatch to front side of pattern. Take swatch at back of head, mark B, and attach to pattern.

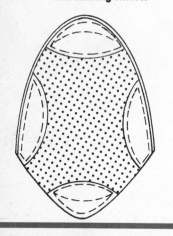

16.17 – Foundation diagram without lace front

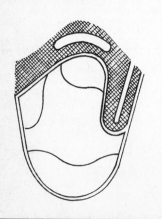

16.18 – Foundation diagram with lace front and side part

Hair Samples

For a hairpiece to look natural, it is of the utmost importance to take samples of client's hair so that it can be matched by the manufacturer. (Figs. 16.14—16.16)

Ordering Hairpieces

Send the measurements or pattern to the manufacturer with instructions covering the following information:

1. Hairpiece without lace front (Fig. 16.17) . . . . ☐
   a) . Without side part . . . . ☐
   b) . With left side part . . . . ☐
   c) . With right side part . . . . ☐
2. Hairpieces with lace front (Fig. 16.18) . . . . ☐
   a) . Without side part . . . . ☐
   b) . With left side part . . . . ☐
   c) . With right side part . . . . ☐
3. Hair color variations:
   a)   Front: Natural   ☐   Percentage of gray   ☐
                Streaked   ☐   Front and top lighter ☐
   b)   Temples: Natural   ☐   Percentage of gray   ☐
   c)   Back: Natural   ☐   Percentage of gray   ☐
4. Complexion:
   a) . Ruddy . . . . ☐
   b) . Dark . . . . ☐
   c) . Light . . . . ☐

5. Miscellaneous—Give details
   a) Partials ☐   Patches ☐   Fill-ins ☐
6. Photograph. A photo would be quite helpful.

PUTTING ON AND STYLING HAIRPIECE WITHOUT LACE FRONT

Applying Hairpiece

Before adjusting a hairpiece to the scalp, clean the entire bald area with a piece of cotton dampened with rubbing alcohol, or soap and water, then dry thoroughly.

Place two-sided tape in a V-shape on the front reinforced area of the foundation. (Fig. 16.19) This tape holds the hairpiece close to the scalp.

Place additional pieces of tape on the reinforced parts of the foundation at the sides and back of the hairpiece.

Place three fingers above the eyebrow, thus locating the hairline (Fig. 16.20); position the hairpiece at the hairline using the center of the nose as a guide. When the hairpiece is in proper position, press down firmly on the various tape areas. (Fig. 16.21)

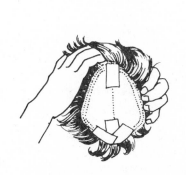

16.19 – Place tape on the foundation as shown.

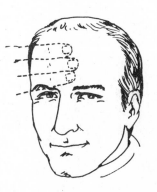

16.20 – Locate hairline.

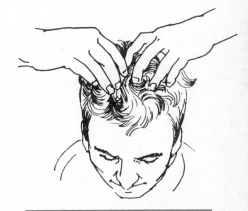

16.21 – Position and secure hairpiece.

Cutting, Tapering, and Blending

Back and sides. When the hair is combed into the desired position, use a razor to taper and blend the hair smoothly at the back of the

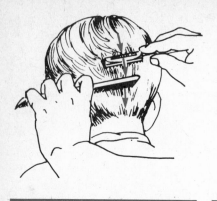

16.22 – Taper and blend the back of the head.

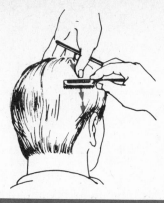

16.23 – Taper and blend the sides.

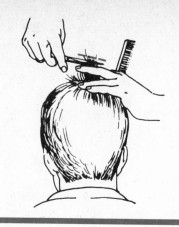

16.24 – Taper with the finger method.

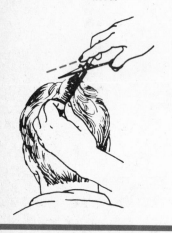

16.25 – Taper with the comb method.

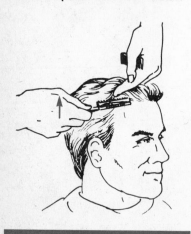

16.26 – Use razor to blend hairpiece with side hair.

head. (Fig. 16.22) Then taper and blend the sides. (Fig. 16.23) The tapering should be done smoothly so that the blending with the client's own hair will be undetectable.

> **NOTE:** A razor should never be used when cutting, tapering, or blending synthetic hairpieces. Blending shears should be used.

> CAUTION: In cutting, tapering, and blending the hairpiece, it is better that less hair be removed than too much. If too much hair is removed, it may destroy the hairpiece.

Top hair. The finger method may be used as in Fig. 16.24. Comb the hair up, bring it slightly forward, and cut. Repeat this operation as needed or utilize the comb method. (Fig. 16.25) Comb up and cut with scissors or thinning shears.

Blend with front side hair. To blend the hairpiece with side hair, cut a small amount of front hair short (Fig. 16.26) to soften the joining of the hairpiece to the client's hair.

Thick front hairline. If the front hairline appears heavy, use a razor for thinning. Be sure to make very narrow partings in order to

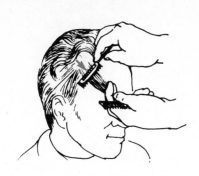

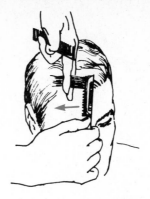

16.27 – Use narrow partings to blend front hairline.

16.28 – Thin hair with razor.

form a natural-looking front hairline (Fig. 16.27). To thin underneath hair, comb the hair forward and thin it with a razor. (Fig. 16.28) When combed back, the hair will lie flat.

> CAUTION: Use this technique only on a hairpiece without a lace front—never on the front area of a lace-front hairpiece.

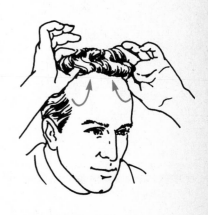

Removing a Hairpiece

Reach up under the hairpiece with the fingertips and detach the tape from the scalp. (Fig. 16.29) Make sure the tape stays on the foundation. This tape is left on the foundation, and it is reactivated with spirit gum or nail polish remover each time the hairpiece is worn.

16.29 – Remove tape from scalp.

PUTTING ON AND STYLING A HAIRPIECE WITH A LACE FRONT

A hairpiece with a lace front is recommended when the hair is worn in an off-the-face style. It is scarcely visible from the front view. The use of a lace-front hairpiece gives the required lightness for a natural-looking hairstyle. This natural effect is impossible to achieve with other types of hairpieces.

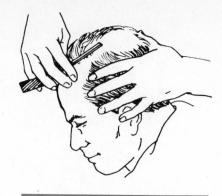

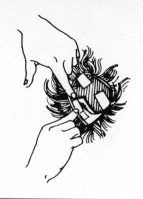

16.30 – Remove hair from head where tape or lace is to be placed.

16.31 – Reinforce foundation with tape.

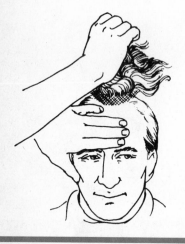

16.32 – Position hairpiece.

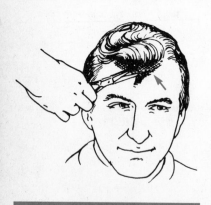

16.33 – Trim lace.

Putting on a Hairpiece

1. Clean the bald area with rubbing alcohol or with soap and water.
2. Remove hair on the scalp where the tape or lace is to be attached. (Fig. 16.30)
3. Attach strips of tape (two-sided) to reinforced parts of the foundation, usually near front, on the sides, and the back part of the hairpiece. (Fig. 16.31) Reinforced areas vary with the design of the foundation and manufacturer's directions.

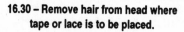

CAUTION: Never use tape directly on the lace.

4. Adjust the hairpiece to the desired position using the three-finger method previously described. Press it down into place. (Fig. 16.32)
5. Cut, taper, and blend the front lace hairpiece to match smoothly with the client's own hair.
6. Trim the lace to within one-quarter of an inch of the hairline (Fig. 16.33), or right down to the contour of the hairline, according to the client's preference. The decision to trim or not to trim should be left until the hairpiece has been worn for a while. In the beginning, leave the small one-quarter inch margin.

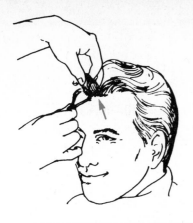

16.34 – Brush spirit gum on scalp.

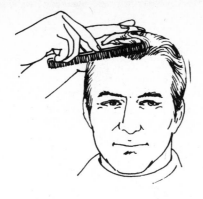

16.35 – Raise front hair with comb.

7. Lift the lace and brush spirit gum sparingly on the scalp under it. (Fig. 16.34) When tacky, press down the front lace with a moist, lint-free cloth.

8. To keep the front hairline from lying too flat, reach in with a comb and twist the comb forward slightly. (Fig. 16.35) This will give the proper lift and make the hair look as if it is really growing out of the scalp.

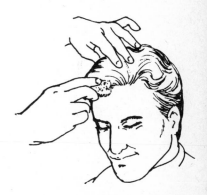

16.36 – Dampen lace with solvent before removing.

Removing a Lace-Front Hairpiece

1. Before removing a lace-front hairpiece, dampen the lace with acetone or solvent in order to loosen it from the scalp. (Fig. 16.36) Do not pull or stretch the lace. To apply solvent, use a piece of cotton or a brush.

2. After the lace becomes loosened, use the fingertips to remove the tape from the scalp (Fig. 16.37). Do not pull off the hairpiece by tugging on the hair.

3. The pieces of tape are not removed from the reinforced areas of the hairpiece. They are reactivated with spirit gum or nail polish remover each time the hairpiece is worn.

NOTE: Instruct the client on how to put on and remove his hairpiece, thereby avoiding possible damage to it.

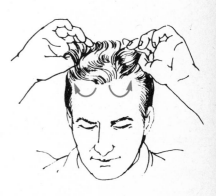

16.37 – Remove tape from scalp.

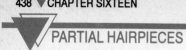

PARTIAL HAIRPIECES

Partial Lace Front Fill-In

For a small degree of hair loss, a partial lace fill-in may be all that is required.

1. Clean the area with soap and water or with rubbing alcohol and allow it to dry. Brush on spirit gum and wait until it gets tacky.
2. Place the hairpiece properly (Fig. 16.38) and press down.
3. Comb into the rest of the hair. If required, taper and shorten the hairpiece to blend in with the client's own hair.

Frontal lace partials are made of very fine lace, and they are excellent for receding hairpart lines.

Partial Crown Hairpiece

For clients who are bald at the crown, a small hairpiece may be used. Measure the diameter of the bald area and send a hair sample when ordering.

To attach a partial crown, clean the area in the usual manner, dry, and apply spirit gum to the outer edges of the bald spot. (Fig. 16.39) Then:

1. Attach a piece of two-sided tape to the center of the hairpiece.

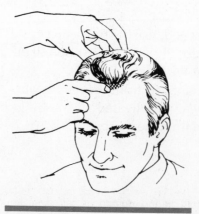

16.38 – Place hairpiece.

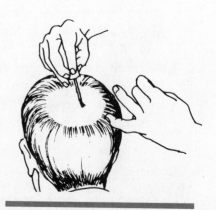

16.39 – Apply spirit gum to bald area.

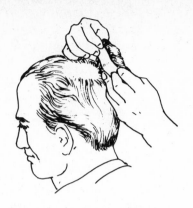

16.40 – Secure hairpiece with tape and/or spirit gum.

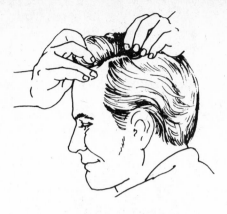

16.41 – Position partial hairpiece.

2. Carefully position the hairpiece over the bald spot, press the center firmly to the scalp, and then press the outer edges into position. Once in position, it may be held in place with two-sided adhesive tape or spirit gum. (Fig. 16.40)
3. Cut, taper, and blend the crown hairpiece with a razor. Comb the hair carefully to blend with the client's own hair.

Partial Top Hairpiece

1. Shave a wide side part so that the tape will adhere to the scalp.
2. Place the partial hairpiece next to the part. (Fig. 16.41)
3. Cut the hair to blend with client's own hair.
4. Comb the hair into the desired style, preferably to conceal the front hairline.

Every time the hairpiece is worn, reactivate the tape with spirit gum or nail polish remover.

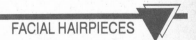

FACIAL HAIRPIECES

Facial hairpieces are attached with spirit gum.

Mustache. Apply spirit gum to the upper lip, wait until it is tacky, position the mustache, and gently press down with a lint-free cloth. Trim the mustache to the desired style.

Beard. Apply spirit gum around the circumference of the area to be covered. Wait until it is tacky. Position the beard and press the edges down with a lint-free cloth. Trim the beard to the desired style.

Sideburns may be applied in the same manner as a mustache.

▼ CLEANING AND STYLING HAIRPIECES

Cleaning Hairpieces

Great care should be exercised when cleaning hairpieces. Remove all old tape (Fig. 16.42) and clean any reinforced areas by rubbing them lightly with solvent or wig cleaner.

Put enough cleaner in an open bowl so that the hairpiece can be submerged. Swish the hairpiece back and forth (or dip it up and down) in the cleaner until all residue is removed from the hair and foundation. Gently press out the cleaner or let it drip into the bowl. (Fig. 16.43) Fasten the hairpiece on a covered head mold to dry naturally.

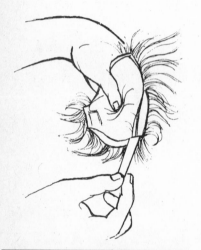

16.42 – Remove tape before cleaning.

> CAUTION: Some cleaning agents are hazardous if not used according to instructions. Be sure to read the label carefully before using any cleaning agent.

Styling Hairpieces on a Head Mold

After the hairpiece has been cleaned, place it on a covered head mold and fasten it securely with T-pins or straight pins. (Fig. 16.44) Set the hair in the desired style while still wet. (Fig. 16.45)

Hairpieces may be dried naturally (Fig. 16.46) or a hand blower may be used, after covering the hairpiece with a hair net. (Fig. 16.47)

> CAUTION: Avoid heat on gray hair. The heat tends to make the hair yellow.

Styling Hairpieces on Client's Head

The hairpiece may also be styled after being placed on the client's head. The scalp must be clean and dry and the foundation of the

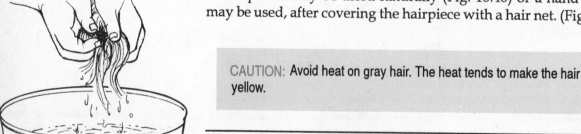

16.43 – Clean with solvent or wig cleaner.

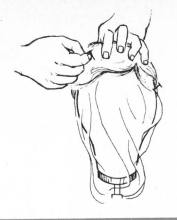

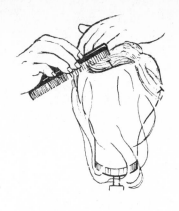

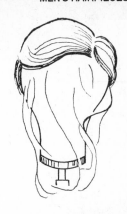

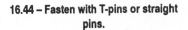

16.44 – Fasten with T-pins or straight pins.

16.45 – Set hair into style while wet.

16.46 – Hairpiece left to dry naturally

hairpiece thoroughly dried on a head mold before attaching it to the client's scalp.

Moisten the hairpiece with a damp comb and style it as desired. Be careful not to dampen the foundation. A styling hair net is then adjusted over the client's head (Fig. 16.48) and the hair thoroughly dried with a hand dryer.

Cleaning Synthetic Hairpieces

Synthetic hairpieces should never be washed in solvent. Attach the hairpiece to a styrofoam head mold with T-pins. Then immerse it in lukewarm water with a mild shampoo. Do not use hot water or the hairpiece will shrink. Swish the hairpiece around in the shampoo solution. Rinse with clean, lukewarm water. Permit the hairpiece to dry naturally, pinned on the mold overnight or if time does not permit, place it under a dryer with cool air. Some hairpieces may be dry cleaned. Follow the manufacturer's instructions.

Special Note About Hairpieces

Hairpieces made of human hair must always be dry cleaned. Never use a shampoo.

Synthetic hairpieces are usually mass-produced, and synthetic fibers are rarely used for lace-type or custom made hairpieces.

When setting hairpieces, use plain water. The use of a small amount of pomade or a similar product will add luster to the hair.

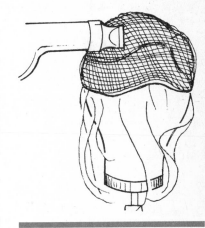

16.47 – Drying hairpiece on block with hand blower

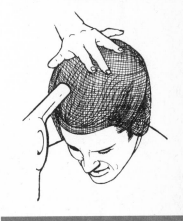

16.48 – Drying hairpiece on client's head with hand blower

COLORING AND RECONDITIONING HAIRPIECES

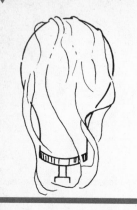

16.49 – Cover block with plastic wrap.

Permanent Hair Coloring

Permanent hair coloring products (aniline derivatives) can be used only on hairpieces made of 100 percent human hair.

Procedure

1. The hairpiece is cleaned with a solvent or cleaner.
2. Cover the head mold with plastic material to prevent damage to the mold by the coloring product. (Fig. 16.49)
3. Secure the hairpiece firmly with T-pins or straight pins in the front, back, and sides. (Fig. 16.50)
4. Give a strand test on a small section of hair to determine the color desired. If using a tint with peroxide, apply it on a dry hair strand.

The following is a suggested procedure for hair coloring:
1. Mix the hair coloring to the desired shade.
2. Apply with a hair coloring brush. (Fig. 16.51)
3. Comb it through lightly, being careful not to saturate the foundation.
4. Test every five minutes until the desired shade is obtained.
5. Rinse with warm water (Fig. 16.52). Do not use soap.

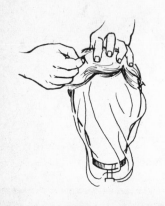

16.50 – Secure hairpiece on block.

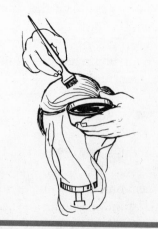

16.51 – Apply hair coloring product to hairpiece.

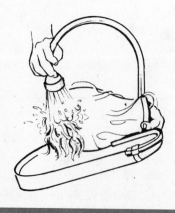

16.52 – Rinse hairpiece after application.

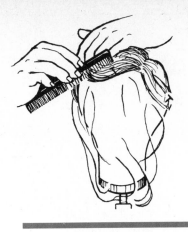

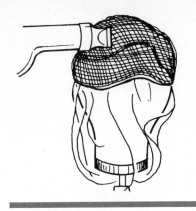

16.53 – Style hairpiece.   **16.54 – Dry hairpiece.**

6. Set into the desired style. (Fig. 16.53)
7. Dry with a hand blower. (Fig. 16.54) (Air should not be too hot. Excess heat causes frizziness.)

Reconditioning Hairpieces

Reconditioning treatments should be given as often as necessary to prevent dryness or brittleness of the hair. Reconditioning treatments may also be used to liven up hairpieces that look dull and lifeless.

A small amount of reconditioner may be used, as directed by the manufacturer or instructor. If a slight color adjustment is necessary due to fading, yellowing, or sun-bleaching, a suitable color rinse is recommended. Be guided by your instructor. Select the rinse carefully so that the color matches that of the client's hair.

> CAUTION: Coloring a hairpiece always does some damage to the foundation. It may not be evident immediately, but it may result in hair loss later on. Do not use strong bleaches since peroxide also tends to damage the foundation of a hairpiece. Synthetic hairpieces should not be colored.

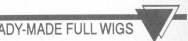

READY-MADE FULL WIGS

Ready-to-wear wigs usually are made of **modacrylic** fibers such as **kanekalon**, **dynel**, and **venicelon**. They meet the personal needs of many clients.

Reasons for Wearing Full Wigs

1. A complete change of style and image
2. To cover natural hair temporarily
3. To hide a balding head

Construction and Fit

Full, ready-made wigs are constructed on a stretch cap made of lightweight elastic. The wig has permanent elastic bands at the sides designed to hold it in place. It should fit comfortably, but tightly enough to maintain its position without slipping, shifting, or lifting. Wigs come in a wide variety of colors and in many different styles.

Cleaning Wigs

Cleaning of ready-made wigs is a fairly quick and easy process. However, manufacturer's cleaning instructions should be carefully followed.

General Cleaning Procedures

1. Brush the wig thoroughly to remove all surface dirt and residue.
2. Mix a solution of warm water and mild shampoo in a bowl.
3. Dip the entire wig into the solution; swish it around in the solution.
4. Rinse the wig in clean, cold water.
5. Blot it dry with a towel.
6. Turn the wig inside out and dry it with a towel.
7. Pin the wig to a head mold of the correct size.
8. Carefully brush the hair into shape.
9. Permit the wig to dry naturally—pinned to the form.
10. If necessary, use cool air to dry it quickly.
11. When dry, brush it into the proper style.

> **NOTE:** If the tape on the wig is not clean, carefully use a liquid solvent to clean it.

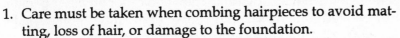

SAFETY PRECAUTIONS AND REMINDERS

1. Care must be taken when combing hairpieces to avoid matting, loss of hair, or damage to the foundation.
2. When combing a hairpiece, use a wide-tooth comb to avoid weakening or damaging the foundation.
3. When dry cleaning a hairpiece, never rub or wring the cleaning fluid from it. Let it dry naturally.
4. When cutting, tapering, and blending a hairpiece, be careful not to cut too much; once the hair has been cut, it cannot grow back.
5. To assure a comfortable and secure fit, correct measurements must be taken or a suitable pattern of the client's head made.
6. Recondition hairpieces as often as necessary to prevent dryness or brittleness of the hair and to liven up the appearance, which may have become dull and lifeless.
7. If required, dry clean hairpieces before styling.
8. Brush and comb hairpieces with a downward movement.
9. To avoid damage to the foundation, never lighten a hairpiece.
10. To avoid damage to the foundation, never give a cold wave to a hairpiece.
11. If hair coloring is necessary, it must be done with care.
12. To reactivate faded hair, a color rinse may be applied.
13. Do not work the tint into the foundation of the hairpiece. This will cause the foundation to deteriorate.
14. Hairpieces made of human hair must be dry cleaned, whereas those made of synthetics may be shampooed or dry cleaned, whichever the manufacturer recommends.

SELLING HAIRPIECES

In order to sell men's hairpieces, it is important to know why men buy them. Often they are purchased in an effort to retain a youthful appearance. Large corporations tend to place younger men in positions offering the most potential for advancement. Men seeking such positions may consider purchasing hairpieces in an effort to advance their careers.

Selling to Older Men

Do not attempt to convince older men that they can recapture the appearance they had in their twenties. It simply cannot be done. An older man's skin coloring is very different from that of his youth. Solid black is not an advisable color choice for an older person. It is better to recommend salt and pepper or medium brown shade. The customer's looks will be more believable.

Demonstration Technique

One or two correctly styled demonstration hairpieces (preferably a lace piece in salt and pepper and a regular hairpiece in dark brown) will help immensely to encourage a client to buy a hairpiece. Make certain that your sample is clean and nicely styled . It should be large enough to cover the average balding area of a man, since most clients will be men with an average amount of hair loss.

Word-of-Mouth Advertising and Window Displays

Word-of-mouth and window displays do a great deal in increasing the sale of hairpieces. It is wise to place before and after illustrations in the shop or shop window to encourage those clients whom you feel cannot be approached directly. However, many clients can be approached directly if tact is used. You might suggest a hairpiece as a solution to a client's problem if, during a consultation, hair loss is discussed. A quick demonstration may convince him of his greatly improved appearance and lead to a sale.

Printed Ads

It is also important to advertise your hairpiece service. In most areas an extra line in the telephone book, mentioning hairpieces, will pay for itself. Your phone book also may contain a special listing for hair goods. This is a good spot to place an advertisement.

In some communities newspaper advertising is inexpensive and profitable. If you do use printed advertising, be sure to secure the model's release for any illustrations that you might use in your ad. Even if the model is your best friend, do not assume that a release is unnecessary.

Personal Experience

If you wear a hairpiece yourself, you can develop an excellent promotional approach. Often, nothing is more convincing than your own before-and-after demonstration. The fact that you wear your hairpiece with assurance and complete ease can make a very strong impression.

HAIR REPLACEMENT TECHNIQUES

There are two hair replacement techniques available at this time. These techniques, which are considered to be either permanent or semi-permanent, are hair transplants and hair weaving.

Hair Transplants

The transplanting of hair is strictly a medical procedure that should be performed only by a trained dermatologist. The process consists of removing hair from normal areas of the scalp, such as the back and sides, and transplanting it into the bald areas. Small sections of hair (about one-eighth of an inch) are surgically removed, including the hair follicle, papilla, and hair bulb, and reset in the bald area. These sections are called plugs. A local anesthetic is used. The transplanted hair grows normally in its new environment. The area from which the hair was removed heals and shrinks in size to a very tiny scar.

The dermatologist must select the hair to be transplanted with care, taking into consideration color, texture, and type. Placement of the hair in the direction of natural growth, to permit proper care and grooming, is also an important factor.

Transplanted hair can last a lifetime if the dermatologist service is performed properly. If the doctor is skilled and the individual cares for the hair as directed, hair transplants can be very successful as a method of permanently eliminating baldness.

Hair Weaving

Hair weaving has been practiced in barber-styling shops for many years. It is another method of covering bald areas of the head.

While there are numerous claims of new techniques and exclusive methods in hair weaving, they all follow generally the same procedure. Hair weaving consists of sewing or weaving a foundation into the remaining hair or on the scalp, and then weaving wefts of human hair to this foundation. The two principal techniques are the suture method and the hair weaving method.

The Suture Method

A perimeter of **anchor-bases**, made of strong, non-reactive, teflon-coated, stainless steel wire, is imbedded or sutured into the scalp by a medical doctor. To this imbedded wire, a network of foundation of siliconized Dacron is attached. This foundation must fit the scalp very tightly and snugly. Wefts of matching human hair are sewn or woven to the foundation in a previously determined pattern and style. Since the foundation wires are imbedded in the scalp, the suture method of hair weaving is not affected by hair growth.

While the suture method seems to offer a hair replacement technique involving some semblance of permanency without constant adjustments, it also presents a number of severe problems. These include, among others, the danger of scalp infection from the teflon wire, the possibility of pain when combing or shampooing the hair, and the danger of injury to the scalp caused by pulling the wire in combing. Clients should be advised to consider carefully all of the possible problems before deciding upon this form of hair replacement.

The Hair Weaving Method

This method consists of firmly sewing or weaving a foundation into the remaining hair on the individual's head with thread and then sewing or weaving wefts of matching human hair to this foundation in a pre-planned pattern. Since the foundation is attached to the remaining hair on the head, as the hair grows the foundation moves out from the scalp. Continual adjustments are required, therefore, in order to maintain the desired natural appearance.

The hair woven on the head requires continuous care and servicing. The foundation must be tightened and brought close to the scalp every six to eight weeks.

The hair must be shampooed carefully, in sections, to avoid pulling and causing damage to the foundation or pain to the client. The hair should also receive periodic conditioning treatments to add luster and to avoid dryness and damage.

REVIEW QUESTIONS

Men's Hairpieces

1. Explain why men would wear hairpieces.
2. List three kinds of hair that are used to make men's hairpieces.
3. In what two ways can head measurements be taken for hairpieces?
4. Why should hair samples be taken for every man's hairpiece?
5. In what two ways are hairpieces usually manufactured?
6. List five kinds of hairpiece bases.
7. What is used to attach a hairpiece to the scalp?
8. What is used to reactivate the pieces of tape attached to the reinforced areas of the hairpiece?
9. How are hairpieces cleaned?
10. To be fully qualified, what points of basic information should the barber-stylist know about men's hairpieces?
11. Why is bleaching (lightening) of a hairpiece not recommended?

12. Why are reconditioning treatments recommended for hairpieces?
13. What should be used in combing a hairpiece to avoid abuse to its foundation?
14. Name five promotional aids for selling of men's hairpieces.
15. Name two categories of hairpieces available to the barber-stylist.

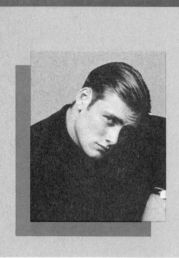

Nails, Nail Disorders, and Manicures

Learning Objectives

After completing this chapter, you should be able to:

1. *Identify the composition and structure of nails.*

2. *Describe and identify nail irregularities and diseases.*

3. *Recognize the four general shapes of nails.*

4. *Identify manicuring implements, equipment, and products.*

5. *Demonstrate the proper use of implements, equipment, and products.*

6. *Demonstrate manicures on female and male models.*

7. *Perform a hand and arm massage properly.*

Many full-service barber-styling shops offer manicuring as one of their services. As a result, it is advisable for the barber-stylist to be acquainted with the manicuring procedure.

In order to perform the service, a basic understanding of nail composition and structure is necessary.

The **nail,** an appendage of skin, is a horny, translucent plate that serves to protect the tips of fingers and toes. **Onyx (ON**-iks) is the technical term for nail.

The condition of the nail, like that of the skin, reflects the general health of the body. The normal, healthy nail is firm and flexible. Its surface should be smooth, curved, and unspotted, without any hollows or wavy ridges. The pink color of the nail bed can be seen through the nail. The horny nail plate contains no nerves or blood vessels. It is composed mainly of keratin.

Nail Structure

The nails consist of three parts: the **nail body,** the **nail root,** and the **free edge.** The nail body, or plate, is the visible portion of the nail which rests upon, and is attached to, the nail bed. The nail body extends from the root to the free edge.

Although the nail plate seems to be made of one piece, it is actually constructed in layers. The readiness with which nails split clearly demonstrates this form of structure.

The nail root is at the base of the nail and is imbedded underneath the skin. It originates from an actively growing tissue known as the **matrix (MAY**-triks).

The free edge is the end portion of the nail that reaches over the fingertips.

The nail bed is the portion of the skin upon which the nail body rests. It is supplied with many blood vessels that provide nourishment for continued growth of the nail. The nail bed is also abundantly supplied with nerves.

The matrix is that part of the nail bed that extends beneath the nail root and contains nerves, lymph, and blood vessels. The matrix produces the nail as its cells reproduce and harden. The matrix will continue to grow as long as it receives nutrition and remains healthy. The growth of nails may be retarded by poor health, a nail disorder or disease, or injury to the nail matrix.

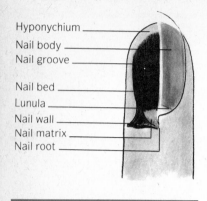

Hyponychium

Nail body

Nail groove

Nail bed

Lunula

Nail wall

Nail matrix

Nail root

17.1 – Diagram of the nail

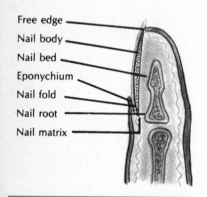

Free edge

Nail body

Nail bed

Eponychium

Nail fold

Nail root

Nail matrix

17.2 – Cross section of the nail

The **lunula** (**LOO**-nyoo-la) or **half-moon** is located at the base of the nail. The matrix is located underneath the lunula. The light color of the lunula may be due to the reflection of light where the matrix and the connective tissue of the nail bed join.

The **cuticle** (**KYOO**-ti-kel) is the overlapping epidermis around the nail. A normal cuticle around the nail should be loose and pliable.

The **eponychium** (ep-o-**NIK**-ee-um) is the extension of the cuticle at the base of the nail body which partly overlaps the lunula.

The **hyponychium** (heye-poh-**NIK**-ee-um) is that portion of the epidermis under the free edge of the nail.

The **perionychium** (**PER**-i-o-nik-ee-um) is that portion of the cuticle surrounding the entire nail border.

The **nail walls** are the folds of skin overlapping the sides of the nail.

The **nail grooves** are slits, or tracks, on the sides of the nail upon which the nail moves as it grows.

The **mantle** (**MAN**-tel) is the deep fold of skin in which the nail root is imbedded. (Figs. 17.1 and 17.2)

Nail Growth

Nail growth is influenced by nutrition, health, and disease. The nail grows forward, starting at the matrix and extending over the fingertip. The average rate of growth in the normal adult is about one-eighth of an inch per month. Nails grow more quickly in summer than in winter. Children's nails grow more rapidly, whereas those of elderly persons grow more slowly. The nail grows most quickly on the middle finger and most slowly on the thumb. Although toenails grow more slowly than fingernails, they are thicker and harder.

Nail Malformation

If the nail is separated from the nail bed through injury, it becomes distorted or discolored. Should the nail bed be injured after the loss of a nail, a badly formed new nail will result.

Nails are not shed in the same way as hair sheds. If a nail is torn off accidentally or lost through an infection or disease, it will be replaced only if the matrix remains in good condition. The replacement nails frequently are shaped abnormally, due to interference at the base of the nail. Replacement of the nail takes about four months.

NAIL DISORDERS

A **nail disorder** is a condition caused by injury to the nail, disease, or chemical or nutritional imbalance. Most, if not all, clients will have had some common nail disorder, and may have one when they are scheduled for a manicure. A nail technician learns to recognize the symptoms of nail disorders and so can make a responsible decision about whether or not to perform a service on the client. In some cases it may be necessary to recommend medical treatment. In others, the disorder may be improved cosmetically.

It is the nail technician's responsibility to know when it is safe to work on a client's nails. It is important, therefore, to learn to recognize the symptoms of nail disorders that would preclude service being provided, as well as to know when to treat nails with extra care and when a disorder can be improved cosmetically. Use the **golden rule** to make a responsible decision: If the nail or skin to be worked on is infected, inflamed, broken, or swollen, a nail technician should not service the client. Instead, refer the client to a doctor. An inflammation is red and sore. An infection will have evidence of pus. Inflammation and infection are not the same thing, although they often occur at the same time. Broken skin or nail tissue is a cut or tear that exposes deeper layers of these structures. Raised or swollen skin will appear fatter than normal skin and rise above the normal level.

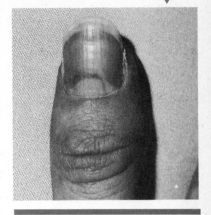

17.3 – Bruised nail

Nail Disorders That Can Be Serviced by a Nail Technician

Bruised nails occur when a blood clot forms under the nail plate. The clot is caused by injury to the nail bed. It can vary in color from maroon to black. In some cases, a bruised nail will fall off during the healing process. Applying artificial nail services to a bruised nail is not recommended. (Fig. 17.3)

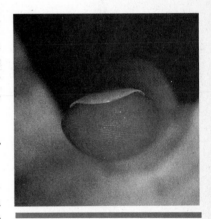

17.4 – Eggshell nail

Discolored nails is a condition in which nails turn a variety of colors including yellow, blue, blue-gray, green, red, and purple. Discoloration can be caused by poor blood circulation, a heart condition, or topical or oral medications. It may also indicate the presence of a systemic disorder. Artificial tips or wraps, or an application of colored nail polish can hide this condition.

Eggshell nails are thin, white, and curved over the free edge. The condition is caused by improper diet, internal disease, medication, or nerve disorders. Be very careful when manicuring these nails. They are fragile and can break easily. Use the fine side of an emery board to file gently and do not use pressure with a metal pusher at the base of the nail. (Figs. 17.4, 17.5)

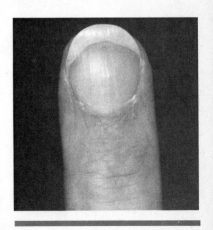

17.5 – Eggshell nail

Furrows, also known as corrugations, are long ridges that run either lengthwise or across the nail. Some lengthwise ridges are normal in adult nails, and they increase with age. Lengthwise ridges can also be caused by conditions such as psoriasis, poor circulation, and frostbite. Ridges that run across the nail can be caused by conditions such as high fever, pregnancy, measles in childhood, and a zinc deficiency in the body. If ridges are not deep and the nail is not broken, the appearance of this disorder can be corrected. Carefully buff the nails with pumice powder to remove or shorten the ridges. The remaining ridges can be filled with ridge filler and covered with colored polish to give a smooth, healthy look. (Fig. 17.6)

Hangnails, also known as agnails, is a common condition in which the cuticle around the nail splits. Hangnails are caused by dry cuticles or cuticles that have been cut too closely to the nail. This disorder can be improved by softening the cuticles with oil and trimming them with nippers. Though this is a simple and common disorder, hangnails can become infected if not serviced properly. (Fig. 17.7)

Leuconychia (loo-ko-**NIK**-ee-ah) is a condition in which white spots appear on the nails. It is caused by air bubbles, a bruise, or other injury to the nail. Leuconychia cannot be corrected, but it will grow out. (Fig. 17.8)

Nevus (**NEE**-vus) is a brown or black stain on the nail caused by a pigmented mole that occurs in the nail. Nail polish or an artificial nail service can hide this disorder.

Onychatrophia (on-i-kah-**TROH**-fee-ah), also known as atrophy, describes the wasting away of the nail. The nail loses its shine,

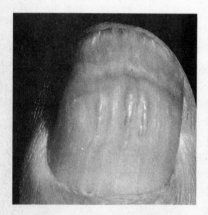

17.6 – Furrows or corrugations

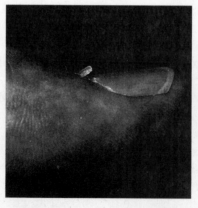

17.7 – Hangnail

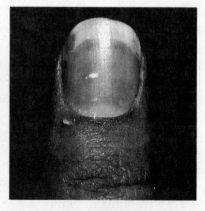

17.8 – Leuconychia

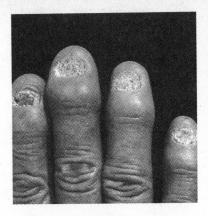

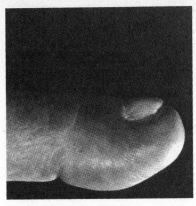

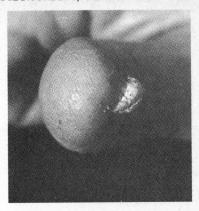

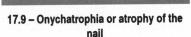

17.9 – Onychatrophia or atrophy of the nail

17.10 – Onychauxis

17.11 – Onychauxis (end view)

shrinks, and falls off. Onychatrophia can be caused by injury to the nail matrix or by internal disease. Handle this condition with extreme care. File the nail with the fine side of the emery board and do not use a metal pusher, strong soaps, or washing powders. If the condition is caused by internal disease and the disease is cured, new nails may grow back. (Fig. 17.9)

Onychauxis (on-i-**KIK**-sis) or **hypertrophy** (hy-**PER**-troh-fee) shows the opposite symptoms of onychatrophia. Onychauxis is the overgrowth of nails. The nails are abnormally thick. The condition is usually caused by internal imbalance, local infection, or heredity. File the nail smooth and buff it with pumice powder. (Figs. 17.10, 17.11)

Onychocryptosis (on-i-ko-krip-**TOH**-sis) or **ingrown nails** is a familiar condition in which the nail grows into the sides of the tissue around the nail. Improper filing of the nail and poor-fitting shoes are causes of this disorder. If the tissue around the nail is not infected and if the nail is not imbedded too deeply in the flesh, trim the corner of the nail in a curved shape to relieve the pressure on the nail groove. If the nail has grown very deeply into the groove, refer the client to a physician. (Fig. 17.12)

Onychophagy (on-i-**KOH**-fa-jee) is the medical term for nails that have been bitten enough to become deformed. This condition can be improved greatly by professional manicuring techniques. Give frequent manicures, using the techniques described in this chapter. (Fig. 17.13)

Onychorrhexis (on-i-kohr-**REK**-sis) refers to split or brittle nails that also have a series of lengthwise ridges. It can be caused by

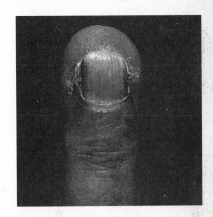

17.12 – Onychocryptosis or ingrown nail

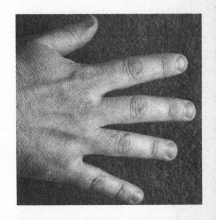

17.13 – Bitten nails or onychophagy

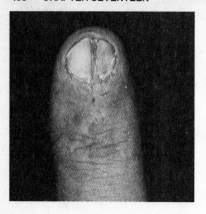

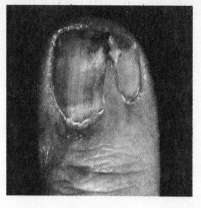

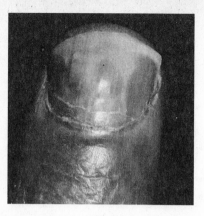

17.14 – Onychorrhexis

17.15 – Pterygium

17.16 – Mold

injury to the fingers, excessive use of cuticle solvents, nail polish removers, and careless, rough filing. Nail services can be performed only if the nail is not split below the free edge. This condition may be corrected by softening the nails with a reconditioning treatment and discontinuing the use of harsh soaps, polish removers, or improper filing. (Fig. 17.14)

Pterygium (te-**RIJ**-ee-um) describes the common condition of the forward growth of the cuticle on the nail. The cuticle sticks to the nail and, if not treated, will grow over the nail to the free edge. This condition can be treated easily by a reconditioning hot oil manicure, which will soften the cuticle so it can be pushed back by the metal pusher and then removed. (Fig. 17.15)

Nail Disorders That Cannot Be Serviced by a Nail Technician

Mold is a fungus infection of the nail that usually is caused by moisture that seeps between an artificial nail and the free edge of the nail. Mold starts with a yellow-green color and darkens to black if not treated by a doctor. A client with mold must be referred to a doctor. (Fig. 17.16)

Onychia (on-**NIK**-ee-ah) is an inflammation somewhere in the nail. The tissue at the base of the nail may be red and swollen, and pus may form. It is often caused by improperly sanitized manicuring implements. (Fig. 17.17)

Onychogryphosis (on-i-koh-greye-**FOH**-sis) is a condition in which the nail curvature is increased and enlarged. The nail becomes thicker and curves, sometimes extending over the tip of the

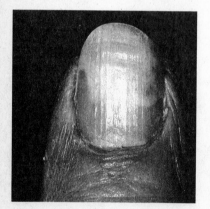

17.17 – Onychia

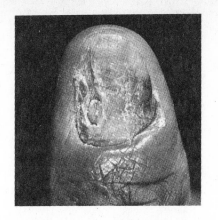

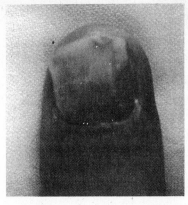

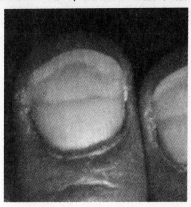

17.18 – Onychomycosis   **17.19 – Onycholysis (caused by trauma)**   **17.20 – Onycholysis**

finger or toe. This condition results in inflammation and pain if the nail grows into the skin. The cause of this disorder is unknown.

Onychomycosis (oni-koh-meye-**KOH**-sis), **tinea unguim** (**TIN**-ee-ah **UN**-gwee-um), of the nails, is an infectious disease caused by a fungus. A common form is whitish patches that can be scraped off the surface. A second form is long, yellowish streaks within the nail substance. The disease invades the free edge and spreads toward the root. The infected portion is thick and discolored. In a third form, the deeper layers of the nail are invaded, causing the superficial layers to appear irregularly thin. These infected layers peel off and expose the diseased parts of the nail bed. (Fig. 17.18)

Onycholysis (on-i-**KOL**-i-sis) is a condition in which the nail loosens from the nail bed, beginning usually at the free edge and continuing to the lunula, but does not come off. It is caused by an internal disorder, trauma, infection, or certain drugs. It can occur on the nails of the hands or feet. (Figs. 17.19, 17.20)

Onychoptosis (on-i-kop-**TOH-**sis) is a condition in which part or all of the nail sheds periodically and falls off the finger. It can affect one or more nails. It occurs during or after certain diseases such as syphilis, as a result of fever, as a reaction to certain prescription drugs, or as a result of trauma.

Paronychia (par-oh-**NIK**-ee-ah) is a bacterial inflammation of the tissue around the nail. The symptoms are redness, swelling, and tenderness of the tissue. It can occur at the base of the nail, around the entire nail plate, or on the fingertip. Paronychia around the entire nail is sometimes referred to as runaround. Chronic paronychia occurs continually over a long period of time and causes damage to the nail plate. It can be caused by the use of unsanitary

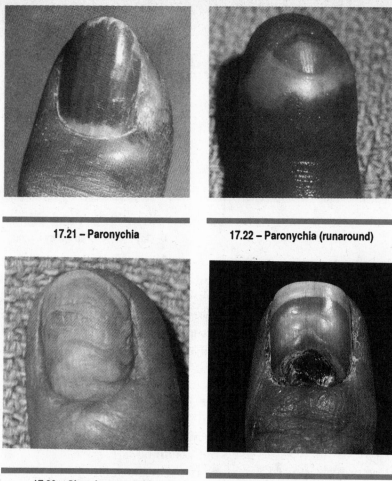

17.21 – Paronychia

17.22 – Paronychia (runaround)

17.23 – Chronic paronychia

17.24 – Pyrogenic granuloma

implements or by aggressive pushing or cutting of the cuticle. (Figs. 17.21, 17.22, 17.23)

Pyrogenic granuloma (pye-ro-**JEN**-ick gran-yoo-**LO**-muh) is a severe inflammation of the nail in which a lump of red tissue grows up from the nail bed to the nail plate. (Fig. 17.24)

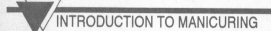

INTRODUCTION TO MANICURING

The ancients regarded long, polished and colored fingernails as a mark of distinction between aristocrats and common laborers. Manicuring, once considered a luxury for the few, is now a service used by many men and women.

The word manicure is derived from the Latin *manus* (hand) and *cura* (care), which means the care of the hands and nails. Its purpose is to improve the appearance of the hands and nails.

A client pleased with a professional manicure is more likely to become a regular client, as well as for other services.

NAIL TECHNOLOGY SUPPLIES

Equipment

Permanent items used in nail technology are called equipment. They can be used for all your services and do not have to be replaced until they wear out.

Manicure table with adjustable lamp. Most standard manicuring tables include a drawer for storing sanitized implements and cosmetics, and an attached, adjustable lamp. The lamp should have a 40 watt bulb. The heat from a higher wattage bulb will interfere with manicuring and sculptured nail procedures. A lower wattage bulb will not warm a client's nails in a room that is highly air conditioned. The warmth from the bulb will help to maintain product consistency.

Client's chair and nail technician's chair or stool.

Finger bowl. A plastic, china, or glass bowl that is shaped specifically for soaking the client's fingers in warm water and anti-bacterial soap. (Fig. 17.25)

Wet sanitizer. A receptacle large enough to hold the disinfectant solution in which objects to be sanitized are immersed. A cover is provided with most wet sanitizers to prevent contamination of the solution when it is not in use. (Fig. 17.26)

Client's cushion. The cushion is usually 8 to 12 inches and especially made for manicuring; a towel that is folded to cushion size can also be used. The cushion or folded towel should be covered with a clean, sanitized towel before each appointment.

Sanitized cotton container. This container will hold clean absorbent cotton.

Supply tray. The tray holds cosmetics such as polishers, polish removers, and creams.

Electric nail dryer. A nail dryer is an optional item used to shorten the length of time necessary for the client's nails to dry.

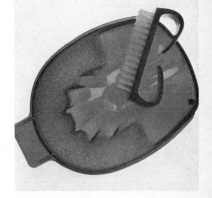

17.25 – Finger bowl filled with warm water and anti-bacterial soap, and nail brush

Implements

Implements are tools that must be sanitized or discarded after use with each client. They are small enough to be sanitized in a wet sanitizer.

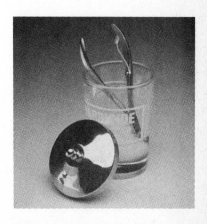

17.26 – Wet sanitizer

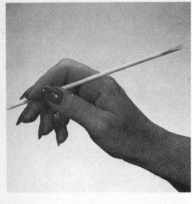

17.27 – Orangewood stick

Orangewood stick. Use the orangewood stick to loosen the cuticle around the base of a nail or to clean under the free edge. Hold the stick similarly to a pencil. For applying cosmetics, wrap a small piece of cotton around the end. (Fig. 17.27)

> CAUTION: If you drop an orangewood stick on the floor, it must be discarded. It is a disposable implement that cannot be sanitized or re-used. The cotton on an orangewood stick needs to be changed after each use.

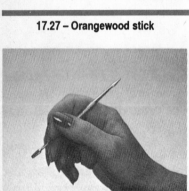

17.28 – Steel pusher

Steel pusher. The steel pusher, also called a cuticle pusher, is used to push back excess cuticle growth. Hold the steel pusher in the same way as the orangewood stick. The spoon end is used to loosen and push back the cuticle. If the pusher has rough or sharp edges, use an emery board to dull them. This prevents digging into the nail plate. (Fig. 17.28)

Metal nail file. A metal nail file is used to shape the free edge of hard or sculptured nails. Most professional nail technicians use seven- or eight-inch nail files because some states do not allow shorter files to be used. Since a nail file is metal and reusable, it must be sanitized after each use. When using a nail file, hold it with the thumb on one side of the handle and four fingers on the other side. (Fig. 17.29)

Emery board. Many nail technicians prefer an emery board to a nail file. It is also a good choice for filing soft or fragile nails, because it is not as coarse as a nail file. An emery board has two sides, a coarse-grained side and a fine-grained side. The coarse side is used to shape the free edge of the nail, and the fine side is used to bevel the nail or smooth the free edge. Hold the emery board in the same manner as a nail file, with the wider end in your hand so you can file with the narrow end. To bevel, hold the emery board at a 45-degree angle and file, using light pressure, on the top or underside of the nail. Most professional nail technicians use seven- or eight-inch emery boards because some states do not allow the use of smaller ones. Emery boards cannot be sanitized—either give it to the client or break it in half and discard it after use. It is not a good idea to save an emery board in a plastic bag for each client. Bacteria

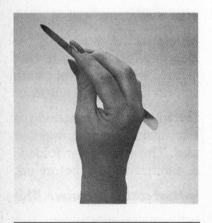

17.29 – Metal nail file

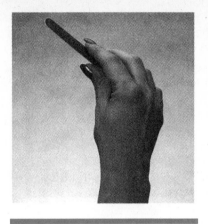

17.30 – Emery board

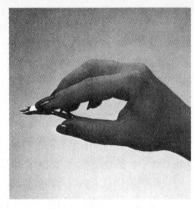

17.31 – Cuticle nippers

can grow on the unsanitized implement before the client's next appointment. (Fig. 17.30)

CAUTION: If you drop an emery board on the floor during a procedure, it must be discarded. This is a disposable item and cannot be reused or sanitized.

Cuticle nipper. A cuticle nipper is used to trim away excess cuticle at the base of the nail. To use the nippers, hold them in the palm of the hand with the blades facing the cuticle. Place the thumb on one handle and three fingers on the other handle, with the index finger on the screw to help guide the blade around cuticle. (Fig. 17.31)

Tweezers. Tweezers are used to lift small bits of cuticle from the nail.

Nail brush. A nail brush is used to clean fingernails and remove bits of cuticle with warm, soapy water. Hold the nail brush with the bristles turned down and away from you. Place the thumb on the handle side of the brush that is facing you, and the fingers on the other side.

Chamois buffer. The chamois (**SHAM**-ee) buffer is used to add shine to the nail and to smooth out corrugations or wavy ridges. There are two types of chamois buffer. The first has an open handle; the second has a closed handle on the top. To use the open-handled buffer, place the fingers around the handle with the thumb on the

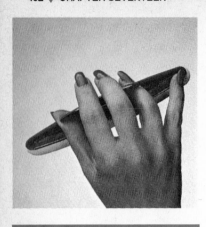

17.32 – Holding a nail buffer

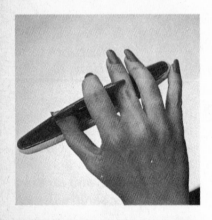

17.33 – Alternative way to hold a nail buffer

side of the handle to help guide it. To use the closed-handled type, rest the thumb along the edge of the buffer to guide and support the implement. Another way to hold a closed-handled chamois buffer is to place the middle and ring fingers through the closed-handled buffer if it has an open slot. Be guided by your instructor on how to hold the chamois buffer. (Figs. 17.32, 17.33)

> CAUTION: A chamois buffer must be designed so that the chamois can be changed for each client. Be sure to discard the used chamois after each use.

Fingernail clippers. Fingernail clippers are used to shorten nails. For very long nails, clipping cuts filing time.

Sanitation for Implements

It is recommended that you have two complete sets of metal implements. By doing so, a complete, sanitized set can be available for each client, with no waiting between appointments. If you have only one set of implements, remember that it takes 20 minutes to sanitize implements after each use. A few sanitation hints are given below:

- Wash all implements thoroughly with soap and warm water and rinse off all traces of soap with plain water. Dry them thoroughly with a sanitized towel.
- Metal implements should be immersed in a wet sanitizer with cotton at the bottom and filled with an approved disinfectant. The required sanitation time is 20 minutes. Dry the implements with a sanitized towel when they are removed from the wet sanitizer.
- Follow state regulations for storage of sanitized manicuring implements. They must be stored in sealed containers, sealed plastic bags, or in a cabinet sanitizer until they are needed.

Materials

Materials are supplies that are used during a manicure and need to be replaced for each client.

Disposable towels or terry cloth towels. A fresh, sanitized terry towel is used to cover the client's cushion before each manicure. Another fresh towel should be used to dry the client's hands after soaking in the finger bowl. Other terry or lint-free disposable towels are used to wipe spills that may occur around the finger bowl.

Cotton or cotton balls. Cotton is used to remove polish, wrap the end of the orangewood stick, and apply nail cosmetics. Some nail technicians prefer to use small, fiber-free squares to remove polish because they don't leave cotton fibers on the nails that might interfere with polish application.

Plastic spatula. The spatula is used to remove nail cosmetics from their containers. Always use a plastic spatula, not the fingers, to remove cosmetics. A closed container of nail cosmetics is a perfect place for bacteria to grow.

Plastic bags. Tape or clip a bag to the side of the manicuring table to hold materials used during a service. Line all trash cans with plastic bags. Be sure to have a generous supply of bags so that they can be changed regularly during the day.

Alcohol. Alcohol is used as a disinfectant for the manicure table and implements. Consult your state health department for information about the required strength.

Powdered alum or styptic powder. Powdered alum, or styptic powder, is used to contract the skin to stop minor bleeding that may occur during a manicure. To use, blot the cut with powdered alum on a cotton-tipped orangewood stick.

Nail Cosmetics

A professional nail technician needs to know how to use each nail cosmetic and what ingredients it contains. It is also important to know when to avoid using a product because of a client's allergies or sensitivities. This section identifies and describes some of the basic nail cosmetics, as well as listing their basic ingredients.

Anti-bacterial soap. This soap is mixed with warm water and used in the finger bowl. It contains a soap or detergent and an anti-bacterial agent to sanitize the client's hands. It comes in four forms: flaked, beaded, cake, and liquid.

Polish remover. Polish remover is used to dissolve and remove nail polish. It usually contains organic solvents and acetone. Sometimes oil is added to offset the drying effect of the acetone. Use non-acetone polish remover for clients who have artificial nails, since acetone will weaken or dissolve the tips, wrap glues, and sculptured nail compound.

Cuticle cream. Cuticle cream is used to lubricate and soften dry cuticles and brittle nails. It contains fats and waxes such as lanolin, cocoa butter, petroleum, and beeswax.

Cuticle oil. Cuticle oil keeps the cuticle soft and helps to prevent hangnails or rough cuticles. It gives an added touch to the finish of a manicure. Cuticle oil contains ingredients such as vegetable oil, vitamin E, mineral oil, jojoba, and palm nut oil. Suggest that your clients use it at bedtime to keep their cuticles soft.

Cuticle solvent or cuticle remover. Cuticle solvent makes cuticles easier to remove and minimizes clipping. It contains 2 to 5 percent sodium or potassium hydroxide, plus glycerin.

Nail bleach. Apply nail bleach to the nail plate and under the free edge to remove yellow stains. It contains hydrogen peroxide. If nail bleach cannot be purchased, use 20 volume (6 percent) hydrogen peroxide.

> CAUTION: Care must be taken not to get nail bleach on cuticles or skin because it can cause irritation.

Nail whitener. Nail whiteners are applied under the free edge of a nail to make the nail appear white. They contain zinc oxide or titanium oxide. Nail whiteners are available in paste, cream, coated string, and pencil form.

Dry nail polish. Dry nail polish, or **pumice** (PUM-is) powder is used with the chamois buffer to add shine to the nail. Some clients prefer it to liquid clear polish. Dry nail polish contains mild abrasives that are used for smoothing or sanding, such as tin oxide, talc, silica, and kaolin. Dry nail polish is available in powder and cream form.

Nail strengthener/hardener. Nail strengthener is applied to the nail before the base coat. It prevents splitting and peeling of the nail. There are three types of nail strengthener:

1. Protein hardener is a combination of clear polish and protein, such as collagen.
2. Nylon fiber is a combination of clear polish with nylon fibers. It is applied first vertically, and then horizontally on the nail plate. It can be hard to cover because the fibers on the nail are visible.
3. Formaldehyde strengthener contains 5 percent formaldehyde.

Base coat. The base coat is colorless and is applied to the nail before the application of colored polish. It prevents red or dark polish from yellowing or staining the nail plate. Base coat is the first polish applied in the polish procedure, unless a nail strengthener is being used. It contains more resin than colored polish to maintain a tacky surface, so the colored polish will adhere better. It contains ethyl acetate, a solvent, isopropyl alcohol, butyl acetate, nitrocellulose, resin, and sometimes formaldehyde.

Colored polish, liquid enamel, or lacquer. Colored polish is used to add color and gloss to the nail. Usually it is applied in two coats. Colored polish contains a solution of nitrocellulose in a volatile solvent such as amyl acetate, and evaporates easily. Manufacturers add castor oil to prevent the polish from drying too rapidly.

CAUTION: All nail polishes are flammable.

Top coat or sealer. The top coat, a colorless polish, is applied over colored polish to prevent chipping and to add a shine to the finished nail. It contains nitrocellulose, toluene, a solvent, isopropyl alcohol, and polyester resins.

Liquid nail dry. Liquid nail dry is used to prevent smudging of the polish. It promotes rapid drying so that the polish is not tacky, and prevents the polish from dulling. It has an alcohol base and is available in brush-on or spray.

Hand cream and hand lotion. Hand lotion and hand cream add a finishing touch to a manicure. Since they soften and smooth the hands, they make the finished manicure as beautiful as possible. Hand cream helps the skin retain moisture. It is thicker than hand lotion and is made of emollients and humectants such as glycerin, cocoa butter, lecithin, and gums. Hand lotion has a thinner consistency than hand cream because it contains more oil. In addition to oil, hand lotion contains stearic acid, water, mucilage of quince seed as a healing agent, lanolin, glycerin, and gum. Hand cream or hand lotion can be used as oil in a reconditioning hot oil manicure.

Nail conditioner contains moisturizers and should be applied at night, before bedtime, to help prevent brittle nails and dry cuticles.

PROCEDURE FOR BASIC TABLE SET-UP

It is important that the manicure table be sanitary and properly equipped with implements, materials, and cosmetics. Anything needed during a service should be readily available. An orderly table gives the client confidence during the manicure. The actual placement of supplies on the manicuring table is a suggestion. Since regulations regarding table set-up vary from state to state, be guided by your instructor. To set up a table, use the following procedure.

NOTE: If you are left-handed, reverse the placement of the equipment.

---

1. Wipe the manicure table with an approved disinfectant.
2. Wrap the client's cushion in a clean, sanitized towel—either terry cloth or disposable. Put it in the middle of the table so the cushion is toward the client and the end of towel is toward the operator.
3. Put cotton in the bottom of the wet sanitizer. Then fill the wet sanitizer with alcohol 20 minutes before the first manicure of the day. Put all metal implements into the wet sanitizer. Place the wet sanitizer to your right.
4. Put all cosmetics except polish on the right side of the table behind the wet sanitizer.
5. Put emery boards and a chamois buffer on the right side of the table.
6. Put a finger bowl and brush in the middle or to the left, toward the client. The finger bowl or hot oil heater should not be moved from side to side of the manicure table. It should stay where it is placed for the duration of the manicure. For a reconditioning hot oil manicure, replace the finger bowl and brush with an electric hot oil heater.
7. Tape or clip a plastic bag to right side of table. This is used for depositing used materials during the manicure.
8. Put polishes to the left.
9. The drawer can be used to keep the following items: extra cotton or cotton balls in their original container or in a fresh plastic bag; pumice stone or powder; extra chamois for buffer; instant nail dry or other supplies. Be sure to wipe the drawer with alcohol before putting supplies in it. Never place used materials in the drawer. Only completely sanitized implements sealed in air-tight containers and extra materials or cosmetics should be placed in this drawer. Always keep it clean and sanitary. (Fig. 17.34)

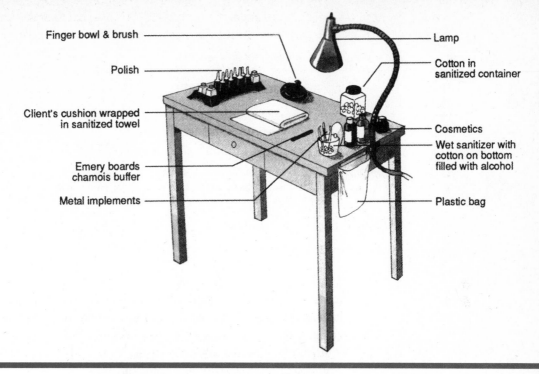

Finger bowl & brush

Polish

Client's cushion wrapped
in sanitized towel

Emery boards
chamois buffer

Metal implements

Lamp

Cotton in
sanitized container

Cosmetics

Wet sanitizer with
cotton on bottom
filled with alcohol

Plastic bag

17.34 – Basic table set-up; your instructor's table set-up is equally correct.

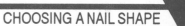

CHOOSING A NAIL SHAPE

Before performing a service on a client, take time to talk with that client. During the conversation, called the **client consultation,** you will discuss issues of general health, the health of nails and skin, the client's lifestyle and needs, and the nail services that you can perform. You will use your knowledge of skin, nails, and each type of nail service to help the client select the most appropriate service. If the client has a nail or skin disorder that prevents you from performing a service, refer that client to a physician and offer to perform a service as soon as the disorder has been treated. A good client consultation can make the difference between being a professional and just *doing nails.*

After the client consultation, discuss with the client the shape of the nails and polish color desired. Consider the shape of the hands, length of the fingers, shape of the cuticles, and the type of work the

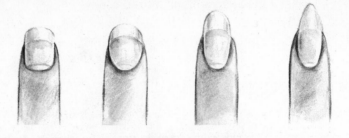

17.35 – The four basic nail shapes: rectangular, round, oval, and pointed

client does. The following are four shapes from which to choose. (Fig. 17.35)

- The rectangular or square nail should extend only slightly past the tip of the finger with the free edge rounded off. This shape is sturdy because the full width of the nail remains at the free edge. Clients who work with their hands—on a typewriter, computer, or assembly line—will need shorter, square nails.
- The round nail should be slightly tapered and extend just a bit past the tip of the finger.
- The oval nail is a square nail with slightly rounded corners. Professional clients whose hands are visible (professional business people, teachers, or salespeople, for example) may want longer oval nails.
- The pointed nail is suited to thin hands with narrow nail beds. The nail is tapered somewhat longer than usual to enhance the slender appearance of the hand; however, these nails are weak and break easily.

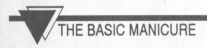

THE BASIC MANICURE

A professional nail technician follows a three-part procedure for all services. The **pre-service** consists of greeting and consulting with the client, and any necessary sanitizing steps. Next, the actual **procedure** will be performed. In the **post-service**, another appointment is scheduled, the client is given the opportunity to purchase any recommended products, and the technician once again sanitizes the work area and implements used.

Manicure Pre-Service

1. Set up a standard manicuring table.
2. Greet the client.
3. The client's hands should be washed with anti-bacterial soap. Thoroughly dry the hands and nails with a sanitized towel.
4. Refer to the client record/health card to record responses and observations during the client consultation. Check for nail disorders and decide if it is safe and appropriate to perform a service on this client. If the client should not receive service, explain the reasons and make a medical referral, if necessary. If it is safe to proceed, discuss the service desired by the client.
5. Begin working with the hand that is not the client's favored hand. The favored hand will need to soak longer, because it is used more often.

Manicure Procedure

During the manicure, talk with the client about the products and procedures being used. Suggest products the client will need to maintain the manicure between visits. These products might include polish, lotion, top coat, and emery boards.

> **NOTE:** The following procedure is written for a right-handed client.

1. **Remove polish.** Begin with the little finger of the client's left hand. Saturate cotton with polish remover. If the client is wearing artificial nails, use non-acetone remover to avoid damaging them. Hold saturated cotton on the nail for approximately 10 seconds. Wipe the old polish off the nail with a stroking motion toward the free edge. If all the polish is not removed, repeat this step until all traces of polish are gone. It may be necessary to put cotton around the tip of an orangewood stick and use it to clean polish away from the cuticle area. Repeat this procedure on each finger. (Fig. 17.36)

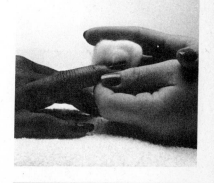

17.36 – Remove polish.

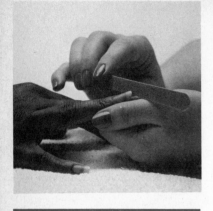

17.37 – Shape nails.

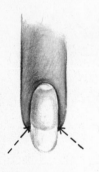

17.38 – Do not file into the corners of the nail.

NOTE: To keep loose cotton fibers from sticking to the nail or finger, roll a piece of cotton between your hands before using it. An alternative method to remove nail polish is to moisten cotton pledgets with nail polish remover and put them on all the nails at the same time. Pledgets absorb and do not leave a polish smear on the cuticles.

2. **Shape the nails.** Using an emery board or nail file, shape the nails. Start with the left little finger, holding it between the thumb and index finger. Use the coarse side of an emery board to shape the nail. File from the right side to the center of the free edge and from the left side to the center of the free edge. (Fig. 17.37) Do not file into the corners of the nails. (Fig. 17.38) File each hand from the little finger to the thumb.
3. **Soften the cuticles.** After filing the left hand, put it in a soap bath while filing the right hand, to soak and soften the cuticles.
4. **Clean the nails.** Brushing the nails and hands with a nail brush cleans the fingers and pieces of cuticle from the nails. Remove the left hand from the soap bath and brush the fingers with a nail brush. Use downward strokes, starting at the first knuckle and brushing toward the free edge. (Fig. 17.39)
5. **Dry the hand** with the end of a fresh towel. Make sure to dry between the fingers. Gently push back the cuticle. (Fig. 17.40)

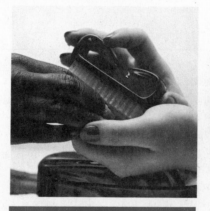

17.39 – Clean nails.

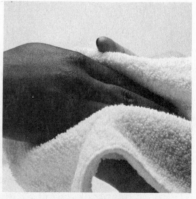

17.40 – Dry hand.

6. **Apply cuticle remover** using a cotton-tipped orangewood stick. Cuticle remover should be applied to the cuticle of each nail on the hand that has just been brushed. (Fig. 17.41) Saturate cotton with cuticle remover and spread the remover generously around the cuticles and under the free edge of each finger. Now, put the right hand into the soap bath to soak and work on the client's left hand. (Fig. 17.42)

7. **Loosen the cuticles.** Use an orangewood stick and/or the spoon end of a steel pusher to push back gently and lift the cuticle off of the nails of the left hand. Use a circular movement to help lift cuticles that cling to the nail plate. The cuticle remover will probably remove enough cuticle so that clipping will be unnecessary. (Fig. 17.43)

8. **Nip the cuticles.** Use a cuticle nipper to nip any ragged, excess cuticle or hangnails. Try to remove the cuticle in one piece. Wipe away excess cuticle remover if necessary to see the cuticle clearly. Be careful not to cut into the mantle—it will hurt the client. (Fig. 17.44)

9. **Clean under the free edge** using a cotton-tipped orangewood stick. Remove the right hand from the soap bath. Hold the left hand over the soap bath and brush a last time, to remove any bits of cuticle and traces of solvent. Then let the client's left hand rest on the sanitized towel. (Fig. 17.45)

10. **Repeat steps 4 through 9 on the right hand.**

11. **Bleach the nails—optional.** If the client's nails are yellow, they can be bleached with a prepared nail bleach or 20 volume (6 percent) hydrogen peroxide. Apply the bleaching agent to the yellowed nail with a cotton-tipped orangewood stick. Be careful not to brush bleach on the client's

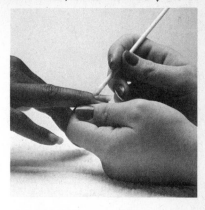

17.41 – Apply cuticle remover.

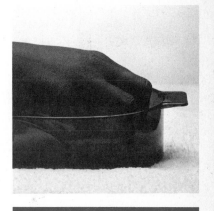

17.42 – Soak hand.

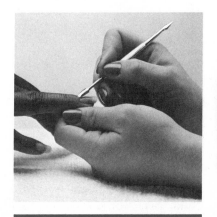

17.43 – Loosen cuticle.

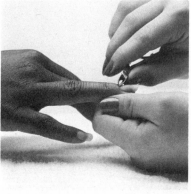

17.44 – Nip cuticles.

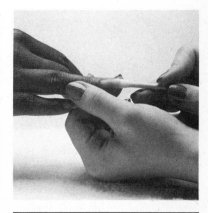

17.45 – Clean under free edge.

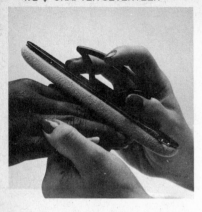

17.46 – Buff nail.

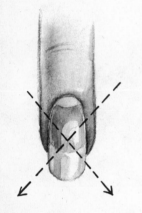

17.47 – Buff nail in an *X* pattern with downward strokes.

skin or cuticle—it will cause irritation. Apply the bleach several times if the nails are extremely yellow. Certain clients' nails will need to be bleached every time as part of each manicure for a period of time, since all the yellow may not fade after one service.

12. **Buff with a chamois buffer—optional.** To buff nails, apply dry nail polish to the nail with an orangewood stick. Buff on a diagonal, from the base of the nail to its free edge. (Fig. 17.46) Buff in one direction, from left to right with a downward stroke and then from right to left with a downward stroke, forming an X pattern. (Fig. 17.47) While buffing, lift the back of the buffer off the nail to prevent friction that will cause a burning sensation. After buffing, the client's hands should be washed to remove any traces of abrasive or dry polish. The chamois buffer also can be used to smooth out wavy ridges or corrugated nails.

> **NOTE:** Spraying the client's nail with water before buffing will reduce the heat generated during buffing.

13. **Apply cuticle oil.** Using a cotton-tipped orangewood stick, apply cuticle oil to each nail. Start with the little finger, left hand, and rub oil into each cuticle in a circular motion. (Fig. 17.48)

14. **Bevel nails.** To bevel (BEH-vel) the underside of the free edge, hold an emery board at a 45-degree angle and file with an upward stroke. This removes any rough edges or cuticle particles. (Fig. 17.49)

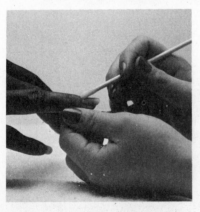

17.48 – Apply cuticle oil.

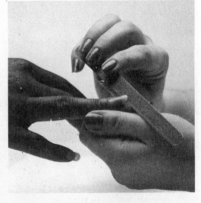

17.49 – Bevel nail.

15. **Apply hand lotion and massage hands and arms.** A hand massage is a pleasant touch before applying polish. Apply lotion or cream to the hand and arm with a sanitary spatula. (Follow the procedure for hand and arm massage on pages 478–481.)

16. **Remove traces of oil.** You must remove any traces of oil so that the polish will adhere to the nail. Use a small piece of cotton saturated with alcohol or polish remover.

17. **Choose a color.** If the client is undecided about a color of nail polish, suggest a shade that complements the skin tone. If the manicure and polish are for a special occasion, pick a color that matches the client's clothing. Generally, darker shades are appropriate for fall and winter, and lighter shades are better for spring and summer. Always have a variety of nail polish colors available. Before applying polish, suggest that the client pay for the service, put on any outer clothing, and get out car keys. This will avoid smudges on the fresh polish.

18. **Apply polish.** Polish is applied in four or five coats. The first, the base coat, is followed by two coats of color and one or two applications of top coat. (Fig. 17.50) Roll the polish bottle in the palms of the hands to mix. Never shake polish. Shaking causes air bubbles to form, which will make the polish application rough.

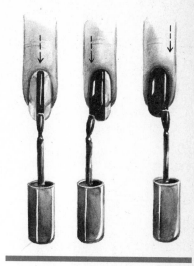

17.50 – Apply polish.

- **Base coat.** Base coat is applied first, to keep polish from staining the nails and to help colored polish adhere to the nail. The base coat will stay tacky to the touch. To apply the base coat, remove the brush from the bottle and wipe one side on the bottle neck so that a bead of polish remains on the end of the brush. Start in the center of the nail, position the brush one-sixteenth of an inch away from the cuticle, and brush toward the free edge. Using the same technique, do left side of nail, then the right side. There should be enough polish on the brush to complete three strokes without having to dip it back into the bottle. The more strokes used the more lines or lumps will show on the client's nail. Any small areas missed with the first color coat can be covered with the second coat.

- **Colored polish.** Apply two coats of colored polish with the same technique used for the base coat. Complete the first color coat on both hands before starting the second coat. Polish on the cuticle should be removed with a cotton-tipped orangewood stick saturated in polish remover. Never use a polish corrector pen—it is unsanitary.

- **Top coat.** Apply one or two coats of top coat to prevent chipping and to give nails a glossy look.
- **Instant nail dry—optional.** Apply instant nail dry on each nail to prevent smudging and dulling.

> **NOTE:** If you use an electric nail dryer, put one of the client's hands in the dryer while polishing the other. The dryer should be set on cool; this helps to dry the polish surface and makes it less likely to smudge.

Five Types of Polish Application

There are five different methods that can be used in applying polish:

1. **Full coverage.** The entire nail plate is polished.
2. **Free edge.** The free edge of the nail is unpolished. This helps to prevent the polish from chipping.
3. **Hairline tip.** The nail plate is polished and one-sixteenth of an inch is removed from the free edge. This prevents polish from chipping.
4. **Slimline or free walls.** Leave one-sixteenth of an inch margin on each side of the nail plate. This makes a wide nail appear narrow.
5. **Half-moon or lunula.** A half-moon shape, the lunula, at the base of the nail is unpolished.

> **NOTE:** If a finished nail becomes smudged, apply polish remover to the smudge before reapplying polish.

Manicure Post-Service

After the manicure is complete, follow the post-service procedure described below.

1. **Make another appointment.** Schedule another appointment with the client either to maintain the manicure or to perform another service.
2. **Sell retail products.** Suggest that the client purchase any products discussed during the manicure. Polish, lotion, top

coat, etc. are valuable tools for maintaining the nails between salon visits.

3. **Clean up around the table.** Take the time to restore the basic table set-up.

4. **Discard used materials.** Place all used materials in the plastic bag at the side of the table. If the bag is full or contains used materials from artificial nail services, discard it in a closed pail.

5. **Sanitize the table and implements.** Perform the complete pre-service sanitation procedure. Implements must be sanitized for 20 minutes before they can be used on the next client.

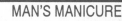

MAN'S MANICURE

A man's manicure is basically the same as a woman's manicure. Table set-up is the same, except that colored polish is not used. Some men like a clear liquid polish, and others prefer a dry polish and a chamois buffer. Using hand cream or lotion is optional.

Procedure

During the procedure, talk with the client about products that will help to maintain the manicure between visits. You might suggest clear polish and hand cream.

1. **Complete manicure pre-service.**
2. **Remove the old polish.** If the client has clear polish from a previous manicure, it must be removed. Begin with the left hand, little finger.
3. **Shape the nails.** Most men keep their nails fairly short. If the nails are long, clip them with fingernail clippers before filing them. (Fig. 17.51)

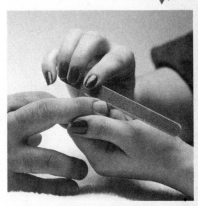

17.51 – Shape nails.

> **NOTE:** Nails that have been soaking are soft and easy to break or split when filed. Therefore, always file nails before soaking them.

4. **Soften the cuticles.** After filing the nails of the left hand, soak them in a soap bath while filing the right hand. (Fig. 17.52)
5. **Clean the nails and hands.** Brushing hands and nails with the nail brush cleans fingers and pieces of cuticle from

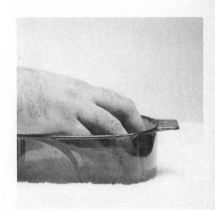

17.52 – Soften cuticles.

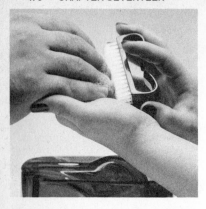

17.53 – Clean nails.

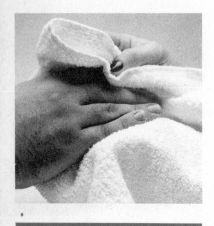

17.54 – Dry hand.

nails. Remove the left hand from the soap bath and brush the fingers with downward strokes, starting at the first knuckle and brushing in one direction toward the free edge. (Fig. 17.53)

6. **Dry the hand.** Use the end of the towel that is wrapped around the cushion, making sure to dry between the fingers. As you dry, gently push back the cuticle. (Fig. 17.54)

7. **Apply cuticle remover.** Use a cotton-tipped orangewood stick to apply cuticle remover to the back of each nail on the hand you've just brushed. Now, put the right hand into the soap bath while you continue to work on the client's left hand. (Fig. 17.55)

8. **Loosen the cuticles.** Men generally have more cuticle than women; therefore, more work may need to be done on them than in a women's manicure. Use the pusher to gently push back and lift the cuticle off the nails of the left hand. (Fig. 17.56)

9. **Nip the cuticles.** If you have to nip excess cuticle or hangnails, try to do so in one piece. (Fig. 17.57)

10. **Clean under the free edge.** Clean under the free edge with a cotton-tipped orangewood stick, hold the left hand over the soap bath and brush a last time, to remove bits of cuticle and traces of solvent that remain on the nail. Then let the client put the left hand on a sanitized towel. (Fig. 17.58)

11. **Repeat steps 5 through 10 on the right hand.**

12. **Bleach nails—optional.** If the client's nails are yellow, they can be bleached with a prepared nail bleach or by applying 20 volume (6 percent) hydrogen peroxide.

13. **Buff with a chamois buffer.** To shine the nails, apply dry

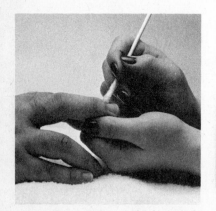

17.55 – Apply cuticle remover.

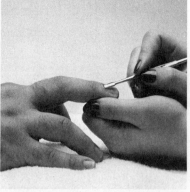

17.56 – Loosen cuticle with pusher.

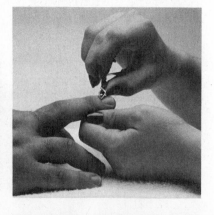

17.57 – Nip cuticles.

nail polish with an orangewood stick, buffing on a diagonal from the base of the nail to its free edge. Buff in one direction, from left to right, with a downward stroke and cross over from right to left with a downward stroke, forming an X pattern. As you buff, lift the back of the buffer off the nail to prevent friction that can cause a burning sensation. After buffing, the client's hands should be washed to remove any traces of abrasive or dry polish. The chamois buffer can also be used to smooth out wavy ridges or corrugated nails. This is done with an abrasive, such as pumice powder, that is applied to the nail with an orangewood stick. (Fig. 17.59)

14. **Apply cuticle oil.** Use a cotton-tipped orangewood stick to apply cuticle oil to each nail. Start with the little finger of the left hand and rub oil into each cuticle, in a circular motion. (Fig. 17.60)

15. **Bevel nails.** To bevel the underside of the free edge, hold an emery board at a 45-degree angle and file with an upward stroke. This removes any rough edges or cuticle particles.

16. **Apply hand lotion and massage the hands and arms—optional.** As a pleasant touch before applying polish, suggest a hand lotion or hand cream massage. Apply lotion or cream to the arm and hand with a sanitary spatula. (Follow the procedure for hand and arm massage on pages 478–481.) (Fig. 17.61)

17. **Remove traces of oil.** Using a small piece of cotton saturated with alcohol or polish remover, wipe off the nail.

18. **Polish the nails.** If the client wants polish, apply a base coat and a clear top coat. Follow with instant nail dry. (Fig. 17.62)

19. **Complete manicure post-service procedure.**

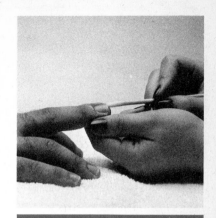

17.58 – Clean under free edge.

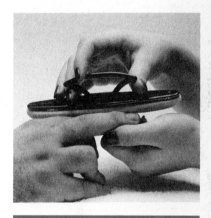

17.59 – Buff nails with chamois buffer.

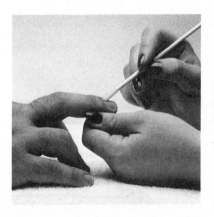

17.60 – Apply cuticle oil.

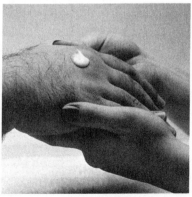

17.61 – Apply hand lotion.

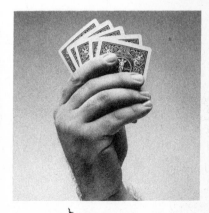

17.62 – Finished man's manicure

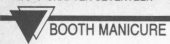

BOOTH MANICURE

In many barber-styling shops, the manicurist performs the manicure at the work station. This procedure is called a **booth** or **chair-side manicure** and requires that the manicurist either balance the supply tray on the lap or have a small table at hand. If manicures are to be performed chair-side, the styling chair should have a small, recessed hole at the end of the armrest to hold the finger bowl. The manicurist must then move around the client, depending on which hand is being manicured.

> **NOTE:** The manicurist who works chair-side should always be considerate of the barber-stylist's position during the haircutting/styling process in order to prevent client discomfort and interference with the stylist's procedure.

HAND AND ARM MASSAGE

Massage is a service that can be offered with any type of manicure. It stimulates blood flow, and relaxes the client.

> **CAUTION:** DO NOT use massage if the client has high blood pressure, a heart condition, or has had a stroke. Massage increases circulation and may be harmful to such clients. Have the client consult a physician first. Be very careful to avoid vigorous massage of joints if the client has arthritis. Talk with the client throughout the massage and adjust your touch to the client's needs.

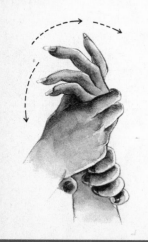

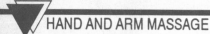

17.63 – Relaxer movement

Hand Massage Techniques

1. **Relaxer movement.** This is a form of massage known as **joint movement.** At the beginning of the hand massage the client has already received hand lotion or cream. Place the client's elbow on a cushion. With one hand, brace the client's arm. With the other hand, hold the client's wrist and bend it back and forth slowly five to ten times, until you feel the client has relaxed. (Fig. 17.63)
2. **Joint movement on fingers.** Bring the client's arm down, brace the arm with the left hand, and with the right hand start with the little finger, holding it at the base of the nail.

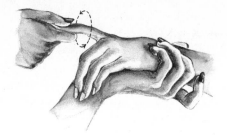

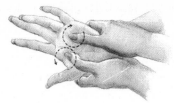

17.64 – Joint movement on fingers

17.65 – Circular movement effleurage (Male clients as well as female clients enjoy massage.)

Gently rotate the fingers to form circles. Work toward the thumb, three to five times on each finger. (Fig. 17.64)

3. **Circular movement in palm.** This is **effleurage (EF-loo-rahzh)**—light stroking that relaxes and soothes. Place the client's elbow on the cushion and, with your thumbs in the client's palm, rotate in a circular movement in opposite directions. (Fig. 17.65)

4. **Circular movement on wrist.** Hold the client's hand with both of your hands, placing your thumbs on top of client's hand, your fingers below the hand. Move the thumbs in a circular motion in opposite directions, from the client's wrist to the knuckle on the back of the client's hand. Move up and down three to five times. At the last rotation, wring the client's wrist by bracing your hands around the wrist and gently twisting in opposite directions. This is a form of friction massage—that is, a deep rubbing action, and very stimulating. (Fig. 17.66)

5. **Circular movement on back of the hand and fingers.** Now rotate down the back of the client's hand using the thumbs. Rotate down the little finger and the client's thumb, and gently squeeze off at the tips of the client's fingers. Go back and rotate down the ring finger and index finger, gently squeezing off. Now do the middle finger and squeeze off at the tip. This restores blood flow to normal. (Fig. 17.67)

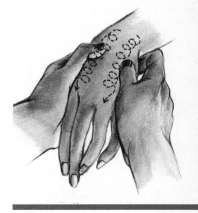

17.66 – Circular movement on wrist

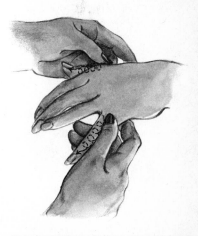

17.67 – Circular movement on back of hand and fingers

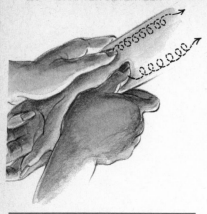

17.68 – Effleurage on arms

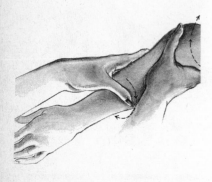

17.69 – Wringing movement on arm friction massage

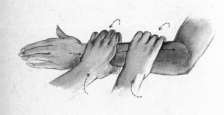

17.70 – Kneading movement on arm

Arm Massage Techniques

1. **Distribute cream or lotion.** Apply a small amount of cream to the client's arm and work it in. Work from the client's wrist toward the elbow, except on the last movement, when work should be from the elbow to the wrist. Finally, squeeze off at the fingertips, as at the end of a hand massage. Apply more cream if necessary.

2. **Effleurage on arms.** Put the client's arm on the table, bracing the arm with your hands. Hold the client's hand palm up in your hand. Your fingers should be under the client's hand, your thumbs side-by-side in the client's palm. Rotate your thumbs in opposite directions, starting at the client's wrist and working toward the elbow. When you reach the elbow, slide your hand down the client's arm to the wrist and rotate back up to the elbow three to five times. Turn the arm over and repeat three to five times on the top side of arm. (Fig. 17.68)

3. **Wringing movement on arm**—friction massage movement. A friction massage involves deep rubbing to the muscles. Bend the client's elbow so the arm is horizontal in front of you, with the back of the hand facing up. Place your hands around the arm with your fingers facing in the same direction as the arm, and gently twist in opposite directions as you would wring out a washcloth, from wrist to elbow. Repeat up and down the forearm three to five times. (Fig. 17.69)

4. **Kneading movement on the arm**. This technique is called the **petrissage** (PE-tre-sahza) kneading movement. It is very stimulating and increases blood flow. Place your thumbs on the top side of the client's arm so they are horizontal. Move them in opposite directions, from wrist to elbow and back down to wrist. This squeezing motion moves the flesh over the bone and stimulates the arm tissue. Do this three to five times. (Fig. 17.70)

5. **Rotation of the elbow**—friction massage movement. Brace the client's arm with your left hand and, with a cotton-tipped orangewood stick, apply cream to the elbow. Cup the elbow with your right hand and rotate your hand over the client's elbow. Repeat three to five times. To finish the elbow massage, move your left arm to the top of the client's forearm. Gently slide both hands down the forearm from the elbow to the fingertips as if climbing down a rope. Repeat three to five times. (Fig. 17.71)

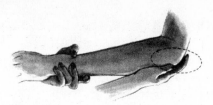

17.71 – Rotation of elbow

1. What are nails?
2. Describe the appearance of a healthy nail.
3. Of what main substance is the nail composed?
4. Locate the following: a) nail root; b) nail body; c) free edge; c) nail bed.
5. What two factors promote the growth of the nails?
6. What three factors retard the growth of the nail?
7. What part of the nail contains the nerve and blood supply?
8. Where does the formation of the nail occur?
9. How does the nail receive its nourishment?
10. What is the average growth of the nail?
11. Define nail disorder.
12. What is the golden rule for dealing with nail disorders?
13. List five nail disorders that can be serviced by a nail technician.
14. List five nail disorders that cannot be serviced by a nail technician.
15. When giving a manicure, equipment, implements, materials, and nail cosmetics are needed. Give three examples of each of these manicuring supplies.
16. What are two reasons for having a manicure table that is sanitary and properly equipped?
17. Describe the four basic nail shapes.
18. List the six steps in the basic manicure pre-service.
19. Briefly describe the basic manicure procedure.
20. Name the five types of polish applications.
21. List the five steps in the basic manicure post-service.
22. What type of polish application is included in a man's manicure?
23. What is a booth or chair-side manicure?
24. Name five hand massage techniques and five arm massage techniques.

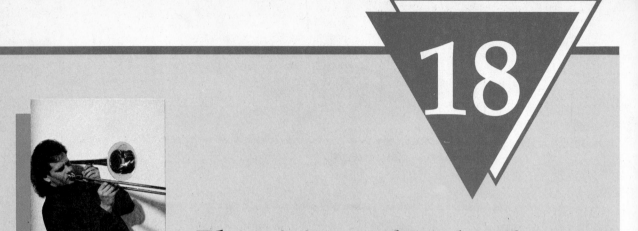

18

Electricity and Light Therapy

Learning Objectives

After completing this chapter, you should be able to:

1. *Define the nature of electricity.*

2. *Name two forms of electricity.*

3. *Identify the four most common types of current used in barber-styling shop services.*

4. *Discuss the procedures and benefits derived from using the four most commonly used currents.*

5. *List and describe electrical appliances available for use in the barber-styling shop.*

6. *Define light therapy.*

7. *List and define the different types of light therapy.*

8. *Explain the proper use of light therapy.*

9. *Demonstrate an understanding of the safety precautions to be practiced when using electrical appliances and light therapy.*

Courtesy of: The National Cosmetology Association's "Encore" release. Joel Moore, Design Team Direction. Jim Douglass, photographer.

ELECTRICITY

Electricity can be a valuable tool for the barber-stylist, provided it is used intelligently and carefully. A considerable amount of time and energy can be saved, and the effectiveness of treatments considerably improved, by the use of electrical energy.

Electricity is a form of energy that, while in motion, produces magnetic, chemical, and heating effects.

Electrical current is a stream of **electrons** (e-**LECK**-trons) (negatively charged particles) moving along a conductor when voltage is applied.

A **conductor** (kun-**DUCK**-tur) is a substance that readily transmits an electrical current. Most metals, carbon, the human body, and watery solutions of acids and salts are good conductors of electricity.

A **non-conductor** or **insulator** (**IN**-su-layt-or) is a substance that resists the passage of an electrical current, such as rubber, silk, dry wood, glass, cement, or asbestos.

An **electric wire** is composed of twisted, fine metal threads as a conductor, covered with rubber or silk as an insulator or non-conductor.

Electrodes are conductors that serve as points of contact when electricity is applied to the body.

An **electrical cycle** is a complete positive and negative wave of an alternating current.

Rheostats are adjustable resistors used for controlling the current in a circuit, such as a light dimmer.

USING ELECTRICITY

There are two types of electricity:

1. **Direct current (D.C.)** is a constant, even-flowing current, traveling in one direction, that produces a chemical reaction. A battery-operated instrument such as a portable radio or a flashlight uses direct current.
2. **Alternating current (A.C.)** is a rapid and interrupted current, flowing first in one direction and then in the opposite direction, that produces a mechanical action. A wall socket utilizes alternating current.

If necessary, one type of current can be changed to the other type by means of a converter or rectifier.

A **converter** (kon-**VER**-ter) is an apparatus used to change a direct current into an alternating current. A **rectifier** (REK-ti-feye-er) is used to change an alternating current into a direct current.

A **complete electrical circuit** is the entire path traveled by the current, from its generating source through various conductors and back to its original source.

Polarity is the negative or positive state of electric current.

Modalities are the currents used in electronic facial and scalp treatments such as **galvanic, sinusoidal, faradic,** and **Tesla high-frequency.**

Phoresis is the process by which chemical solutions are introduced into tissues through the skin by the use of galvanic current.

Electrical Measurements

The following terms designate electrical measurement units:

A **volt (V)** is a unit for measuring the pressure that forces the electrical current forward. A higher voltage increases the strength of the current. If the voltage is lower, the current is weaker.

An **amp (A)**, short for **ampere** (AM-pere), is the unit of measurement for the amount of current running through a wire. A cord must be heavy-duty enough to handle the amps put out by the appliance. For example, an appliance that puts out 40 amps of current requires a cord that is thicker than the one for an appliance that puts out 20 amps of current. If the current—or number of amps—is too strong, an appliance can overheat or the wires can burn out. If the current is not strong enough, the appliance will not operate correctly.

A **milliampere** (mil-i-AM-pere), is 1/1000 part of an ampere. The current for facial and scalp treatments is measured in milliamperes by a milliamperemeter (mil-i-AM-pere-mee-ter); an ampere current would be much too strong.

An **ohm (O)** is a unit for measuring the resistance of an electrical current. Unless the force (volts) is stronger than the resistance (ohms), current will not flow through the wire.

A **watt (W)** measures how much electric energy is being used in one second. A 40–watt bulb uses 40 watts of energy per second.

A **kilowatt (K)** equals 1000 watts. The electricity in a house is measured in kilowatt hours (kwh).

Safety Devices

A **fuse** is a safety device that prevents the overheating of electrical wires. It blows or melts when the wire becomes too hot from overloading the circuit with too much current from too many appliances, or if faulty equipment is used. To re-establish the circuit, the appliance must be disconnected and a new fuse inserted.

> CAUTION: When replacing a blown fuse be sure to use a new fuse with the proper rating; stand on a dry surface; and keep your hands dry.

Circuit Breakers

Modern building construction requires the use of circuit breakers to replace the old fuse box. Circuit breakers supply the same safety control as fuses against overloaded lines and faulty electrical apparatus. When wires become too hot because of overloading or a faulty piece of equipment, the breaker will click off or disengage, thus breaking the circuit.

If an electric appliance malfunctions while in operation, disconnect the appliance from the wall plug without delay.

A **ground fault circuit interruptor (GFCI)** is a device that provides protection. It is designed both to prevent dangerous electrical shocks and to provide over-current protection.

Safety of Electrical Equipment

The protection and safety of the client is the primary concern of the barber-stylist. All electrical equipment should be inspected regularly to determine whether or not it is in safe working condition. Carelessness in making electrical connections or using the right amount of current can result in a shock or a burn. Safety precautions help to eliminate accidents and ensure greater client satisfaction. (Figs. 18.1–18.4) Here is a list of safety hints about electricity:

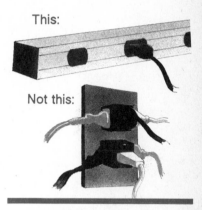

This:

Not this:

18.1 – Use only one plug to each outlet. Overloading, as in illustration on the bottom, may cause a fuse to blow out.

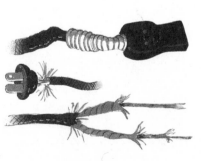

18.2 – Examine cords regularly.

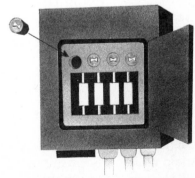

18.3 – Carefully replace blown-out fuses.

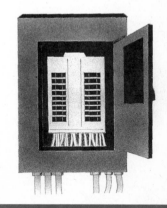

18.4 – Circuit breakers automatically disconnect any current from a defective appliance.

1. Study the instructions before using any electrical equipment.
2. Disconnect appliances when you have finished using them.
3. Keep all wires, plugs, and equipment in good repair.
4. Inspect all electrical equipment frequently.
5. Avoid wetting electrical cords.
6. When using electrical equipment, protect the client at all times.
7. Do not touch any metal while using an electrical appliance.
8. Do not handle electrical equipment with wet hands.
9. Do not allow the client to touch any metal surfaces while being treated with electrical equipment.
10. Do not leave the room when the client is connected to an electrical device.
11. Do not attempt to clean around an electric outlet while equipment is plugged in.
12. Do not touch two metallic objects at the same time if either is connected to an electric current.
13. Do not step on or set objects on electrical cords.
14. Do not allow electrical cords to become twisted or bent; the fine wires inside the cord will break and the insulation will wear away from the wires.
15. Disconnect the appliance by pulling on the plug, not the cord.
16. Do not repair electrical appliances unless you are qualified to do so.

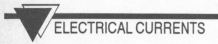

ELECTRICAL CURRENTS

Galvanic Current

The most commonly used modality is the **galvanic** current. It is a constant and direct current (DC), reduced to a safe, low-voltage level. Chemical changes are produced when this current is used. Galvanic current produces two different chemical reactions, depending on the polarity used on the area treated. A positive electrode is called an **anode**. It is red and is marked with a P or a plus (+) sign. A negative current is called a **cathode**. It is black and is marked with an N or a minus (-) sign.

Test for Polarity

If the electrodes are not marked with negative or positive indicators, a simple test can be used.

1. Separate the tips of two conducting cords from each other and immerse them into a glass of saltwater. Turn the selector switch of the appliance to galvanic current, and then turn up the intensity. As the water is decomposed, more active bubbles will accumulate at the negative pole than at the positive pole.
2. Place the tips of two conducting cords on two separate pieces of blue moistened litmus paper. The paper under the positive pole will turn red, while the paper under the negative pole will stay blue. If you use red litmus instead of blue, the positive pole will keep the red litmus the same and the negative pole will turn the red litmus blue.

CAUTION: Do not let the tips of the cords touch or you will cause a short circuit.

The effects of the positive pole on the body are the opposite of those produced by the negative pole.

The positive pole:

Produces acidic reactions

Closes the pores

Soothes nerves

Decreases blood supply

Contracts blood vessels

Hardens (firms) tissues

Forces alkaline solutions into the skin

The negative pole:

Produces alkaline reactions

Opens the pores

Stimulates (irritates) the nerves

Increases the blood supply to the skin

Expands the blood vessels

Softens tissues

Softens and liquifies grease deposits in the hair follicles and pores

Cataphoresis (**kat**-ah-fo-**REE**-sis) is the use of the positive pole to pull a positively charged substance (an acid pH astringent solution) into the skin. **Anaphoresis** (**an**-o-foh-**REE**-sis) is the use of the negative pole to force, or push, a negatively charged substance (an alkaline pH solution) into the skin.

CAUTION: Do not use a negative galvanic current on skin with broken capillaries, pustular acne conditions, or on a client with high blood pressure or metal implants.

The effects of galvanic current by using a galvanic machine are experienced by a client as the current passes through the body from one electrode to the other and completes a circuit. Both the active and inactive (positive and negative) poles must be functioning to complete the circuit. Both the active and inactive carbon (ball and cylinder) electrodes must be lightly wrapped with a moistened cotton pledget.

The **active electrode** is the electrode used on the area to be treated. For instance, if negative reactions (e.g., opened pores, softened tissue) are desired on the face, the negative pole is the active electrode. Apply the carbon ball or carbon roller to the active electrode.

The **inactive electrode** is the opposite pole from the active electrode. Either the client can hold the carbon stick (inactive electrode) wrapped in a moistened cotton pledget, or it can be placed somewhere on the client's body.

Procedure to Close Pores

1. Wrap the carbon ball electrode (active) in cotton moisturized with astringent.
2. Wrap the cylinder electrode (inactive) in cotton moisturized with water.
3. Have the client hold the inactive electrode or place the wet pad on a comfortable spot on the client's body.
4. After a good contact is established with the two electrodes, slowly turn up the current to the desired strength.
5. When the treatment is completed, slowly turn down the current before breaking contact with the client.

Faradic Current

Faradic (FAR-ad-ik) current is an alternating and interrupted current capable of producing a mechanical reaction without a chemical effect. It is used principally to cause muscular contractions.

When faradic current is applied to the body, the muscles are toned, circulation is improved, and metabolism is increased. It can be used during scalp and facial manipulations. The massage action of faradic current is beneficial because it invigorates the area receiving treatment.

Application

Two electrodes are required to complete the faradic circuit. The barber-stylist wears a wrist electrode with a moistened pad and the client holds a carbon electrode wrapped in damp absorbent cotton. Before turning on the current, contact is established with the client's forehead. During treatment the current is applied with the fingertips. At the completion of the treatment, the current is turned off slowly before breaking contact with the client.

It is as important to know when not to use faradic current as to know when to use it.

Benefits derived from the use of the faradic current include:

1. Improved muscle tone.
2. Removal of waste products.
3. Increased circulation of the blood.
4. Relief of congested blood.
5. Increased glandular activity.
6. Stimulated hair growth.

CAUTION: Do not use faradic current if it causes pain or discomfort, or if the face is very florid. If the client has many gold-filled teeth, any indication of high blood pressure, broken capillaries, or a pustular condition of the skin, treatment with faradic current should not be given.

Sinusoidal Current

Sinusoidal (si-nu-SOID-al) current, which resembles faradic current in many respects, may be used during scalp and facial manipulations. It is an alternating current that produces mechanical contractions in the muscles. Application is the same as for faradic current, requiring an electrode on the barber-stylist's wrist while the client holds the carbon electrode.

Advantages of using sinusoidal current include:

1. Greater stimulation, deeper penetration, and less irritation than faradic current.

2. Soothing of the nerves and penetration into the deeper muscle tissue.

Do not use the sinusoidal current if the face is flushed or if the client has broken capillaries in the skin, high blood pressure, or any pustular skin condition.

Faradic and sinusoidal currents are never used for longer than 15 to 20 minutes.

High-Frequency Current

High-frequency current is characterized by a high rate of oscillation. Of chief interest to the barber-stylist is **Tesla current**, commonly called **violet-ray**, used for both scalp and facial treatments.

The primary action of this current is thermal, or heat-producing. Due to its rapid oscillation, there are no muscular contractions. The physiological effects are either stimulating or soothing, depending on the method of application.

The electrodes for high-frequency current are made of glass or metal. Their shapes vary—the facial electrode is flat and the scalp electrode is rake-shaped. As the current passes through the glass electrode, tiny violet sparks are emitted. All treatments given with high-frequency current should be started with mild current and gradually increased to the required strength. Approximately five minutes should be allowed for a general facial or scalp treatment, depending upon the condition being treated. Follow manufacturer's directions.

Application

There are three methods of using the Tesla current:

1. **Direct surface application.** The barber-stylist holds the electrode and applies it over the client's skin. In facial treatments, the electrode is applied directly over facial cream.
2. **Indirect application.** The client holds the metal or glass electrode, while the barber-stylist manually massages the area receiving treatment.
3. **General electrification.** By holding a metal electrode in the hand, a client's body becomes charged with electricity without being touched by the barber-stylist.

To obtain sedative, calming, or soothing effects with a high-frequency current, the general electrification treatment is used, or the electrode is kept in close contact with the areas treated by the use of direct surface application.

To obtain a stimulating effect, lift the electrode from the area and apply the current through the clothing or a towel.

NOTE: When applying high-frequency current along with skin and scalp lotions containing alcohol, apply the electricity first, then the lotion.

CAUTION: The client should avoid any contact with metal, such as chair arms or stools. A burn may occur if such contact is made.

Benefits derived from the use of Tesla high-frequency current are as follows:

1. Stimulated blood circulation.
2. Increased glandular activity.
3. Aid to elimination and absorption.
4. Increased metabolism.
5. Germicidal action.

Tesla current may be used to treat shedding hair, itchy scalp, tight scalp, and excessively oily or dry skin and scalp.

LIGHT THERAPY

Light therapy refers to treatment by means of light rays. In barber-styling we are concerned with the white rays of the visible spectrum, those producing heat, known as infrared rays, and ultraviolet rays which produce chemical and germicidal reaction. When the white light of the visible spectrum is passed through a glass **prism** it produces the seven colors of the rainbow, arrayed in the following manner: red, orange, yellow, green, blue, indigo, and violet. These colors,

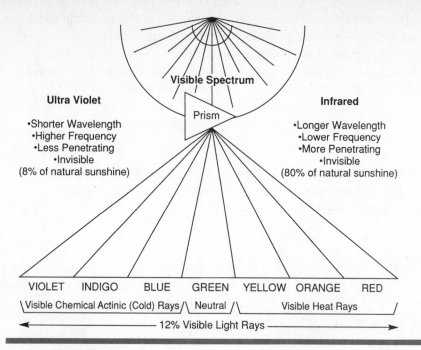

18.5 – Dispersion of light rays by a prism

which are visible to the eye, constitute the visible rays, or visible spectrum which makes up 12 percent of natural sunlight. (Fig. 18.5)

How Light Rays Are Reproduced

Artificial light rays are produced by using an electrical apparatus called a **therapeutic** (ther-a-**PYOO**-tik) **lamp**. These lamps or bulbs are capable of producing the same rays that are originated by the sun. The lamp used to reproduce these light rays is usually a dome-shaped reflector mounted on a pedestal with a flexible neck. The dome usually has a highly polished metal lining capable of reflecting the rays from the different types of light.

There are separate lamps for ultraviolet and infrared rays.

Ultraviolet Lamps

There are three general types of ultraviolet lamps: the glass bulb, the hot quartz, and the cold quartz.

The **glass bulb lamp** is used mainly for cosmetic or tanning purposes.

The **hot quartz lamp** is a general, all-purpose lamp suitable for tanning, tonic, cosmetic, or germicidal purposes.

The **cold quartz lamp** produces mostly short ultraviolet rays. It is used primarily in hospitals.

Infrared rays give no light whatsoever—only a rosy glow when active. Special glass bulbs are used to produce infrared rays. The visible rays, or dermal lights, are reproduced by carbon or tungsten filaments in clear glass bulbs, which give the white light; or in colored bulbs, which give red or blue colors.

> CAUTION: The client's eyes should always be protected by cotton pads saturated with a boric acid or witch hazel solution and placed on the eyelids during final treatments. The barber-stylist and client should always wear safety eye goggles when using ultraviolet rays.

Visible Light Rays

The lamp used to reproduce visible lights is usually also a dome-shaped reflector mounted on a pedestal with a flexible neck. The dome is finished with a highly polished metal lining capable of reflecting heat rays. The bulbs used with this lamp come in various colors for different purposes. As with all other lamps, the client's eyes must be protected from the glare and heat of the light. For proper eye protection, the client's eyes are covered with cotton pads saturated with boric acid or witch hazel solution.

Uses and Effects of White Light:

1. Relieves pain, especially in congested areas, and more particularly around the nerve centers, such as the back of the neck and across the shoulders.

Uses and Effects of Blue Light:

1. Has a tonic effect on the bare skin.
2. Is deficient in heat rays.
3. Has a soothing effect on the nerves.
4. To obtain the desired result, it is always used over the bare skin. Cream, oil, or powder must not be present on the skin.

Uses and Effects of Red Light:

1. Has strong heat rays.
2. Has a stimulating effect when used over the skin.
3. Penetrates more deeply than blue light.
4. Heat rays aid the penetration of lanolin creams into the skin.

5. Is recommended for dry, scaly, and shriveled skin.

6. Is used over creams and ointments to soften and relax body tissue.

Ultraviolet Rays

Scientists have discovered that at either end of the visible spectrum are rays of the sun that are invisible to us. The rays beyond the violet are the ultraviolet rays, also known as the **actinic** (ack-TIN-ick) rays. They are the shortest and least penetrating rays of the spectrum, comprising about 8 percent of sunshine. The action of these rays is both chemical and germicidal.

Ultraviolet (UV) rays are divided into three categories: UVA, UVB, and UVC. The farther away from the visible light spectrum, the shorter and less penetrating the ultraviolet rays. UVC rays are the most germicidal and chemical of the ultraviolet rays, as well as being the farthest away from the visible spectrum. These rays cause the most burning to the skin. UVC rays are destructive to bacteria, as well as to skin tissue if the skin is exposed to them for too long a period of time.

UVB rays are the therapeutic rays in the middle of the UV range, which produce some effects from both ends of ultraviolet rays. This ray will also burn if the skin is left exposed too long. The UVA ray is the tonic UV ray. It is closest to the visible spectrum, penetrates most deeply, and is the longest of all the UV rays. The UVA ray is used in tanning booths. This ray does not burn the skin but penetrates deeply into the skin tissue, and can destroy the elasticity of the skin, causing premature aging and wrinkling.

It was once thought that the slightest obstruction would keep ultraviolet rays from reaching the skin. Recent studies have proven that ultraviolet rays can penetrate up to three feet below the water and that approximately 50 percent of ultraviolet rays can penetrate to the skin through a wet T-shirt. In order to receive full benefit from ultraviolet rays, the area treated should be bare and no cream or lotion should be applied.

Application of Ultraviolet Rays

Ultraviolet rays are applied with a lamp at a distance of 30 to 36 inches from the skin. If shorter rays are needed, the lamp can be used as close as 12 inches from the skin. Extra precautions must be used when the lamp is held at such a close range, to avoid damage to skin tissue.

Time Limit

The average exposure can produce redness of the skin; overdoses will cause blistering. It is well to start with a short exposure of two to three minutes and gradually increase the exposure over a period of days to seven to eight minutes.

Benefits of Ultraviolet Rays

Ultraviolet rays increase resistance to diseases by increasing iron and vitamin D content and the number of red and white cells in the blood. They also increase elimination of waste products, restore nutrition where needed, and stimulate the circulation by improving the flow of blood and lymph. The rays also have a tendency to increase the fixation of calcium in the blood. Ultraviolet rays are used to treat acne, tinea, seborrhea, and to combat dandruff. They also promote healing and can stimulate the growth of hair, as well as produce a tan by increasing skin pigment if the skin is exposed in short doses over a long period of time.

Disadvantages of Ultraviolet Rays

Ultraviolet rays destroy hair pigment. Continued exposure to the sun's rays causes premature aging of the skin, painful sunburn, and a higher risk of skin cancer, especially for fair- or light-skinned individuals.

Infrared Rays

Beyond the red rays of the spectrum are the infrared rays. These are pure heat rays, comprising about 80 percent of sunshine.

Infrared rays are long, have the greatest (deepest) penetration, and can produce the most heat. The infrared lamp produces a reddish glow when turned on. Infrared lamps can be red or white.

The lamp should be operated at an average distance of 30 inches. Check the client's comfort frequently.

CAUTION: Never leave the client unattended during the exposure time or permit the light rays to remain on the body tissue for more than a few seconds at a time. Move your hand back and forth across the ray's path to break constant exposure. Length of exposure should be about five minutes.

Uses and Effects of Infrared Ray Treatment

1. Heats and relaxes the skin without increasing the temperature of the body as a whole.
2. Dilates blood vessels in the skin, thereby increasing blood circulation.
3. Increases metabolism and chemical changes within skin tissues.
4. Increases the production of perspiration and oil on the skin.
5. Relieves pain in sore muscles.
6. Soothes nerves.

REVIEW QUESTIONS

Electricity

1. What is electricity?
2. What is a conductor? What metal serves as a conductor in an electric wire?
3. What is a non-conductor or insulator? Give two examples.
4. What are electrodes?
5. What is a direct current (D.C.)?
6. What is an alternating current (A.C.)?
7. Which apparatus changes a direct current into an alternating current?
8. Which apparatus changes an alternating current into a direct current?
9. What is a volt?
10. What is an ampere?
11. What is an ohm?
12. What is polarity?
13. What is phoresis?
14. Name four electrical currents used in facial and scalp treatments.

High-Frequency or Violet Ray

1. What is a high-frequency current?
2. Which type of high-frequency current is commonly used in the barber-stylist shop?
3. What effects does the Tesla current produce on the body?
4. Name three kinds of electrodes used with high-frequency.
5. Name three methods of applying the Tesla current.
6. Briefly describe how to use direct surface application.
7. Briefly describe how to use indirect application.
8. Briefly describe how to use general electrification.
9. Which method of application produces soothing results?
10. How are stimulating effects produced?

11. How long should a general facial or scalp treatment take to administer?
12. What safety precaution should be observed when using hair tonics having a high alcoholic content?
13. List four benefits obtained by using the Tesla current.
14. List five scalp conditions that may be treated with the Tesla current.

1. What is light therapy?
2. Which rays of the sun are invisible?
3. What is a therapeutic lamp?
4. Name three types of therapeutic lamps that produce ultraviolet rays.
5. Which ultraviolet lamps are desirable for the barber-stylist shop?
6. Which four blood constituents are increased by exposure to ultraviolet rays?
7. What effects do ultraviolet rays have on body functions?
8. Which skin and scalp disorders are helped by ultraviolet rays?
9. What benefit does the hair receive from ultraviolet rays?
10. What is the shortest distance the ultraviolet lamp should be kept from the skin?
11. Why should the eyes of both barber-stylist and client be covered with safety goggles during exposure to ultraviolet rays?
12. How long should the skin be exposed for the first time?
13. To how many minutes can exposure be gradually increased?
14. Why should prolonged exposure be avoided?
15. What causes the skin to tan?
16. Why should the skin be cleaned before exposure to ultraviolet rays?
17. Which types of therapeutic lamps produce infrared rays?
18. How should the client's eyes be protected during exposure to infrared rays?
19. How far should the infrared lamp be kept from the skin?
20. Why should infrared light rays be broken with a hand movement?
21. What are the six effects of infrared rays on the body?
22. Which types of therapeutic lamps produce visible lights?
23. Why should the client's eyes be protected during exposure to therapeutic lamps?
24. What is the benefit of using a white light?
25. Which visible light lacks heat rays?
26. What are the benefits of using a blue light?
27. What are the three benefits of using a red light?

Light Therapy

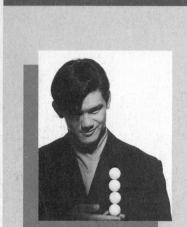

19

Chemistry

Learning Objectives

After completing this chapter, you should be able to:

1. *Define organic and inorganic chemistry.*

2. *Define matter and its states.*

3. *Describe the composition of elements, compounds, and mixtures.*

4. *Describe the parts of an element.*

5. *Discuss the four classes of compounds.*

6. *Define physical and chemical changes in matter.*

7. *Discuss the properties of matter, elements, compounds, and mixtures.*

8. *Describe the chemistry of water.*

9. *Define pH.*

10. *Discuss chemistry as applied to cosmetics.*

Courtesy of: The Ice Cream Collection. NCA's S/S '92 Fashion Release. Danny Ewert, Design Team Director. Jim Douglass, photographer.

The professional barber-stylist works with chemicals and performs services that change the hair chemically and physically. An understanding of the health and safety standards of the chemicals used will help to protect both the barber-stylist and the client.

A basic knowledge of modern chemistry is essential for an intelligent understanding of the various products and cosmetics used in the barber-hairstyling shop. Through advances in chemistry, new and better products are being developed constantly. It is, therefore, important that the professional technician understand these products and learn how to use them for the maximum benefits.

SCIENCE OF CHEMISTRY ▼

Chemistry (KEM-i-stree) is the science that deals with the composition, structure, and properties of matter and how matter changes under different chemical conditions. The subject of chemistry is divided into two areas: organic and inorganic chemistry.

Organic Chemistry

Organic (or-**GAN**-ik) **chemistry** is that branch of chemistry that deals with all substances in which carbon is present. Carbon can be found in all plants, animals, petroleum, soft coal, natural gas, and in many artificially prepared substances. Most organic substances are not soluble in water, but they are soluble in organic solvents, such as alcohol and benzene.

Organic substances are slow in their chemical reactions. Examples of organic substances are grass, trees, gasoline, oil, soaps, detergents, plastics, and antibiotics.

Inorganic Chemistry

Inorganic chemistry deals with all substances that do not contain carbon. Inorganic substances will not burn and are usually soluble in water. They are usually quick in their chemical reactions. Examples are water, air, iron, lead, iodine, and bones.

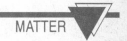

It is not the purpose of this text to train scientists, but to help barber-styling students learn enough about matter to help them in their professional work. It is, therefore, advisable that we briefly examine the nature and the structure of matter.

Matter may be defined as anything that occupies space. It exists in three physical forms: solids, liquids, and gases.

Look around the classroom and note what you see: hair, students, teachers, desks, chairs, walls. These are all matter in a solid state. In the clinic area of the school you see water, shampoos, lotions, hair tonics. These are matter in a liquid state. Take a deep breath. The air you have just brought into your lungs is also matter. It is in a gaseous state.

Matter exists in the form of elements, compounds, and mixtures. A substance is a unit or part of matter that is defined by a particular set of qualities. Elements and compounds are pure substances.

Elements

An element is the basic unit of all matter. It is a substance that cannot be made by the combination of simpler substances and the element itself cannot be reduced to simpler substances. There are 103 elements that are now known, of which some of the more common are iron, sulphur, oxygen, zinc, and silver.

Each element is given a letter symbol. Iron is Fe; sulphur, S; oxygen, O; zinc, Zn; and silver, Ag.

Atoms

An atom is the smallest part of an element that possesses the characteristics of the element. Therefore, an atom of hydrogen has the properties of hydrogen. Should this atom be smashed, it would no longer possess those properties and would no longer resemble a hydrogen atom.

Molecules

A molecule is the smallest part of an element or compound that possesses all the properties of the element or compound. If the molecule is of an element, the atoms are the same. If it is of a compound, the atoms are different. For example, a molecule of hydrogen contains two or more atoms of hydrogen, whereas a molecule of the compound of water is composed of two atoms of hydrogen and one atom of oxygen (H_2O).

Chemical Activities

In general, when we talk about the chemical activity of an element, we refer to the tendency of its atoms to combine with other elements. For example, hydrogen is a very active element and readily combines with other elements, while neon is completely inactive and does not combine with other elements.

Compounds

When two or more elements unite chemically, they form a compound. Each element loses its characteristic properties and the new compound develops its own individual properties. For example, iron oxide (rust) has different properties than the two elements of which it is comprised—iron and oxygen. The new substance, which is a compound, cannot be altered by mechanical means, but only by chemical methods.

Compounds can be divided into four classes:

1. Oxides are compounds of any element combined with oxygen. For example, one part carbon and two parts oxygen equal **carbon dioxide.** One part carbon and one part oxygen equal **carbon monoxide.**

2. Acids are compounds of hydrogen, a non-metal such as nitrogen and, sometimes, oxygen. For example, hydrogen + sulphur + oxygen = **sulphuric acid** (H_2SO_4). Acids turn blue litmus paper red, providing a quick way to test a compound.

ELEMENTS AND COMPOUNDS

Matter	Types and Definition	Smallest Particle
Solids Gases Liquids	Elements: Simplest form of matter	Atom: [Cannot be broken down by simple chemical reactions.] About 100 different kinds.
	Compounds: Formed by combination of elements.	Molecule: [Consists of two or more atoms chemically combined.] Unlimited kinds possible.

Elements Found in Skin or Hair	Compounds Used on Skin or Hair
Carbon	Water
Nitrogen	Hydrogen peroxide
Oxygen	Ammonium thioglycolate
Sulfur	Alcohol
Hydrogen	Alkalis
Phosphorus	

3. Bases, also known as alkalis, are compounds of hydrogen, a metal, and oxygen. For example, sodium + oxygen + hydrogen = **sodium hydroxide** (NaOH), which is used in the manufacture of soap. Bases will turn red litmus paper blue.

4. Salts are compounds that are formed by the reaction of acids and bases, with water also produced by the reaction. Two common salts and their formulas are **sodium chloride** (table salt) (NaCl), which contains sodium and chloride; and **magnesium sulphate** (Epsom salts) ($MgSO_4.7H_2O$), which contains magnesium, sulphur, hydrogen, and oxygen.

Mixtures

A mixture is a substance that is made up of two or more elements combined physically rather than chemically. The ingredients in a mixture do not change their properties, as they do in a compound, but retain their individual characteristics. For example, concrete is composed of sand, gravel, and cement. While concrete is a mixture having its own functions, its ingredients never lose their characteristics.

In a compound, the resulting properties from the chemical union, such as density, color, solubility, etc., are generally completely different from those of the substances combined. Every particle looks and acts like every other particle in the compound. A compound may never be separated by purely mechanical means. In making a compound, there are always energy and matter changes.

In a mixture, the resulting properties are the same as they were originally. The particles of one substance differ from another. Mixtures may be separated by mechanical means. In making a mixture, there are no changes in energy.

Changes in Matter

Matter may be changed either physically or chemically. **Physical change** refers to an alteration of the properties without the formation of a new substance. For example, ice, a solid, melts at a certain temperature and becomes water, a liquid. Conversely, water, a liquid, freezes at a certain temperature and becomes a solid. There is no change in the inherent nature of the substance—merely a change in form.

In a **chemical change** a new substance or substances is formed, having properties different from the original substance. For example, soap is formed from the chemical reaction between an alkaline substance, potassium hydroxide, and an oil or fat. The soap resembles neither the alkaline substance nor the oil from which it is formed.

Properties of Matter

The **properties of matter** refers to how one form of matter is distinguished from another. These properties are broken down into two categories—physical and chemical properties.

Physical Properties

These refer to properties, such as density, specific gravity, odor, color, taste.

1. Density of a substance refers to its weight divided by its volume. For example, the volume of one cubic foot of water weighs 62.4 pounds. Therefore, its density is its weight, 62.4 pounds divided by its volume, 1 cubic foot, equalling a density of 62.4 pounds per cubic foot.

2. Specific gravity of a substance is also referred to as its relative density. This means that substances are referred to as more or less dense than water. For example, copper is 8.9 times as dense as water; therefore, its specific gravity or relative density is 8.9.

3. A substance's odor helps to identify it. For example, the characteristic odor of ammonium thioglycolate is one of its distinguishing characteristics.

4. Color also helps in the identification of many substances. Gold, silver, copper, brass, and coal, for instance, are identified in part by their color.

5. Taste is an identifying trait, as well. For example, oil of wintergreen can be identified by its peppermint taste.

Chemical Properties

The chemical properties of a substance refer to the ability of the substance to react, and the conditions under which it reacts. Two such chemical properties are combustibility and the ability to support combustion. For example, phosphorus is a highly combustible substance. For that reason, it is used on the tips of matches. The heat produced by rubbing the match tip against a surface is enough to cause it to burst into flames.

One of the chemical properties of wood is its ability to support combustion. It is, therefore, used in the manufacture of matches. The phosphorous tip starts the fire and the wood supports the fire.

Properties of Common Elements, Compounds, and Mixtures

Knowledge of some of the properties of the most common elements, compounds, and mixtures is helpful to understand the reasons for certain chemical reactions.

Oxygen (O) is the most abundant element, being found both free and in compounds. It composes about 50 percent of the earth's crust and rock, 20 percent of air, and 90 percent of the water. It is a colorless, odorless, tasteless, gaseous substance, combining with most other elements to form an infinite variety of compounds called oxides. One of the chief characteristics of this element is that substances burn more readily in oxygen than in air.

Hydrogen (H) is also a colorless, odorless, and tasteless gas. It is the lightest element known, being used as a unit of weight. It is inflammable and explosive when mixed with air. It is found in chemical combination with oxygen in water, and with other elements in acids, bases, and organic substances such as wood, meat, fish, sugar, and butter.

Air is the gaseous mixture that makes up the earth's atmosphere. It is odorless and colorless, and consists of approximately one part by volume of oxygen and four parts of nitrogen. These proportions vary somewhat, according to conditions. It also contains a small amount of carbon dioxide, ammonia, nitrates, and organic matter, which are essential to plant and animal life.

Hydrogen peroxide (H_2O_2) is a compound of hydrogen and oxygen. It is a colorless liquid with a characteristic odor and a slightly acid taste. Organic matter, such as silk, hair, feathers, and nails, are bleached by hydrogen peroxide because of its oxidizing power. Hydrogen peroxide solution is used as a bleaching agent for the hair in solutions of 20 to 40 volume. A 3 to 5 percent solution of hydrogen peroxide possesses antiseptic qualities.

Oxidizing agents are substances that readily give up their oxygen. Hydrogen peroxide releases oxygen which in turn oxidizes the hair pigment to a colorless compound. The bleaching agent is reduced and the pigment is oxidized.

When oxygen is taken away from any substance, it is known as reduction. The substance that attracts the oxygen is the reducing agent. Oxidation is always accompanied by reduction.

Nitrogen (N) is a colorless, gaseous element found free in the air. It constitutes part of the atmosphere, forming about four-fifths of air. It is necessary to life because it dilutes the oxygen. It is found in nature chiefly in the form of ammonia and nitrates.

Acidity and Alkalinity

You may recall from the chapter **Treatment of the Scalp and Hair** that the pH of a solution is a chemical measure of its acidity or alkalinity. The pH scale ranges from 0 to 14. Pure water is considered neutral and represented by the number seven in the middle of the scale. Recall that if a solution has a pH of less than seven, it has an acid pH; if a solution has a pH of more than seven, it has an alkaline pH. Also remember that an alkaline solution softens and swells hair while an acid solution contracts and hardens hair.

There are meters and other indicators such as **nitrozine paper** that measure the pH of the products you use as a barber-stylist. If a product is more alkaline, the paper turns dark; if it is more acid, there is not much, if any, change in color.

If hair is wet with water and the pH balance is tested, the result is normally between 4.4 and 4.5; it is slightly acid. Most shampoos have a pH of about eight (more alkaline); chemical waving solutions have a pH of about nine (also more alkaline). Color rinses have a pH of about two and neutralizers about three. Unless a barber-stylist is familiar with a client's hair and history, it is wise to use solutions that are close to a pH balance of seven. Otherwise, a client's hair can be damaged inadvertently.

CHEMISTRY OF WATER

Water (H_2O) is the most abundant of all substances, composing about 75 percent of the earth's surface and about 65 percent of the human body. It is the universal solvent. De-mineralized or distilled water is used as a non-conductor of electricity, while water containing certain mineral substances is an excellent conductor of electricity.

Only water of known purity is fit for drinking purposes. Suspended or dissolving impurities render water unsatisfactory for cleaning objects and for use in shops.

Impurities can be removed from water by:

1. **Filtration** (fil-**TRAY**-shun): passing it through a porous substance, such as filter paper or charcoal.
2. **Distillation** (dis-ti-**LAY**-shun): heating in a closed vessel arranged so that the resulting vapor passes off through a tube and is cooled and condensed to a liquid. This process purifies water used in the manufacture of cosmetics.

Boiling water at a temperature of 212 degrees fahrenheit or 100 degrees celsius will destroy most microbic life.

It is very important that soft water be used for shampooing, lightening, or tinting the hair. Rain water is the softest water. Hard water contains mineral substances such as calcium and magnesium salts, that curdle or precipitate soap instead of permitting a permanent lather to form. Hard water may be softened by distillation or by use of sodium carbonate (washing soda) or sodium phosphate. To effectively soften hard water in barber-styling shops, **zeolite tanks** are used.

A good test for soft water uses a soap solution made by dissolving three-quarters of an ounce of pure, powdered castile soap in a pint of distilled water. A pint bottle is half-filled with fresh water and 0.5 ml. (about seven drops) of the soap solution is added. The bottle is then shaken vigorously. If a lather forms at once and persists, the water is very soft. If a lather does not appear at once, another 0.5 ml. of soap solution is added and the shaking repeated. If an additional 0.5 ml. of the soap solution is needed to produce a good lather, the water is hard and must be softened.

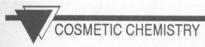

COSMETIC CHEMISTRY

Cosmetic chemistry is the scientific study of the cosmetics used in the barber-styling industry. An understanding of the chemical composition, preparation, and use of cosmetics that are intended to cleanse and improve external hygiene will better equip the barber-stylist to serve the public.

Cosmetics are classified according to their physical and chemical characteristics.

The physical and chemical classification of cosmetics are:

1. Powders
2. Solutions
3. Suspensions
4. Emulsions
5. Soaps
6. Ointments

Powders

Powders are a uniform mixture of insoluble substances (inorganic, organic, and colloidal) that have been properly blended, perfumed, and/or tinted. These cosmetics are mixed and sifted to ensure that they are free from coarse or gritty particles.

Solutions

A solution is made by dissolving a solid, liquid, or gaseous substance in another substance, usually liquid.

A solute (**SOL**-yoot) is a substance dissolved in a solution.

A solvent (**SOL**-vent) is a liquid used to dissolve a substance.

Solutions are clear and permanent mixtures of solute and solvent that do not separate upon standing. Since a good solution is clear and transparent, filtration is often necessary, particularly if the solution is cloudy.

Solutions are easily prepared by dissolving a powdered solute in a warm solvent and stirring at the same time. The solute may be separated from the solvent by applying heat and evaporating the solvent.

Water is a universal solvent. It is capable of dissolving more substances than any other. Grain alcohol and glycerine also are used frequently as solvents. Water, glycerine, and alcohol readily mix with each other; therefore they are miscible (**MIS**-e-bel) (mixable). On the other hand, water and oil do not mix with each other; hence they are immiscible (unmixable).

The solute may be either a solid, liquid, or gas. For example, boric acid solution is a mixture of a solid in a liquid; glycerine and rose water is a mixture of two miscible liquids; ammonia water is a mixture of a gas in water.

Solutions containing volatile substances such as ammonia and alcohol should be stored in a cool place; otherwise the substance will evaporate.

There are various kinds of solutions:

A **dilute** (deye-**LOOT**) **solution** contains a small quantity of the solute in proportion to the quantity of solvent.

A **concentrated** (kon-sun-**TRAY**-ted) **solution** contains a large quantity of the solute in proportion to the quantity of solvent.

A **saturated** (**SACH**-u-rayt-ed) **solution** will not dissolve or take up more solute than it already holds at a given temperature.

Suspensions

Suspensions are mixtures of one type of matter in another type of matter. The particles have a tendency to separate upon standing, making it necessary to shake or stir the product before use. Some skin lotions, such as calamine lotion, are suspensions.

Emulsions

Emulsions (e-**MUL**-shuns) (creams) are permanent mixtures of two or more immiscible substances (oil and water) which are united with the aid of a **binder** or an **emulsifier** (soap). They are usually milky white in appearance. If a suitable emulsifier is chosen and the proper technique used, the emulsion will be stable. A stable emulsion can hold as much as 90 percent water. Depending on the amount of water and wax present, the cream may be either liquid or semi-solid in character. The amount of emulsifier used depends on its efficiency and the amount of water or oil to be emulsified.

Emulsions are prepared either by hand or with the aid of a grinding and cutting machine called a colloidal mill. In the process of preparing the emulsion, the emulsifier forms a protective film around the microscopic globules of the oil or water. The smaller the globules, the thicker and more stable the emulsion.

Emulsions are classified as either oil-in-water (O/W) or water-in-oil (W/O).

Oil-in-water (O/W) emulsions are comprised of oil droplets suspended in a water base. In addition to the emulsifier, which coats the oil droplets and holds them in suspension, there may be a number of additional ingredients that are designed to cause certain reactions in the hair. Examples of O/W emulsions are permanent wave solutions, lighteners, neutralizers, and tints.

Water-in-oil (W/O) emulsions are formed with drops of water suspended in an oil base. These are usually much thicker and oilier than the O/W emulsions. Examples of W/O emulsions are hair grooming creams, cleansing creams, cold creams, and similar products. (Fig. 19.1)

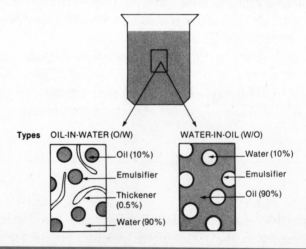

19.1 – Types of emulsions

TYPICAL FORMULA OF AN O/W EMULSION

In an emulsion, the following substances may be found:

oil type conditioner	light mineral oil or lanolin
emulsifier	a joining agent between the water and the conditioner, usually a form of soap
thickener	to control the thickness of the emulsion or to make it look richer
clouding agent	to give a pearly-white, attractive appearance
perfume and water	to disguise unpleasant odors and impart a pleasing odor to the skin

Important Features

OIL-IN-WATER (O/W)

Break on contact to release the following:
1. Moisture to enter skin (softens, helps overcome dryness)
2. Oils remain on skin surface (reduces loss of moisture, lubricates skin)
Can be easily diluted by water

WATER-IN-OIL (W/O)

Help to prevent moisture loss from the skin
Useful for removing grime from skin
Cannot be diluted by added water
(Test for W/O emulsions)

Examples

moisturizing lotion
cleansing lotion
suntan lotion
vanishing creams

cleansing creams
cold creams
night creams
massage creams

NOTE: The percentage of water and oil in a product will vary, depending on the formulation of the product and the texture (such as cream or liquid) that is desired.

Soaps

Soaps are compounds formed in a chemical reaction between alkaline substances and the fatty acids in the oil or fat. Besides soap, glycerine is also formed. Potassium hydroxide produces a soft soap, whereas sodium hydroxide forms a hard soap. A mixture of the two alkalis will yield a soap of intermediate consistency.

A good soap does not contain excess free alkali and is made from pure oils and fats.

The soaps currently used in the industry fall into three classifications: deodorant, beauty, and medicated.

Deodorant soaps include a bactericide that remains on the body to kill the bacteria responsible for odors. The most common antiseptic and anti-bacterial agent is probably triclocarban. Triclocarban, often listed in the ingredients as TCC, is prepared from aniline. Aniline additives have been known to increase the skin's sensitivity to the sun.

Beauty soaps are intended for the more delicate tissues of the face. They have a more acid pH and are less drying to the skin, yet able to remove dirt and debris from the skin's surface. Many beauty soaps are transparent and contain large quantities of glycerine. Other beauty soaps contain larger amounts of oils that leave an emollient film on the skin.

Medicated soaps are designed to treat skin problems such as rashes, pimples, and acne. Many contain small percentages of **cresol, phenol,** or other antiseptics. **Resorcinol** is often used as a drying agent in medicated products designed to treat oily conditions. The strongest medicated soaps can be obtained only with a doctor's prescription.

Shaving Soaps

Shaving soaps can be purchased in various forms and shapes. Hard shaving soaps include those sold in cake, stick, or powdered form, and are similar in composition to toilet soaps. They are also available as soft soap as in shaving cream in a tube, jar, or press-button container. Liquid soap can also be used by a barber-stylist.

Whatever form of shaving soap is used, it usually contains animal and vegetable oils, alkaline substances, and water. The presence of coconut oil improves the lathering qualities of shaving soap.

Sticks are similar to ointments. They are a mixture of organic substances (oils, waxes, petrolatum) that are poured into a mold to solidify. Sticks are a little harder than ointments, since they contain no water. Lipstick is an example of a cosmetic stick.

Pastes are soft, moist cosmetics, with a thick consistency. They are bound together with the aid of gum, starch, and water. If oils and

Kinds of Soaps

Soaps	Common Ingredients	Uses
Castile soap (pure)	Olive oil and soda.	Best for the skin—produces little lather.
Castile soap (other kinds)	Synthetic detergents, olive or other oils.	Used for normal skin.
Green soap	Made from potash and olive or linseed oil and glycerine.	A medicinal liquid soap used for oily skin.
Tincture of green soap	Mixture of green soap in about 35% alcohol and a small amount of perfume.	Used for correcting oily skin and scalp. Very drying, if used on normal or dry skin over a period of time.
Medicated soap	Contains a small percent of cresol, phenol, and other anti-septics.	Used for acne conditions.
Shaving soap	Contains alkalies, coconut oil, vegetable and animal fats, and a small amount of gum.	Used for shaving. The alkalinity softens the hair. The thick lather keeps the hair erect.
Shaving soap in pressure can	Shaving soap and gas under pressure.	Used the same as shaving soap.
Carbolic soap	A disinfectant soap containing 10% phenol.	Used for oily skin and acne infection.
Transparent soap	Contains glycerine, alcohol, and sugar, which render it transparent.	Used for normal skin.
Super-fatted soap	Contains a fatty substance, such as lanolin or cocoa butter.	Recommended for dry or sensitive skin. Keeps the skin soft after washing. Not suitable for hard water.
Naphtha soap	Contains naphtha, obtained from petroleum.	Do not use on face or scalp. Used mainly for laundry purposes.
Hard water soap	Contains coconut oil, varying amounts of washing soap or borax, sodium silicate, and a phosphate.	Used only on oily skin. The alkaline substances will dry the skin.

fats are present, water is absent. The colloidal mill assists in the removal of grittiness from the paste.

Ointments

Ointments (OINT-ments) are semi-solid mixtures of organic substances such as lard, petrolatum, or wax, and a medicinal agent. No water is present. For the ointment to soften, its melting point should be below that of the body temperature (98.6 degrees fahrenheit).

Ointments are prepared by melting the organic substances and mixing them with the medicinal agent.

Depilatories

Depilatories (de-PIL-uh-to-rees) are preparations used for the temporary removal of superfluous hair by dissolving it at the skin line. Depilatories contain detergents to strip the sebum from the hair and adhesives to hold the chemicals to the hair shaft for the 5 to 10 minutes necessary to remove the hair. During the application time swelling accelerating agents such as urea or melamine expand the hair, helping to break hair bonds. Finally, chemicals such as sodium hydroxide, potassium hydroxide, thioglycolic acid, or calcium thioglycolate destroy the disulfide bonds. These chemicals turn the hair into a soft, jelly-like mass of hydrolyzed protein that can be scraped from the skin. Although depilatories are not commonly used in salons, familiarity with them is necessary.

Epilators

Epilators (ep-i-LAY-tors) remove hair by pulling it out of the follicle. Two types of wax are currently used for professional epilation: cold and hot. Both products are made primarily of resins and beeswax. Beeswax has a relatively high incidence of allergic reaction; therefore it is advisable to give a small patch test of the product to be used. Recently, an electrical apparatus made for the home market has become available.

Cosmetics for Skin and Face

The cosmetic industry has made available a vast array of products designed to improve the condition and appearance of the skin.

Creams

The creams used for professional skin treatments fall into four main categories: cleansing, wrinkle treatments, moisturizers, and massage cream.

The action of **cleansing cream** is caused in part by the oil content of the cream, which has the ability to dissolve other greasy substances. Older formulas such as cold cream contain relatively few ingredients: vegetable or mineral oil, beeswax, water, preservatives, and emulsifiers. The newer cleansing formulations are much more complicated and may contain additional de-greasers such as lemon juice, synthetic surfactants, emollients, and humectants.

Wrinkle treatments are designed to conceal lines on aging skin in two ways. One is with a crease-filling capacity and the other is through a plumping up of the tissues. Among the many possible ingredients in these treatments are **hormones, hyaluronic acid,** and **collagen.** Some are made of herbs and other natural ingredients; others are entirely synthetic.

Moisturizing creams are designed to treat dryness. They contain humectants, which create a barrier that allows the natural water and oil of the skin to accumulate in the tissues. This barrier also works to protect the skin from air pollution, dirt, and debris. Moisturizers contain a variety of emollients ranging from simple ingredients such as peanut, coconut or a variety of other oils, to more complex chemical compounds such as **cetyl alcohol, cholesterol, dimethicone,** or **glycerine derivatives.**

Massage creams are used to help the hands to glide over the skin. They are formulations of cold cream, lanolin or its derivatives, and possibly **casein** (a protein found in cheese).

Lotions

Lotions are used professionally in a variety of hair and facial treatments and generally are available in clear or lightly tinted solutions.

Cleansing lotions serve the same purposes as cleansing creams but are of a lighter oil content. They come in formulations for dry, normal, and oily skin. Some ingredients common to cleansing lotions are **cetyl alcohol, cetyl palmitate,** and **sorbitol** combined with perfumes and colorings to enhance their marketing value.

Astringent lotions are designed to remove oil accumulation on the skin. The alcohol content of the product also irritates the skin, causing it to swell slightly and appear to close the pores. Astringent lotions contain a large percentage of alcohol and small percentages of some or all of the following: alum, boric acid, sorbitol, water, camphor, and perfumes.

Freshener lotions are similar to astringent lotions; however, they are designed to be gentler for dry and normal skin types. The formulation of a freshener typically includes some or all of the following: **witch hazel, alcohol** and **camphorated alcohol, citric**

acid, boric acid, lactic acid, phosphoric acid, aluminum salts, menthol, chamomile, and floral scents.

Eye lotions are generally formulas of boric acid, bicarbonate of soda, zinc sulfate, glycerine, and herbs. They are designed to soothe and brighten the eyes.

Medicated lotions are prescribed by a physician for skin problems such as acne, rashes, or other eruptions.

Suntan lotions are designed to protect the skin from the harmful ultraviolet rays of the sun. They are rated with a sun protection factor (SPF) that enables sunbathers to calculate the time they can remain in the sun before the skin begins to burn. Suntan lotions are emulsions that might contain **para-aminobenzoic acid** (PABA), a variety of oils, petrolatum, sorbitan stearate, alcohol, ultraviolet inhibitors, acid derivatives, preservatives, and perfumes.

Miscellaneous Cosmetics

Greasepaint is a mixture of fats, petrolatum, and a coloring agent that is used for theatrical purposes.

Cake or **pancake makeup** is generally composed of kaolin, zinc, talc, titanium oxide, mineral oil, fragrances, precipitated calcium carbonate, finely ground pigments, and inorganic pigments such as iron oxides. Cake makeup is used to cover scars and pigmentation defects.

Masks and **packs** are available to serve many purposes and skin conditions—deep cleansing, pore reduction, tightening, firming, moisturizing, and wrinkle reduction. Clay masks typically contain varying combinations of **kaolin** (china clay), **bentonite, purified siliceous (fuller's) earth** or **colloidal clay, petrolatum, glycerine, proteins, SD alcohol,** and water. The prime ingredients typically found in peel-off masks are **SD alcohol 40, polysorbate-20,** and polymers such as **polyvinyl alcohol** or **vinyl acetate.**

Scalp Lotions and Ointments

Scalp lotions and ointments usually contain medicinal agents for active correction of a scalp condition such as itching or flakiness. An astringent lotion may be applied to the scalp before shampooing to control oiliness as well as the itching and flakiness of dry scalp conditions. Medicated lotions and ointments for severe scalp conditions must be prescribed by a physician.

Hair Dressings

Hair dressings give shine and manageability to dry or curly hair. They may be applied to either wet or dry hair. Such dressings typically consist of lanolin or its derivatives, petrolatum, oil emulsions, fatty acids, waxes, mild alkalis, and water.

Styling Aids

A professional barber-stylist utilizes a variety of styling gels and mousses. Both of these products are typically polymer and resin formulations designed to give the hair body and texture. Many incorporate the same ingredients found in hair sprays (see below) but add moisturizers and humectants, such as **cetyl alcohol, panthenol, hydrolyzed protein, quats,** or a variety of oils to the ingredient list.

Hair Sprays

Hair spray is used to hold the finished style. Many new formulations for hair spray contain a variety of polymers, such as **acrylic/acrylate copolymer, vinyl acetate, crotonic acid copolymer, PVM/MA copolymer,** and **polyvinylpyrrolidone (PVP),** and **plasticizers** such as **acetyl triethyl citrate,** benzyl alcohol, and silicones as stiffening agents. Additional ingredients might include silicone, shellac, perfume, lanolin or its derivatives, vegetable gums, alcohol, sorbitol, and water.

> CAUTION: Careless use of hair spray can cause eye and lung damage and throat irritation.

UNITED STATES PHARMACOPEIA (U.S.P.) ▼

A barber-stylist should be familiar with the United States Pharmacopeia (U.S.P.), a book defining and standardizing drugs. The following are some of the terms of interest to barber-stylists:

Alcohol, also known as grain or ethyl alcohol, is a colorless liquid obtained by the fermentation of certain sugars. It is a powerful antiseptic and disinfectant; a 70 percent solution is usable for sanitizing instruments, and a 60 percent solution can be applied to the skin. It is widely used in perfumes, lotions, and tonics.

Alum is an aluminum potassium or ammonium sulphate, supplied in the form of crystals or powder, which has a strong astringent action. It is used in skin tonics and lotions. It is also used in powder form as a styptic.

Ammonia water, as commercially used, is a colorless liquid with a pungent, penetrating odor. It is a by-product of the manufacture of coal gas. As it readily dissolves grease, it is used as a cleansing agent and is also used with hydrogen peroxide in lightening hair. A 28 percent solution of ammonia gas dissolved in water is available commercially.

Boric acid is used for its bactericidal and fungicidal properties in baby powder, eye creams, mouthwashes, soaps, and skin fresheners. It is a mild healing and antiseptic agent although the American Medical Association warns of possible toxicity. Severe irritation and poisonings have occurred after application to open skin wounds.

Ethyl methacrylate (**ETH**-il-meth-u-**KRYE**-layt) is an **ester** (compound) of ethyl alcohol and **methacrylic** acid used in the chemical formulation of many sculptured nails. Inhalation of the fumes is not recommended.

Formaldehyde is a colorless gas manufactured by an oxidation process of methyl alcohol. It is used as a disinfectant, fungicide, germicide, and preservative as well as an embalming solution. In the industry, formaldehyde is used in soap, cosmetics, nail hardeners and polishes. It should be used with caution because National Cancer Institute studies indicate that it is toxic, can lead to DNA damage, and can react with other chemicals to become carcinogenic.

Glycerine is a sweet, colorless, odorless, syrupy liquid formed by the decomposition of oils, fats, or molasses. It is used as a skin softener in cuticle oil, facial creams and a variety of lotions.

Petrolatum, commonly known as vaseline, petroleum jelly, or paraffin jelly, is a yellowish to white, semi-solid, greasy mass that is almost insoluble in water. It is used in wax epilators, eyebrow pencils, lipsticks, protective creams, cold creams, and many other cosmetics for its ability to soften and smooth the skin.

Phenylenediamine (**FEN**-i-leen-**dye**-uh-meen), derived from coal tar, has a succession of derivatives known to penetrate the skin. It is believed to cause cancer.

Potassium hydroxide (puh-**TAS**-ee-um high-**DROCK**-side) (caustic potash) (**KAWS**-tick **POT**-ash) is prepared by electrolysis of potassium chloride. It may be used for its emulsifying abilities in the formulas for hand lotions, liquid soaps, protective creams, and cuticle softeners.

Quaternary ammonium compounds (quats) are found in many antiseptics, surfactants, preservatives, sanitizers, and germicides. Quats are synthetic derivatives of ammonium chloride. Although quats can be toxic, they are considered safe in the proportions used in the industry.

Sodium bicarbonate (baking soda) is a precipitate made by passing carbon dioxide gas through a solution of sodium carbonate. The resulting white powder is used as a neutralizing agent and, when mixed in shampoo, to remove hair spray buildup.

Sodium carbonate (soda ash or washing soda) is found naturally in ores and lake brines or sea water. It is used in shampoos and permanent wave solutions. Sodium carbonate absorbs water from the air.

Witch hazel is a solution of alcohol, water, and powder ground from the leaves and twigs of the **Hamamelis virginiana.** It works as an astringent and skin freshener. Because of the alcohol content it should not be applied directly to an open wound or the delicate membranes of the eye.

Zinc Oxide is a heavy white powder that is insoluble in water. It is used cosmetically in face powder and foundation creams for its ability to impart opacity.

REVIEW QUESTIONS

Chemistry

1. Why is a basic knowledge of chemistry important to the barber-stylist?
2. What is organic chemistry? Give five examples of organic substances.
3. In what type of liquids are organic substances soluble? Give two examples.
4. What is inorganic chemistry? Give five examples of inorganic substances.
5. What is matter?
6. In what three physical forms does matter exist?
7. What is an element? How many are there?
8. What is the smallest part of an element?
9. What is a molecule?
10. What do we mean by the chemical activities of an element?
11. What is a compound?
12. Name and describe the four classes of compounds.
13. What is a mixture?
14. What are the two ways in which matter may be changed? Give an example of each.
15. What is a physical change?
16. What is a chemical change?
17 List the five properties of matter.
18. What is meant by pH?
19. How do acids register on the pH scale?

20. How do alkalines register on the pH scale?
21. What is the most abundant of all substances?
22. What two methods are employed to remove impurities from water?
23. What two types of water are found?
24. Why is hard water unsuitable for shop use?
25. What is the chemical symbol for water?

20

Anatomy and Physiology

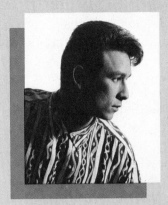

Learning Objectives

After completing this chapter, you should be able to:

1. *Define the functions of human cells.*

2. *Define metabolism.*

3. *Describe the various types of tissues.*

4. *Describe the structures and functions of the human body.*

5. *Demonstrate an understanding of the organs and systems of the human body and how they function.*

Courtesy of: The Ice Cream Collection. NCA's S/S '92 Fashion Release. Danny Ewert, Design Team Director. Jim Douglass, photographer.

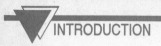

INTRODUCTION

Anatomy and physiology are subjects of importance in the practice of barber-styling. A knowledge of the structure and functions of the human body provides the barber-stylist with a scientific and professional approach when analyzing and performing services.

The body is composed of cells, tissues, organs, and systems that assimilate into one-fourth solid matter and three-fourths liquid in the human organism.

Anatomy (ah-**NAHT**-o-mee) is the study of the structure of the body and its components—muscles, bones, arteries, veins, and nerves. The barber-stylist is concerned with those parts being treated in the barber-styling shop such as the head, face, and neck.

Histology (hi-**STOL**-o-jee) is the study of the minute structure of the various parts of the body. The barber-stylist is particularly concerned with the histology of the skin and its appendages (hair, sweat and oil glands).

Physiology (fiz-i-**OL**-o-jee) is the study of the functions or activities performed by the various parts of the body.

CELLS

Cells are the basic units of all living things. Every part of the body is composed of cells, which differ from each other in size, shape, structure, and function.

In order to understand anatomy and physiology, it is necessary to study the structure and activities of cells. The human body is composed of millions of specialized cells performing the various functions required for living.

Nucleus   Nucleoli   Nuclear membrane

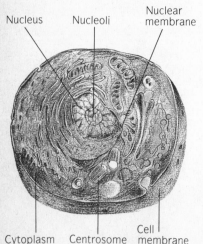

Cytoplasm   Centrosome   Cell membrane

20.1 – Structure of the cell

Structure of the Cell

A cell is a minute portion of living substance containing **protoplasm** (**PROH**-toh-plaz-em), a colorless, jelly-like substance in which food elements and water are present. The protoplasm of the cell contains the following important structures: (Fig. 20.1)

The **nucleus** (**NOO**-klee-us), found in the center, plays an important part in the reproduction of the cell. It is made up of dense protoplasm.

The **cytoplasm** (**SEYE**-toh-plaz-em) is found outside of the nucleus. It is made up of protoplasm less dense than that of the nucleus. It contains food materials necessary for the growth, reproduction, and self-repair of the cell.

The **centrosome** (**SEN**-tro-sohm) is a small, round body in the cytoplasm, which also affects the reproduction of the cell.

The **cell membrane** encloses the protoplasm. It permits soluble substances to enter and leave the cell.

Cell Growth and Production

As long as the cell receives an adequate supply of food, oxygen, and water, eliminates waste products, and is favored with proper temperature, it will continue to grow and thrive for the duration of its life cycle. If these requirements are not fulfilled, and the presence of **toxins** (poisons) or pressure is evident, the growth and health of the cell is impaired. Most body cells are capable of growth and self-repair during their life cycle.

When a cell reaches maturity in the human body, reproduction takes place by indirect division. This is a process in which a series of changes occur in the nucleus before the entire cell divides in half. (Fig. 20.2)

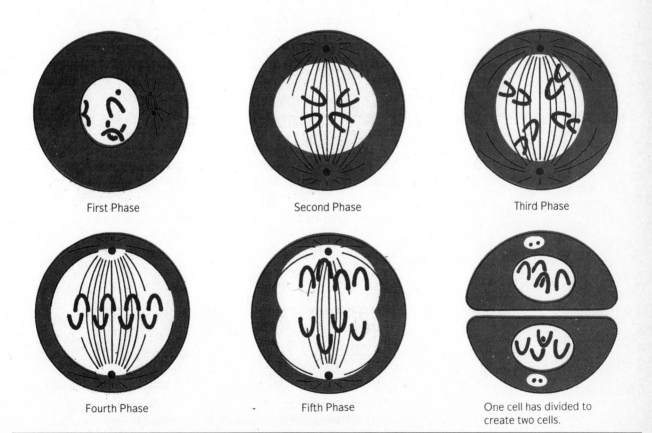

First Phase   Second Phase   Third Phase

Fourth Phase   Fifth Phase   One cell has divided to create two cells.

20.2 – Indirect division of the human cell

Metabolism

Metabolism (meh-**TAB**-o-lis-em) is a complex chemical process whereby the body cells are nourished and supplied with the energy needed to carry on their many activities.

There are two phases to metabolism:

1. **Anabolism** (ah-**NAB**-o-lizm) builds up cellular tissues. During anabolism, the body cells absorb water, food, and oxygen for the purpose of growth and repair.
2. **Catabolism** (kah-**TAB**-o-liz-em) breaks down cellular tissues. During catabolism, the cells consume what they have absorbed in order to perform specialized functions such as muscular effort, secretions, or digestion.

Cells have various duties. They create and renew all parts of the body; they assist in blood circulation by carrying food to the blood and waste matter from the blood; and they control all body functions.

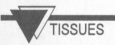

TISSUES

Tissues are composed of groups of cells of the same kind. Each tissue has a specific function and can be recognized by its characteristic appearance. Body tissues are classified as follows:

1. **Connective tissue** serves to support, protect, and bind together other tissues of the body. Bone, cartilage, ligament, tendon, and fat tissue are examples of connective tissue.
2. **Muscular tissue** contracts and moves various parts of the body.
3. **Nerve tissue** carries messages to and from the brain, and controls and coordinates all body functions.
4. **Epithelial** (ep-i-**THEEL**-ee-ul) **tissue** is a protective covering on body surfaces such as the skin, mucous membranes, linings of the heart, digestive and respiratory organs, and glands.
5. **Liquid tissue** carries food, waste products, and hormones by means of the blood and lymph.

Organs are structures containing two or more different tissues that are combined to accomplish a specific function. The most important organs of the body are:

1. The brain, which controls the body
2. The heart, which circulates the blood
3. The lungs, which supply oxygen to the blood
4. The liver, which removes toxic products of digestion
5. The kidneys, which excrete water and other waste products
6. The stomach and intestines, which digest food

Systems are groups of organs that cooperate for a common purpose, namely the welfare of the entire body. The human body is composed of the following important systems:

Skeletal (**SKEL**-e-tahl) System—Bones
Muscular (**MUS**-kyoo-lahr) System—Muscles
Nervous (**NUR**-vus) System—Nerves
Circulatory (**SUR**-kyoo-lahr-tohr-ee) System—Blood supply
Endocrine (**EN**-doh-krin) System—Glandular organs
Excretory (**EK**-skre-tohr-ee) System—Organs of elimination
Respiratory (**RES**-pi-rah-tohr-ee) System—Lungs
Digestive (deye-**GES**-tiv) System—Stomach and intestines
Reproductive (ree-proh-**DUK**-tiv) System—Reproducing

All these systems are closely interrelated and dependent upon each other. While each forms a unit specially designed to perform a specific function, that function cannot be performed without the complete cooperation of other systems.

The **skeletal system** is the physical foundation of the body. It is composed of differently shaped bones that are connected by moveable and immovable joints.

Bone, except for the tissue that forms the major part of the tooth, is the hardest tissue of the body. It is composed of connective tissues consisting of about one-third animal matter such as cells and blood, and two-thirds mineral matter, mainly calcium carbonate and calcium phosphate. The scientific study of bones, their structure and functions is called **osteology** (os-tee-**OL**-oh-jee). **Os** is the technical term for bone.

The following are the primary functions of the bones:

1. Give shape and support to the body
2. Protect various internal structures and organs
3. Serve as attachments for muscles and act as levers to produce body movement
4. Produce various blood cells in the red bone marrow
5. Store various minerals such as calcium, phosphorus, magnesium, and sodium

Bones of the Skull

The **skull** is the skeleton of the head. It is an oval, bony case that shapes the head and protects the brain. It is divided into two parts: the eight bones of the cranium and the 14 facial bones. They are involved with scalp and facial manipulations. (The bones listed below are numbered to correspond with the bones shown on Fig. 20.3.)

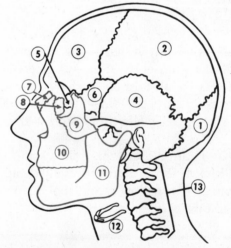

20.3 – Diagram of the cranium, face, and neck bones

1. The **occipital** (ok-**SIP**-i-tal) bone forms the lower back part of the cranium.
2. The two **parietal** (pa-**REYE**-e-tal) bones form the sides and top (crown) of the cranium.
3. The **frontal** (**FRUNT**-al) bone forms the forehead.
4. The two **temporal** (**TEM**-po-rahl) bones form the sides of the head in the ear region, below the parietal bones.

5. The **ethmoid** (**ETH**-moid) bone is a light, spongy bone between the eye sockets. It forms part of the nasal cavities.
6. The **sphenoid** (**SFEEN**-oid) bone joins all of the bones of the cranium together.
7. The two **nasal** (**NAY**-zal) bones form the bridge of the nose.
8. The two **lacrimal** (**LAK**-ri-mahl) bones are small, fragile bones located at the front part of the inner wall of the eye sockets.
9. The two **zygomatic** (zeye-goh-**MAT**-ik) or **malar** (**MAY**-lur) bones form the prominence of the cheeks.
10. The two **maxillae** (mak-**SIL**-ee) are the upper jawbones, which join to form the whole upper jaw.
11. The **mandible** (**MAN**-di-bel) is the lower jawbone and is the largest and strongest bone of the face. It forms the lower jaw.

The following bones do not appear on Fig. 20.3: Two **turbinal** (**TUR**-bi-nahl) bones are thin layers of spongy bone situated on either of the outer walls of the nasal depression. The **vomer** (**VOH**-mer) is a single bone that forms part of the dividing wall of the nose. The two **palatine** (**PAL**-i-teyen) bones form the floor and outer wall of the nose, roof of the mouth, and floor of the eye socket.

Bones of the Neck

12. The **hyoid** (**HEYE**-oid) bone, a U-shaped bone, is located in the front part of the throat and is commonly called the Adam's Apple.
13. The **cervical vertebrae** (**SUR**-vi-kal **VER**-te-bray) form the top part of the spinal column located in the neck region.

Bones of the Chest (Thorax)

The **thorax** (**THO**-racks) or chest is an elastic, bony cage made up of the breast bone, the spine, the ribs, and connective cartilage. It serves as a protective covering for the heart, lungs, and other delicate internal organs. This framework is held in place by 24 ribs, 12 on each side.

Bones of the Shoulder, Arm, and Hand

These descriptions correspond to the numbers on Fig. 20.4.

1. Each **shoulder** consists of one clavicle and one scapula, which forms the back of the shoulder.

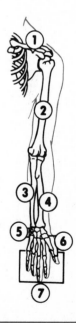

20.4 – Bones of the shoulder, arm, and hand

2. The **humerus (HYOO**-mo-rus) is the largest bone of the upper arm.
3. The **ulna (UL**-nah) is the large bone on the little finger side of the forearm.
4. The **radius (RAY**-dee-us) is the small bone on the thumb side of the forearm.
5. The **wrist** or **carpus (KAHR**-pus) is a flexible joint composed of eight small, irregular bones held together by ligaments.

The hand is divided into two regions:

6. The **palm** or **metacarpus** (met-a-**KAHR**-pus) consists of five long, slender bones, called **metacarpal** bones.
7. The **fingers** or **digits (DIJ**-its) consist of three **phalanges** (fa-**LAN**-jeez) in each finger and two in the thumb, totalling 14 bones.

NOTE: In chapter 8 you were introduced to the muscles, nerves, and arteries of the head, face, and neck that are affected during facial and scalp massage treatments. In the following sections, you will be presented with specific scientific data relating to the muscular, nervous, and circulatory systems of the human body. A thorough understanding of this material will enhance your awareness, knowledge, and overall skills as a professional barber-stylist.

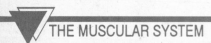

THE MUSCULAR SYSTEM

The **muscular (MUS**-kyu-lar) **system** covers, shapes, and supports the skeleton. Its function is to produce all movements of the body.

Myology (mi-**OL**-o-jee) is the study of the structure, functions, and diseases of the muscles. No outward sign of human life is more distinctive than that of muscular movement.

The muscular system consists of five hundred muscles, large and small, comprising 40 to 50 percent of the weight of the human body. Muscles are made up of contractile, fibrous tissue on which various movements of the body depend for their variety and action. The

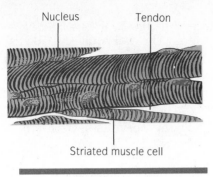

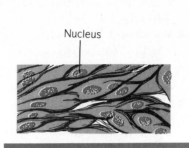

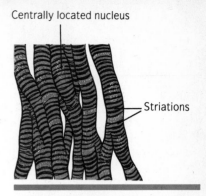

20.5 – Striated (striped) muscle cells

20.6 – Non-striated muscle cells

20.7 – Cardiac (heart) muscle cells

muscular system relies upon the skeletal and nervous systems for its activities.

There are three kinds of muscular tissues:

1. **Striated** (**STRY**-ay-ted) **(striped)** or **voluntary**, which are controlled by will, such as those of the face, arms, and legs. (Fig. 20.5)
2. **Non-striated (smooth)** or **involuntary**, which function without the action of the will, such as those of the stomach and intestines. (Fig. 20.6)
3. **Cardiac**, which is the heart itself and is not duplicated anywhere else in the body. (Fig. 20.7)

Origin, Insertion, and Belly of Muscles

As explained in chapter 8, when a muscle contracts and shortens, one of its attachments usually remains fixed and the other one moves.

The **origin** of a muscle is the term applied to the more fixed attachment, such as muscles attached to bones or some other muscle. Muscles attached to bones are usually referred to as **skeletal muscles.**

The **insertion** of a muscle is the term applied to the more movable attachment, such as muscles attached to the movable muscle, to a movable bone, or to the skin.

The **belly** of a muscle is the part between the origin and the insertion.

THE NERVOUS SYSTEM

Neurology (nu-**ROL**-o-jee) is the study of the structure, function, and pathology of the nervous system. The **nervous** (**NUR**-vus) **system** is one of the most important systems of the body. It controls and coordinates the functions of all the other systems and makes them work harmoniously and efficiently. Every square inch of the human body is supplied with fine fibers that we know as **nerves.**

The two main purposes in studying the nervous system are to understand:

1. How to correctly administer scalp and facial services.
2. What effects these treatments have on the nerves in the skin and scalp, and on the body as a whole.

Divisions of the Nervous System

The nervous system is composed of the brain, spinal cord, and their nerves. It consists of three main divisions:

1. The **cerebro-spinal** (ser-**EE**-broh **SPEYE**-nahl) or **central** nervous system
2. The **peripheral** (pe-**RIF**-er-al) nervous system
3. The **sympathetic** (sim-pah-**THET**-ik) nervous system

The cerebro-spinal nervous system consists of the brain and spinal cord. It performs the following functions:

1. Controls consciousness and all mental activities
2. Controls voluntary functions of the five senses
3. Controls voluntary muscle actions

The peripheral system is made up of the sensory and motor nerve fibers which extend from the brain and spinal cord and are distributed to all parts of the body. Their function is to carry messages to and from the central nervous system.

The sympathetic nervous system is related structurally to the cerebro-spinal (central) nervous system, but its functions are independent of the will. The sympathetic nervous system is also referred to as the autonomic nervous system, meaning self-control, by some anatomists.

The sympathetic nervous system is very important in the operation of internal body functions such as breathing, circulation, digestion, and glandular activities. Its main purpose is to regulate these internal operations, keeping them in balance and working properly.

Nerves

A **neuron (NOOR**-on), or **nerve cell**, is the structural unit of the nervous system. It is composed of a cell body and long and short fibers called **cell processes.** The short processes, called **dendrites,** carry impulses to the cell body. The longer processes, called **axons,** carry impulses away from the cell body to the muscles and organs. The cell body stores energy and food for the cell processes, which convey the nerve impulses throughout the body. Practically all the nerve cells are contained in the brain and spinal cord. (Fig. 20.8)

Nerves are long, white cords made up of fibers that carry messages to and from various parts of the body. Nerves have their origin in the brain and spinal cord, and distribute branches, which furnish both sensation and motion to all parts of the body.

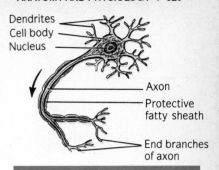

20.8 – A neuron or nerve cell

Types of Nerves

Sensory nerves, called **afferent (AF**-fer-ent) nerves, carry impulses or messages from sense organs to the brain, where sensations of touch, cold, heat, sight, hearing, taste, smell, and pain are experienced.

Motor nerves, called **efferent (EF**-fer-rent) nerves, carry impulses from the brain to the muscles. The transmitted impulses produce movement.

Sensory nerves are situated near the surface of the skin. Motor nerves are in the muscles. As impulses pass from the sensory nerves to the brain and back over the motor nerves to the muscles, a complete circuit is established and movements of the muscle result.

A **nerve reflex** is the path traveled by a nerve impulse through the spinal cord and brain, in response to a stimulus. (Example: the quick removal of the hand from a hot object.) A reflex act does not have to be learned.

The Brain

The brain is the largest mass of nerve tissue in the body. It is contained in the cranium. The weight of the average brain is 44 to 48 ounces. It is the central power station of the body, sending and receiving messages. Twelve pairs of cranial nerves originate in the brain and reach various parts of the head, face, and neck.

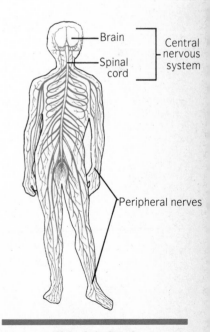

The Spinal Cord

The spinal cord is composed of masses of nerve cells with fibers running upward and downward. (Fig. 20.9) It originates in the

20.9 – Spinal cord

brain, extends down to the lower extremity of the trunk, and is enclosed and protected by the spinal column.

Thirty-one pairs of spinal nerves, extending from the spinal cord, are distributed to the muscles and skin of the trunk and limbs. Some of the spinal nerves supply the internal organs controlled by the sympathetic nervous system.

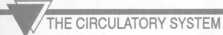

THE CIRCULATORY SYSTEM

The **circulatory** (SUR-kyoo-lah-tohr-ee) or **vascular** (VAS-kyoo-lahr) **system** is vitally related to the maintenance of good health. Proper circulation is essential to the entire body.

The vascular system is made up of two divisions:

1. The **blood-vascular system** consists of the heart and blood vessels (arteries, capillaries, and veins) for the circulation of the blood.
2. The **lymph-vascular**, or **lymphatic** (lim-FAT-ik) **system** consists of lymph glands and vessels through which the lymph circulates.

These two systems are intimately linked with each other. The blood vascular system controls the circulation of the blood through the body in a steady stream by means of the heart and blood vessels. Lymph is derived from the blood and is gradually shifted back into the bloodstream.

The Heart

The heart is a muscular, conical-shaped organ, about the size of a closed fist. It is located in the chest cavity and enclosed in a membrane, the **pericardium** (per-i-KAHR-dee-um). The 10th cranial nerve and nerves from the sympathetic nervous system regulate the heartbeat. In a normal adult the heart beats between 72 and 80 times a minute.

The interior of the heart contains four chambers and four valves. The upper, thin-walled chambers are the **right atrium** (AY-tree-um) and **left atrium**. The lower, thick-walled chambers are the **right ventricle** (VEN-tri-kel) and **left ventricle**. **Valves** allow the blood to flow in only one direction. With each contraction and relaxation of the heart, the blood flows in, travels from the **atria** (AY-tri-a) to the ventricles, and is then driven out, to be distributed all over the body. The atrium is also called **auricle** (OR-ik-kel) (Fig. 20.10)

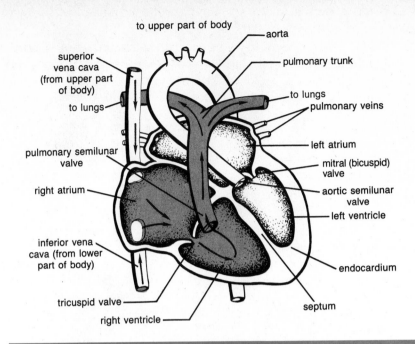

20.10 – Diagram of the heart

Blood Vessels

The arteries, capillaries, and veins are tube-like in construction. They transport blood to and from the heart and to various tissues of the body.

Arteries are thick-walled, muscular and elastic tubes that carry pure blood from the heart to the capillaries.

Capillaries are minute, thin-walled blood vessels that connect the smaller arteries with the veins. Through their walls, the tissues receive nourishment and eliminate waste products.

Veins are thin-walled vessels that are less elastic than arteries. They contain cup-like valves to prevent back-flow, and carry impure blood from the various capillaries back to the heart. Veins are located closer to the outer surface of the body than the arteries. (Fig. 20.11)

Circulation of the Blood

The blood is in constant circulation from the moment it leaves, until it returns to the heart. There are two systems that control this circulation:

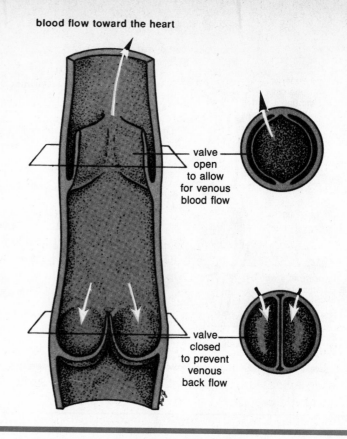

blood flow toward the heart

valve
open
to allow
for venous
blood flow

valve
closed
to prevent
venous
back flow

20.11 – Cross-sections of veins

1. **Pulmonary (PULL-mo-ner-ee) circulation** is the blood circulation that goes from the heart to the lungs to be purified, and then returns to the heart.
2. **General circulation** is the blood circulation from the heart throughout the body and back again to the heart.

The Blood

Blood is the fluid circulating through the circulatory system. It is a sticky, salty fluid, with a normal temperature of 98.6 degrees fahrenheit, and it makes up about one-twentieth of body weight. An adult has from eight to ten pints of blood.

Color of blood. Blood itself is bright red in color in the arteries (except in the pulmonary artery) and dark red in the veins (except in the pulmonary vein). This change in color is due to the gain or loss of oxygen as the blood passes through the lungs.

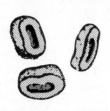 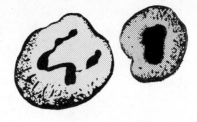 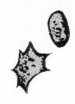

20.12 – Red corpuscles   **20.13 – White corpuscles**   **20.14 – Platelets**

Composition of blood. Blood is composed of one-third cells (red and white **corpuscles** and blood **platelets**) and two-thirds **plasma**. The function of red corpuscles is to carry oxygen to the cells. White corpuscles or **leucocytes** destroy disease-causing germs. (Figs. 20.12, 20.13)

Blood platelets are much smaller than the red blood cells. They cause blood to clot over a wound. (Fig. 20.14)

Plasma is the fluid part of the blood in which the red and white blood cells and blood platelets flow. It is straw-like in color. Plasma is made up of about nine-tenths water. It carries food and secretions to the cells, and carbon dioxide from the cells.

Blood performs the following functions:

1. Carries water, oxygen, food, and secretions to body cells.
2. Carries carbon dioxide and waste products from the cells to be eliminated through the lungs, skin, kidneys, and large intestine.
3. Helps to equalize body temperature, thus protecting the body from extreme heat and cold.
4. Helps to protect the body from harmful bacteria and infections, through the action of the white blood cells.
5. Causes wounds to close, or be sealed off, by the process of clotting.

The Lymph-Vascular System

The **lymph-vascular system**, also called **lymphatic system**, consists of lymph spaces, lymph vessels, lymph glands, and **lacteals** (LAK-teels). It acts as an aid to the blood system.

Lymph is a colorless, watery fluid that is derived from blood plasma, mainly by filtration through the capillary walls into the tissue spaces. By bathing all cells, the tissue fluid acts as a medium of exchange, trading its nutritive materials to the cells in return for the waste products of metabolism. This fluid is absorbed into the lymphatics or lymph capillaries to become lymph, and is then filtered and detoxified as it passes through the lymph nodes and is eventually reintroduced into the bloodstream.

The following are the primary functions of lymph:

1. Reaches the parts of the body not reached by blood and carries on an interchange with the blood.
2. Carries nourishment from the blood to the body cells.
3. Acts as a bodily defense against invading bacteria and toxins.
4. Removes waste material from the body cells to the blood.
5. Provides a suitable fluid environment for the cells.

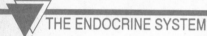

THE ENDOCRINE SYSTEM

Glands are specialized organs that vary in size and function. The circulatory and nervous systems are intimately connected with the glands. The nervous system controls the glands' functional activities. Glands are able to remove certain constituents from the blood and to convert them into new compounds.

There are two main sets of glands. One group is called the **duct glands**, possessing canals that lead from the gland to a particular part of the body. Sweat and oil glands, and intestinal glands belong to this group. The secretions of the other group, known as **ductless glands**, are thrown directly into the bloodstream, which in turn influences the welfare of the entire body.

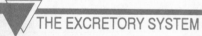

THE EXCRETORY SYSTEM

The **excretory (EK-skre-tohr-ee) system**, including the kidneys, liver, skin, intestines, and lungs, purifies the body by elimination of waste matter. Each plays the following part:

1. The kidneys excrete urine.
2. The liver discharges bile pigments.
3. The skin eliminates perspiration.
4. The large intestine evacuates decomposed and undigested food.
5. The lungs exhale carbon dioxide.

Metabolism creates various toxic substances which, if retained, would have a tendency to poison the body. The excretory system disposes of those poisons.

THE RESPIRATORY SYSTEM

The **respiratory** (RES-pi-rah-tohr-ee) **system** is situated within the chest cavity, which is protected on both sides by the ribs. The **diaphragm** (DI-a-fram), a muscular partition that controls breathing, separates the chest from the **abdominal** (ab-DOM-i-nal) region.

The **lungs** are spongy tissues composed of microscopic cells into which the inhaled air penetrates. These tiny air cells are enclosed in a skin-like tissue. Behind this, the fine capillaries of the vascular system are found.

With each respiratory cycle an exchange of gases takes place. During **inhalation** (in-ha-**LAY**-shun) oxygen is absorbed into the blood, while carbon dioxide is expelled during **exhalation** (eks-ha-**LAY**-shun).

Oxygen is required to change food into energy. It is more essential than either food or water. Although a human being may live more than 60 days without food and a few days without water, life cannot continue without air for more than a few minutes.

The rate of breathing depends on the activity of the individual. Muscular activities and energy expenditures increase the body's demands for oxygen. As a result, the rate of breathing is increased. A person requires about three times as much oxygen when walking as when standing.

Nose breathing is healthier than mouth breathing because the air is warmed by the surface capillaries, and the bacteria in the air are caught by the hairs that line the **mucous** (**MYOO**-kus) membranes of the nasal passages.

Abdominal breathing is of value in building health. Abdominal breathing means deep breathing, which brings the diaphragm into action. The greatest exchange of gases is accomplished with abdominal breathing. **Costal breathing** involves light, or shallow, breathing without action of the diaphragm.

THE DIGESTIVE SYSTEM

The **digestive** (deye-**GES**-tiv) **system** changes food into a **soluble** (**SOL**-yu-bel) form, suitable for use by the cells. Digestion begins in the mouth and is completed in the small intestine. From the mouth, the food passes down the **pharynx** (**FAR**-ingks) and the **esophagus** (i-**SOF**-a-gus), or food pipe, into the stomach. The food is completely digested in the small intestine. The large intestine, or colon, stores the refuse for elimination through the rectum. The complete digestive process of food takes about nine hours. (Fig. 20.15)

Digestive enzymes (EN-zeyems) present in the digestive secretions are chemicals that change certain kinds of food into a form capable of being used by the body.

Intense emotions, excitement, and fatigue may disturb digestion. On the other hand, happiness and relaxation may promote good digestion.

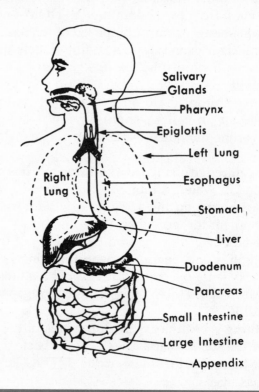

20.15 – Diagram of the human alimentary canal with its principle digestive glands

REVIEW QUESTIONS

Anatomy and Physiology

1. Why should barber-stylists study those parts of anatomy on which they give services?
2. On what parts of the body are barber-styling services applied?
3. Define anatomy and give examples.
4. Define physiology.
5. Define histology and give four examples.

Cells

1. Why should the structure and activities of the cell be studied?
2. What is a cell?
3. Why is knowledge of cellular activities important to the barber-stylist?
4. Of what substance are cells composed?
5. Name four important structures found in the protoplasm.
6. Give the function of the four structures found in protoplasm.
7. How does reproduction of cells take place?
8. Where does indirect cell division occur?
9. What is metabolism?
10. Name two phases of metabolism.
11. Which activities occur during anabolism or construction process of the cells?
12. What activities occur during catabolism or destructive process of the cells?
13. What is tissue?
14. List five classifications of body tissues.
15. What is the function of liquid tissue? Give two examples.
16. What is an organ?
17. List seven important organs of the body.
18. What are systems?
19. Name nine body systems.

The Skeletal System

1. What is the hardest structure of the body?
2. List four functions of the bones.
3. Define the term skull.
4. Into how many parts is the skull divided? Name them.
5. The cranium consists of how many bones?
6. List the skull bones affected by scalp massage.
7. Locate the occipital bone.
8. Locate the parietal bones.
9. Which bone forms the forehead?
10. What bones are located in the ear region?
11. Which bone joins together all the cranial bones?
12. How many bones are found in the face?
13. List the facial bones affected by facial massage.
14. What is formed by the maxillae?
15. Which bony structure is formed by the mandible?
16. Which bones form the prominence of the cheek?
17. Where is the hyoid bone located?
18. Locate the cervical vertebrae.

The Muscular System

1. Define muscle.
2. What are the important functions of the muscles?
3. Name three kinds of muscular tissue.
4. Distinguish between voluntary and involuntary muscles.
5. On which two systems of the body is the muscular system dependent for its activities?
6. Briefly define a) origin of muscle; b) insertion of muscle.

The Nervous System

1. Give two reasons why the barber-stylist should study the nervous system.
2. What are the three principal parts of the nervous system?
3. Name the three main divisions of the nervous system.
4. Name the three functions of the cerebro-spinal nervous system.
5. Explain the peripheral system and its function.
6. Name the main function of the sympathetic (autonomic) nervous system.
7. What is a neuron?
8. Of what is a neuron, or nerve cell, composed?
9. Define nerves.
10. Name two kinds of nerves that are found in the body.
11. What is the function of sensory nerves?
12. What is another name for: a) sensory nerves; b) motor nerves?
13. What is the function of motor nerves?
14. Give an example of nerve reflex.

The Circulatory System

1. Why is it necessary for the barber-stylist to understand the functions of the circulatory system?
2. What are the five important functions of the blood-vascular system?
3. What is the function of the heart?
4. Name three kinds of vessels found in the blood-vascular system.
5. Which blood vessels carry pure blood from the heart to the body?
6. Which blood vessels are nearest to the skin's surface?
7. What is the function of the veins?
8. Which two systems take care of blood circulation throughout the body?
9. What is the composition of the blood?
10. What is the normal temperature of the blood?
11. What is the composition of blood plasma?
12. What is the most important function of the red blood cells?
13. What is a function of the white blood cells?
14. What is lymph?
15. List the important functions of lymph.
16. From what source is the lymph derived?

1. What are the two main types of glands in the human body?
2. Name the five important organs of the excretory system.
3. Describe a respiratory cycle.
4. Name the important organs of the digestive system.

21

The Job Search

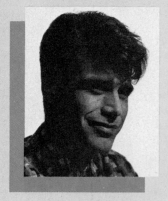

Learning Objectives

After completing this chapter, you should be able to:

1. *Explain the guidelines of goal setting.*
2. *Discuss student attitude.*
3. *List the ways in which a student can enhance marketability.*
4. *List four possible part-time barber-styling shop positions for the barber-styling student.*
5. *Discuss the reasons that employment in a shop or salon is beneficial for the student.*
6. *Define the portfolio.*
7. *List the components of a resumé.*
8. *List seven resources for the job search.*
9. *List nine points the stylist must consider before accepting a position.*

Courtesy of: The Ice Cream Collection. NCA's S/S '92 Fashion Release. Danny Ewert, Design Team Director. Jim Douglass, photographer.

INTRODUCTION

INTRODUCTION

This chapter has been provided to assist you in your search for employment in the barber-styling field. Many aspects of the job search will be addressed, from resumés to employer expectations. First, however, let's discuss what you can do now, as a student, to enhance the marketability of your personal and professional skills.

GOAL SETTING

At some point during your education as a barber-stylist, the subject of setting or determining goals will be discussed. Goal setting provides a useful road map for the professional journey.

1. Be realistic. Too often expectations are set so high that regardless of the outcome, the reality is a disappointment. For example, it is unrealistic to think or expect that a newly licensed barber-stylist will be booked solid during his or her first week of employment. When planning goals, be realistic.
2. Look before you leap is an old but accurate expression. Apply this principle whenever a major decision must be made. Be cautious in business dealings, and always seek legal counsel when contracts are involved.
3. Keep an open mind. Doing so can create more opportunities and probable successes. Personal and professional growth can be the result of keeping an open mind in a field that is technically and professionally advancing each year. There is always something new to learn, new interests to develop, and new roads to explore.
4. Be flexible. Timing can be extremely important. Being flexible can assist you in applying the preceeding guidelines. Time and timing, combined with realistic goals and expectations, may produce a very workable plan that allows you to realize your full potential in a steady progression of insight, experience, and skill.
5. Believe in yourself. While being realistic, have a clear knowledge that by allowing for circumstances and contingencies, and keeping a flexible but cautious open mind, most of your goals can be achieved.

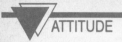

ATTITUDE

Two of the strongest marketing tools are personality and attitude. As indicated in the discussion of a professional image earlier in the book, confidence and the ability to communicate effectively are extremely important skills. Attitude affects not only other people, but also the way one views life in general. A positive attitude generates a positive response in those you meet, and self-confidence bolsters the confidence your clients will have in you as a professional.

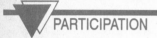

PARTICIPATION

There will be many opportunities while still in school to attend special events relating to barber-styling. Attendance at trade shows and educational seminars enhances a student's product knowledge, technical skill, and overall understanding of the industry. In addition, trade shows are fun, stimulating, and a good way to get a feel for the profession. Seminars are offered on a myriad of subjects and topics, and platform demonstrations educate in the hands-on arena.

Becoming a member of an industry association or organization on a student level is one of the best ways of getting involved. Trade organizations are usually involved in all aspects of the profession, including the hosting of trade shows and the representation of the industry in legislative circles. The benefits to a student of membership in such groups may include discounted trade show and educational tickets, student competitions, leadership training, and other related interests.

Student competitions offer yet another opportunity for students to experience a thrilling aspect of the profession. Competitions may be sponsored by vocational or professional organizations; distributors, manufacturers, and suppliers; or other education-oriented groups. Participation in competition hones the student's professional image, skills, and sense of self-esteem while laying the foundation for future professional performance.

Your school also may offer other opportunities for self-growth and industry awareness. Many instructors use students as teachers' aides. The duties vary, and may include office and/or classroom assistance, either of which will be noted and appreciated by the instructor and create a learning experience for the student. If your school does not have such a program, consider approaching the instructor with the idea.

Participation in any of the preceeding or similar activities is of value to a potential employer. It indicates a student's initiative and interest in the profession. Such activities also may illustrate a willingness to be a team player, the ability to be a leader, or the drive of an achiever.

A job search for a part-time position can begin as soon as a student has mastered basic skills for which licensing is not required. These skills may include communication and human relation skills, the shampoo service, and in many states, performing a manicure (check with your state board). A student with any of the above skills is a potential employee for a barber-styling shop in the capacity of a receptionist, stylist's assistant, shampoo technician, or manicurist.

The opportunity to assist a professional barber-stylist while still in school provides one of the best learning experiences for a student of barber-styling. Participation in the actual day-to-day operations of a shop or salon can benefit the student by providing:

- Exposure to the overall duties, responsibilities, and services of the shop
- Understanding of the individual tasks and responsibilities of shop personnel
- Experience in communicating with clients and co-workers
- Experience in perfecting service skills
- Observing advanced services, techniques, and skills
- Familiarity with shop procedures and standards
- Opportunity to lay the foundation for future employment
- Financial gain.

Clearly, the above experiences would enhance appreciably a student's understanding and ability regarding the profession.

THE PORTFOLIO

A portfolio is a collection of photographs depicting your ability to provide hair care services. The concept of creating a portfolio for the purpose of marketing a skill or talent is not new to individuals in the fields of art, photography, and modeling. Until recently, however, its application to the barber-styling job search has been limited, if not non-existent. Presentation of a portfolio is a graphic way to demonstrate your full range of talent, creativity, and skill to a prospective employer.

As a marketing tool, a portfolio should represent a stylist's best work. Consider keeping an inexpensive camera and film in your kit. After obtaining a client's permission, take before and after photographs, or simply the finished result. Keep a log of the dates, names, and services performed so that the pictures can be labeled. To avoid the possibility of any future complaints or conflicts, ask the client to sign a permission card or waiver.

Sample Card:

I, _____ hereby grant permission to _____ , student barber-stylist, to photograph the hair services rendered to me on _____ 19___ for the purpose of creating a portfolio of his/her work.

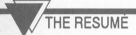

THE RESUMÉ

Another effective marketing tool is the resumé, which should contain the following information: name, address, and phone number; a professional objective; accomplishments or experience; work history; education; and availability. If your school has a student employment office, ask if it has sample resumés to use as guides for format and presentation.

There are many forms and types of resumés. Customize it to suit your needs. Visualize the impression it will make on a prospective employer and go for it!

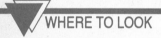

WHERE TO LOOK

Your school is one of the best places to begin a job search. Most barber-styling schools maintain contact with shops and salons and, in fact, usually post openings at a central location in the school.

Use any resource available to locate shops and salons in your area, including:

- Fellow students and instructors
- Suppliers who visit the school
- Distributor seminars and classes
- Trade shows
- Newspaper classified section
- Telephone book (yellow pages)

It is preferable, if at all possible, to know the name of the owner or manager and to have been referred by someone they know. In the event that this ideal situation does not present itself, you may have to do some cold calling. Although it may not be the most desirable way to seek a position, it can work.

Job hunting and interviewing is a familiar exercise for most people. The unfamiliar element is that you are seeking a position as a barber-stylist. Review of the material on a professional image will give some insight into what a shop owner or manager is looking for in an employee. Many employers require that a potential employee perform a haircut on a live model. This is standard practice. Don't feel intimidated by it.

If the interview and demonstration result in a job offer, there is certain information an applicant needs to consider. This includes:

- Percentage scale—wages
- Pay schedule
- Percentage scale—retail sales
- Benefits (health, life, and dental insurance)
- Sick leave/vacation policies
- Dress code
- Equipment and supplies provided by shop
- Hours
- New client policies

We hope that this chapter has provided some innovative ideas and useful suggestions for your job search in the field of barber-styling. Good luck and happy job hunting!

REVIEW QUESTIONS

The Job Search

1. Name five guidelines to use when setting personal and professional goals.
2. Name two of your best marketing tools.
3. List four areas of industry participation in which a barber-stylist student may get involved.
4. List four shop or salon positions available to the student of barber-styling.
5. Identify two marketing tools that require preparation.
6. List seven resources available to locate shops and salons when job searching.
7. List nine questions to which the barber-stylist should seek answers prior to accepting a position in a shop or salon.

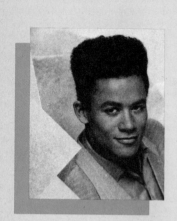

22

Selling in the Barber-Styling Shop

Learning Objectives

After completing this chapter, you should be able to:

1. *Discuss the importance of sales ability in the barber-styling shop.*

2. *Define the psychology of selling.*

3. *List some buying motives of clients in the barber-styling shop.*

4. *List some additional services a client might purchase.*

5. *Sell additional services and products.*

6. *Explain why the barber-stylist is the most qualified to sell grooming supplies.*

7. *List the basic groups of grooming supplies a barber-styling shop should have available for retail sales.*

8. *Discuss the importance of the barber-stylist's attitude in regard to selling additional services and products.*

Courtesy of: Matrix Essentials, Inc.

546

INTRODUCTION

The success of any barber-styling business is based upon the professional skill and selling ability of its personnel. Revenue is derived from both the performance of the various services and the sale of grooming aids. In both of these areas the ability of the professional barber-stylist to sell additional services and/or grooming supplies will greatly influence earnings.

The professional barber-stylist has the important advantage not only of giving professional services, but also of being trained to advise clients on the selection and application of proper grooming supplies.

As more products are added to the marketplace, selling is becoming an increasingly important responsibility for the barber-stylist. Those who are equally proficient as a stylist and a salesperson are the most likely to succeed in business. Advising clients about the proper products to use not only will increase your income, but also will enable clients to maintain the look you worked so hard to achieve.

The keynote of the modern shop is personal service. The professional who gives the best and most complete service has the greatest opportunity to succeed.

PSYCHOLOGY OF SELLING

Successful selling in a barber-styling shop is dependent upon a number of elements, a very important one of which is an understanding of the psychology of selling. This concept consists of establishing a clear and definite understanding of the client's needs and desires. To overcome sales resistance and to be able to satisfy clients, the barber-stylist should have a working knowledge of the psychological factors that control a client's actions and behavior.

It does not matter how good a service or a grooming aid may be. Unless the client feels a need for it, there will be no sale. Thus, in order to sell a product, the barber-stylist must create a need or a desire for a particular item or service. The client must be made to realize that the service or product is necessary.

The Motivation to Buy

Before a barber-stylist can sell properly, a thorough understanding is needed of what motivates a client to purchase a product or a service. Some of these motivating factors are:

1. The desire to improve appearance
2. The wish to improve social relationships

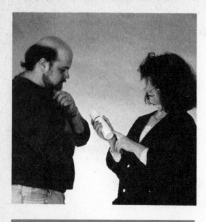

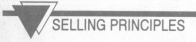

22.1 – A knowledge of good selling practices is necessary for success in the barber-styling shop.

3. The desire to retain a youthful appearance
4. The desire to get the most value for the money
5. The desire for a feeling of well being.

Never Use High-Pressure Tactics

Client's usually resent high-pressure selling tactics. The barber-stylist must be careful not to create antagonism instead of confidence. The approach must be subtle and friendly. Building up a client's confidence in a practitioner's judgment creates a reservoir for many future sales. This can only be done with honesty and sincerity.

Psychology in selling can be as important in the barber-styling shop as it is in the financial and trading world. A basic knowledge and understanding of the few simple principles set forth above may mean the difference between financial success and failure for the professional barber-stylist. (Fig. 22.1)

▼ SELLING PRINCIPLES

The barber-stylist's selling power increases as the client becomes aware of a personal interest in the client's welfare. Treat each client with friendliness and courtesy. Attention to little details for the client's added comfort will be greatly appreciated. Barber-styling services may be obtained in many places; however, the personality behind the service is the factor that brings the client back.

The barber-stylist's own good grooming serves to influence and arouse the client's interest in styling and grooming services. The stylist should be a living example of the services and products available in the shop.

The barber-stylist's manner should reflect dignity, charm, courtesy, and cleanliness. Loud and boisterous laughter, arguments, loss of temper, profanity, and gossip should always be avoided.

▼ SELLING ADDITIONAL SERVICES

The primary function of the barber-styling shop is to sell service. Shop income, to a large degree, depends upon the quantity and quality of the service being given. The professional barber-stylist can increase personal income, as well as that of the shop, by courteously selling as many services as possible to each client.

It is difficult for a barber-styling shop to be financially successful through haircutting services alone. There are additional services that should be offered to clients that will create additional revenue.

Such additional income may mean the difference between just getting along and financial success.

In order to sell additional services to clients, the barber-stylist must have a thorough knowledge of the services available. The stylist not only must be aware of each service, but also must know how to administer it and the benefits to be derived from it. It is also important to be observant and alert enough to know when a client is in need of added service and be able to explain the reasons.

Additional services can be suggested diplomatically. First, engage a client in conversation in which you point out an additional treatment or service and explain the benefits to be received.

The client considers the barber-stylist to be an expert in good grooming and so looks to the stylist for suggestions and advice. It is the responsibility of the barber-stylist to be well informed on all grooming matters so that the advice given will be correct.

The modern trend in haircutting is to develop new styles and methods more suitable to the individual's lifestyle. The barber-stylist can easily recommend a new hairstyle, haircut, or chemical service to achieve the desired result.

Facials

The professional barber-stylist observes the condition of the client's skin while performing hair care services, and tactfully may suggest one of the following:

1. Plain facial—beneficial for stimulating action on skin and for toning facial muscles
2. Facial for correcting dry skin
3. Facial for correcting oily skin
4. Facial for correcting acne
5. Facial to remove blackheads
6. Hot oil mask for correcting dry skin
7. Clay pack to prevent wrinkling of the skin

Mustache and/or Beard

If the client wears a mustache and/or beard, the best policy is to ask if he would like a trim. Some clients prefer to trim their own facial hair while others expect the barber-stylist to offer the service.

Shampooing

Today, most shops and salons include a shampoo as part of the haircutting service. Clean hair allows the barber-stylist greater precision while cutting and styling, and helps to maintain a standard of sanitation in the shop.

Scalp Treatments

After observing the client's hair and scalp, one of the following treatments might be desirable for certain scalp conditions.

1. Normal scalp treatment which is invigorating, prevents dandruff, and retards hair loss
2. Treatment for dry scalp and hair
3. Treatment for oily scalp and hair
4. Treatment for dandruff
5. Treatment for alopecia (baldness)
6. Series of corrective treatments (once a week for several weeks)

Rinses

One of the following rinses may be suggested in connection with a shampoo:

1. If hard water is used, an acid rinse should be recommended.
2. If the client has dandruff, recommend that the shampoo be finished with a dandruff rinse.
3. If the client has discolored gray hair, recommend a bluing rinse.

Hair Coloring

A client with gray hair may welcome the suggestion of a color rinse that would match the client's natural shade, and which can be rinsed out if not satisfactory. Mention that there will be a charge only if the rinse is left on.

If the client likes the color rinse, semi-permanent color may be a next step . . . and then, eventually permanent color.

The colorist should consult tactfully with the client to determine lifestyle and expectations for this color service. Never force the issue of a change of hair color if the client seems to prefer to remain with his or her natural hair color.

Hairpieces

Men are becoming increasingly interested in the use of hairpieces. Carefully suggesting to a client that a hairpiece might make him look younger, and even having him try one on, may result in a sale.

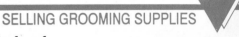

SELLING GROOMING SUPPLIES

The sale of grooming aids and supplies should go hand in hand with the sale of services. The purchase of such items as shaving creams, powders, lotions, and styling aids is a natural extension of the barber-styling shop as a center for good grooming.

Barber-styling shops should maintain a wide assortment of good quality grooming aids to meet the demands and tastes of their clients. (Fig. 22.2) Clean, tasteful display cabinets should be placed in strategic areas in the shop to attract attention. Very little additional effort is required for the stylist to call a client's attention to the variety of grooming supplies available. The stylist should mention proper products to clients and point out new products and the qualities of each. (Fig. 22.3)

No one is better able to explain to a client various products and the benefits to be received from their use than the barber-stylist. The stylist, however, should acquire a complete knowledge of each

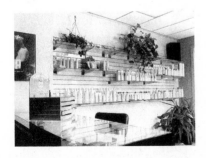

22.2 – Product display setup

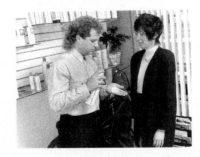

22.3 – Selling products in the barber-styling shop

product, its contents and its reaction on skin and hair. Thus, he or she may give expert advice to clients as to the proper products for their use. Clients soon learn to look for and appreciate the expert advice they receive from the professional barber-stylist.

The sale of one item inevitably leads to the sale of others. Once the client begins to buy grooming supplies in the barber-styling shop, the habit will continue as long as high-quality products and services are available.

The inventory should be properly maintained at all times. Reorder regularly to assure a fresh and complete stock. Display cabinets must be kept attractive-looking to create client interest.

List of Grooming Supplies

The well-equipped barber-styling shop should have available the following items to supply the grooming requirements of all clients.

A. **Shaving Supplies**
  1. **Razors**
    a) Safety razors
    b) Razor blades
  2. **Creams**
    a) Brushless shaving cream
    b) Aerosol shaving cream
    c) Brush lather cream
    d) Lather brushes
  3. **Lotions**
    a) Pre-shave lotion
    b) After-shave lotion
    c) Bay rum
  4. **Powders and Styptics**
    a) After-shave powder
    b) Styptic powder
    c) Styptic pencils
    d) Liquid styptics
B. **Shampoos**
  1. Regular shampoo
  2. Dry hair shampoo
  3. Oily hair shampoo
  4. Dandruff shampoo
C. **Hair Conditioners**
  1. Regular formula
  2. Dry hair formula
  3. Oily hair formula
  4. Dandruff formula
D. **Styling Supplies**
  1. Styling lotions, gels, and mousse
  2. Hair spray
  3. Butch wax sticks and jars
E. **Mustache and Beard Supplies**
  1. Mustache wax
  2. Mustache combs and scissors
  3. Electric trimmer
F. **Hairpiece Accessories**
  1. Spirit gum 2. Cleaners
    a) Jars, bottles, or cans
    b) Aerosol containers
  3. Double-sided tape
G. **Hair Supplies**
  1. Combs
  2. Brushes
  3. Blow-dryers and attachments

Atmosphere

It is in the interest of all shop personnel to maintain an attractive and comfortable atmosphere in the shop.

It should be furnished with the most modern equipment available. Even if the service is efficient, antiquated equipment may tempt the client to go elsewhere. It is natural for clients to be attracted to the shop where comfort, convenience, and speed are the policy. (Fig. 22.4)

Satisfied clients will not hesitate to recommend it to others.

Sanitation

A barber-styling shop must be kept clean and sanitary at all times. Shampoo basins must be kept clean. Hair caught around the sprays or in the drain must be cleaned regularly.

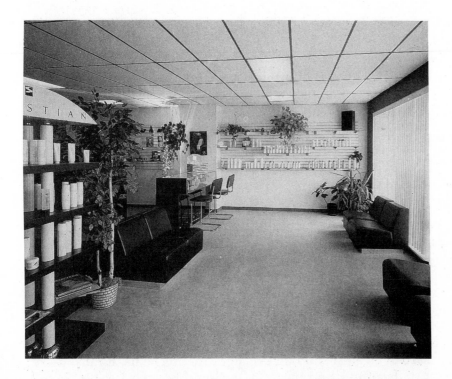

22.4 – The barber-styling shop should have a clean, contemporary atmosphere.

Floors must be swept frequently during the course of the day. Solutions and supplies must be kept covered, and each client furnished with clean towels. Combs, brushes, and all implements must be sanitized after each use.

Attitude

In addition to protecting the physical well-being of clients, the barber-styling shop should be a place for relaxation and rest. In order to retain and increase clientele, it is important to eliminate all disagreeable and grating noises.

The overall atmosphere of the shop is most important. A shop with personnel who create an unfriendly, cold, or disagreeable atmosphere cannot retain clients. If repeat business is desired, all barber-stylists in the shop should be friendly and receptive. They should smile and mean it.

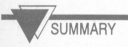

SUMMARY

The financial success of the barber-styling shop is dependent upon many factors.

The barber-stylist must have a definite and complete understanding of the psychology of selling in the shop.

Before a professional barber-stylist can operate successfully in the shop, the stylist must sell himself or herself to clients—as to personal appearance and proper grooming.

It requires more than competent professional skills to attain financial success as a barber-stylist. The stylist must be capable of selling needed additional services to clients. This is best accomplished with tact, friendliness, and honesty. The sale of additional services means additional income.

A great deal of additional income may be generated by the sale of grooming supplies. Employees should make a sincere effort to promote and sell such supplies. This type of business brings additional income to the barber-styling shop instead of diverting it to drug stores and supermarkets.

In order to build a successful barber-styling business, it is necessary to create a shop that is appealing to clients. It must be attractive, healthful, and pleasant. It should be an enjoyable experience for a person to receive barber-styling services in a modern and pleasant environment.

1. What is meant by *psychology of selling*?
2. List five factors that motivate a client to purchase either a product or a service.
3. Name three important factors necessary to promote the shop.

23

Barber-Styling Shop Management

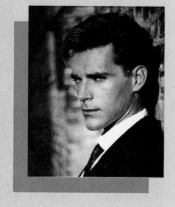

Learning Objectives

After completing this chapter, you should be able to:

1. *List the management functions of a barber-styling shop owner or manager.*
2. *Discuss the aspects of a business plan.*
3. *Identify and define types of business ownership.*
4. *Discuss the importance of location.*
5. *Describe the factors to be considered in the barber-styling shop layout.*
6. *Define different types of advertising.*
7. *List the most common reasons for business failure.*
8. *List the types of records to be kept in a barber-styling shop.*
9. *List the operating expenses of a barber-styling shop.*
10. *Demonstrate good telephone techniques.*
11. *Demonstrate how to handle customer complaints.*
12. *Discuss business law for the barber-styling shop.*
13. *Develop a barber-styling shop business plan.*

Courtesy of: Hair: Kristen LaMorte for Robert Jeffrey Hair Studios, downtown and suburban Chicago. Photo: Havriliak.

INTRODUCTION

Many opportunities exist for a successful career as the owner or manager of a barber-styling shop. In order to be successful, however, a shop must be planned carefully and managed efficiently.

Barber-styling shop management concerns the direct control and coordination of all operational activities. It also includes the proper planning, location, and physical arrangement of the shop.

It would be impossible to present a detailed study in management in a single chapter. This chapter will introduce those business principles and management techniques necessary to satisfactorily operate a barber-styling shop. A more detailed and broader coverage would require special texts and training in business management.

Going into business is a big responsibility. An understanding of business principles, bookkeeping, business laws, insurance, salesmanship, and psychology are all very important for a successful operation. In addition to a thorough knowledge and understanding of the practice of barber-styling, it is important to be able to manage employees and to get along well with clients. Shop management includes all the principles, sensitivities, methods, and understanding of the techniques by which a business is conducted.

MANAGEMENT FUNCTIONS

There are twelve initial functions performed by every barber-styling shop owner/manager. They are:

1. Determining the services to be offered
2. Creating a business plan including financial projections, budgets, sales estimates, etc.
3. Deciding the theme, mood, and decor of the premises
4. Arranging for financing or capital investment
5. Finding the best location for the shop
6. Purchasing equipment, furniture, and fixtures
7. Establishing and maintaining systematic records
8. Establishing and enforcing shop policies
9. Developing sales techniques for shop services and saleable merchandise
10. Arranging for the best and widest publicity for the shop
11. Recruiting and managing employees
12. Developing good public relations with clients and encouraging new clients

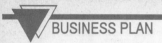

BUSINESS PLAN

A business plan is a necessary tool to obtain financing and to provide a blueprint for future growth. It should be developed before a shop is opened. The plan should include a general description of the business and the services it will provide; the number of personnel to be hired; their salaries and other benefits; an operations plan including price structure, expenses such as equipment, supplies, repairs, advertising, taxes, and insurance; and a financial plan that includes a profit and loss statement. Professional guidance should be sought if there are questions about how to create a business plan.

In addition, it is important to have enough working capital. It often takes time to build up a clientele. Enough money must be available to meet expenses.

How much money is enough money? The answer can be determined in part by considering some individual circumstances, including:

- The clientele and their willingness to move to another location.
- The availability of stylists with a following that will be working in the shop.
- Personal status and financial situation, i.e. single, married, single with dependents, previous debt, etc.
- The availability and type of financing, and its source.

As a general rule, no less than six months worth of operating expenses should be available. If you have no existing clientele, a year to 18 months worth of operating capital is not an unrealistic requirement.

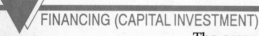

FINANCING (CAPITAL INVESTMENT)

The organization and type of business depends largely upon the amount of capital available. There are three types of business organizations to be considered: sole proprietor, partnership, and corporation.

Sole Proprietor

If the individual has enough money to finance the cost of setting up and operating the barber-styling shop, individual ownership (sole proprietor) should be considered.

A sole proprietorship has certain advantages over a partnership or corporation.

1. The owner is the boss and manager.
2. The owner can determine policies and decisions.
3. The owner receives all profits.

It also has the following disadvantages:

1. The owner's expenditures are limited by the amount of capital investment.
2. The owner is personally liable for all business debts.

Partnership

A lack of sufficient capital could necessitate the formation of a partnership.

A partnership has certain advantages over individual ownership.

1. More capital is made available to equip and operate the shop.
2. Work, responsibilities, and losses are shared.
3. The combined ability and experience of the partners assist in the solution of business problems.

The chief disadvantages of a partnership are:

1. Each partner is responsible for the business actions of the other.
2. Disputes and misunderstandings may arise between partners.
3. Each partner is personally liable for all debts of the business.

There should always be a written agreement defining the duties and responsibilities of each member.

Corporation

When three or more individuals intend to operate a barber-styling shop, a corporation is probably the best form of organization.

A corporation has the advantage over a partnership in that its stockholders are not legally responsible in case of loss or bankruptcy. The earning capacity is in proportion to the profits and the number of stocks the individual has in the corporation. Although the corporation has considerable financial backing, it may only do what is authorized specifically in the charter and approved by the board of directors. The corporation is subject to taxation and regulation by the state.

Federal tax laws allow some types of small corporations to be taxed on a partnership basis. Barber-styling shops fall into this category. An accountant should be consulted on all matters.

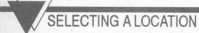

SELECTING A LOCATION

Careful consideration must be given to the selection of a location. The selection of a desirable site is just as important as the capital investment.

The shop should be located in an area large enough to support it. It should be near other active businesses which attract people. In a residential neighborhood, the main source of clients will be from the immediate vicinity. In a transient area, clients will come from surrounding and distant places.

Before selecting a location, consult the local bank, real estate agents, and other local merchants. Find out the earning capacity and the living standards of the people in the particular neighborhood. This information will help in deciding policies and prices.

In judging the merits of a particular site, consider the entrance, the window space, the inside area of the store, a good water supply, lighting and heating facilities, the presence of adequate toilet facilities, a sufficient number of windows, and parking facilities.

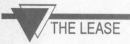

THE LEASE

After the site has been selected, it is advisable to check local zoning ordinances. Before signing a lease, make certain that the area is zoned to permit the operation of a barber-styling shop.

After all facts have been checked and all obstacles removed, a lease should be negotiated for the premises. A lease protects the barber-styling shop owner against unexpected increases in rent. It also protects the right of continued occupancy, and it sets forth clearly the rights and obligations of both the landlord and the barber-styling shop owner.

The lease should contain provisions concerning alterations, decorating, heating, and water supply. Before signing the lease, it should be read carefully and understood clearly to avoid future controversies. In fact, the barber-styling shop owner should have the lease reviewed by an attorney.

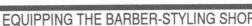

LEGAL REGULATIONS

In conducting a business and employing help, it is necessary to comply with local, state, and federal regulations and laws.

Local regulations may include building renovations (local building code) and zoning laws.

Federal law includes social security, unemployment insurance, cosmetics and luxury tax payments, and OSHA safety and health standards.

State laws cover sales taxes, licenses, and workers' compensation.

Income tax laws are governed by both the state and federal governments. Some localities have local income tax laws.

Insurance includes malpractice, premises liability, fire, burglary and theft, and business interruption.

EQUIPPING THE BARBER-STYLING SHOP

When the location of the shop has been determined, the premises rented, and the lease signed, it is ready to be furnished.

Shop layout takes a considerable amount of planning in order to achieve maximum efficiency and economy.

The barber-styling shop should be planned to provide:

1. Maximum efficiency of operation.
2. Adequate aisle space.
3. Enough space for each piece of equipment.
4. Furniture, fixtures, and equipment chosen on the basis of cost, durability, utility, and appearance. The purchase of standard, durable, and guaranteed equipment, either new or renovated, is a worthwhile investment. If, in the future, equipment must be replaced, repaired, or matched, it is fairly easy to duplicate standard fixtures.
5. Premises that are painted and decorated in colors which are restful and pleasing to the eye.
6. Adequate restrooms and handicap facilities.
7. Good plumbing and sufficient lighting for adequate services.
8. Air conditioning and heating.
9. Proper electrical outlets and current to adequately service all equipment.
10. The reception or waiting area is not to be overlooked. An attractive, adequately furnished, and comfortable waiting area can be one of the best promotional devices. It should make the client comfortable and relaxed, and give the im-

pression that the barber-stylist is really interested in the client's comfort.

The most important requisites for a barber-styling shop are cleanliness and comfort. The equipment should be easily accessible, arranged in an orderly manner, and maintained in good working condition. The electric lighting must be neither too dull nor too bright. Sanitation and sanitary rules must be strictly enforced.

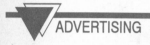

ADVERTISING

Advertising includes all activities that attract attention to the barber-styling shop. The personalities and ability of the owner or manager and the staff, the quality of the work performed, and the attractiveness of the shop are all natural advertising assets.

The right kind of publicity is important because it acquaints the public with the various services offered. To be effective, advertising must attract and hold the attention of those individuals to whom it is directed. It must create a desire for the services or merchandise offered.

The choice of an advertising medium is based on which form will accomplish the desired objective most effectively. For advertising to be effective, it must be repeated. Advertising media to be considered are:

1. Newspaper advertising
2. Distribution of circulars
3. Direct mail
4. Classified advertising
5. Yellow pages
6. Radio advertising
7. T.V. advertising
8. Attractive window display

Once clients are attracted to the barber-styling shop, courteous and efficient service will encourage their return and recommendation of the shop to others. Regardless of where advertising dollars are spent, remember that a pleased and satisfied client is the best form of advertising.

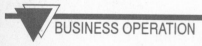

BUSINESS OPERATION

Business problems are numerous, especially when a new barber-styling business is organized. Contributing causes to shop failures are:

1. Inexperience in dealing with the public and employees.

2. Insufficient capital to carry on the business until established.
3. Poor location.
4. High cost of operation.
5. Lack of proper basic training.
6. Careless bookkeeping methods.
7. Business neglect.
8. Lack of qualified personnel.

The owner or manager of the barber-styling shop must have good business sense, knowledge, ability, good judgment, and diplomacy. Smooth management of a barber-styling shop depends on:

1. Sufficient investment capital.
2. Efficiency of management.
3. Cooperation between management and employees.
4. Use of good business judgment.
5. Trained and experienced personnel.

RECORD KEEPING

Good business administration demands a simple and efficient record system. Records are of value only if they are correct, concise, and complete. Bookkeeping means keeping an accurate record of all income and expenses. Income is usually classified as income from services and retail sales. Expenses include rent, utilities, salaries, advertising, supplies, equipment, and repairs. The assistance of an accountant will prove valuable. Retain check stubs, cancelled checks, receipts, and invoices.

Proper business records are necessary to meet the requirements of local, state, and federal laws regarding taxes and employees. All business transactions must be recorded in order to maintain proper records. These are required for the following reasons:

1. For efficient operation of the barber-styling shop.
2. For determining income, expenses, profit, and loss.
3. For proving the value of the barber-styling shop to prospective buyers.
4. For arranging a bank loan.
5. For reports such as income tax, social security, unemployment and disability insurance, wage and hour law, accident compensation, and labor taxes.

One of the causes for business failure is the lack of complete and systematic records. All business transactions must be recorded in order to judge the condition of the business.

Keeping daily records enables the owner or manager to know how the business is progressing. A weekly or monthly summary helps to:

1. Make comparisons with other years.
2. Detect any changes in demand for different services.
3. Order necessary supplies.
4. Check on the use of materials according to the type of service rendered.
5. Control expenses and waste.

Each expense item affects the total gross income. Accurate records show the cost of operation in relation to income.

Keep daily sales slips, appointment book, and petty cash book for at least one year. Payroll records, cancelled checks, monthly and yearly records are usually held for at least seven years. Service and inventory records also are important to keep. Sales records help to maintain a perpetual inventory. An organized inventory system can be used to:

1. Prevent overstocking.
2. Prevent running short of supplies.
3. Help to establish net worth at the end of the year.

If a barber-styling shop is to operate profitably, a simple system of bookkeeping is required. An easy plan is to keep a daily account of income and expenses. The cash register indicates the daily income, whereas the receipts and cancelled checks constitute proof of payments. By adding the daily total income and expense, the weekly and monthly totals can be obtained. The difference between the total income and the total expense is the net profit. A profit accrues when the income is greater than the expense. When the expense is greater than the income, a loss occurs. Continued profits spell success and continued losses may result in bankruptcy.

A budget must be kept in order for sufficient income to cover the expenses. The following list of expenses are commonly met in the barber-styling shop:

Operating and Administrative Expenses

Salaries	Insurance
Taxes	Cleaning
Repair	Sundry supplies, such as
Advanced education and training	soaps, tonics, towels, etc.
Advertising and printing	Heat, light, and water
Telephone	Miscellaneous
Rent	

The payments made on debts, equipment, and fixtures are not classified as expenses, but are considered as a reduction in indebtedness which in turn adds to the value of the barber-styling shop, except when considering depreciation on equipment for income tax purposes.

From time to time, an inventory must be taken of all supplies in the barber-styling shop. This record will show what supplies have been consumed and what new supplies are needed. It is better to have a slight excess of materials than a deficiency.

Service Records

A service record should be kept of treatments given and merchandise sold to each client. A card file system or memorandum book kept in a central location should be used for these records.

All service records should include the name and address of the client, date of each purchase or service, amount charged, products used, and results obtained. Also, note the client's preferences and tastes.

OPERATING TIPS

Hiring Staff

The success of a shop depends on the quality of the work done by the staff. When interviewing potential employees, consider their personality, level of skill, personal grooming, and the clients they will bring with them.

Pricing of Services

Cost of services is generally established according to the location of the shop and the type of clientele. A price list should be posted in a place where it can be seen by all clients—probably at the reception desk.

The Reception Area

First impressions count, and since the reception area is the first thing clients see, it should be attractive, appealing, and comfortable. The receptionist, phone system, and retail merchandise may be located in this area. There should be a supply of business cards with the address and phone number of the shop on the reception desk. This is also the place where the client's financial transactions are handled. (Fig. 23.1) Space will need to be allocated for a cash register or computer monitor. (Fig. 23.2)

Booking Appointments

Booking appointments must be done with care. Services are sold in terms of time on the appointment page. Appointments must be scheduled so that the time of all personnel is used efficiently. A client should not have to wait for service and a barber-stylist should not have to wait for the next client.

The size of the shop determines who books the appointments. This can be done by a full-time receptionist, the owner or manager, or any of the barber-stylists working in the shop. (Fig. 23.3)

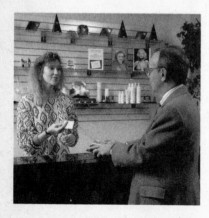

23.1 – Financial transaction being made at the reception desk

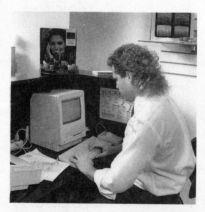

23.2 – Computer terminal in the reception area

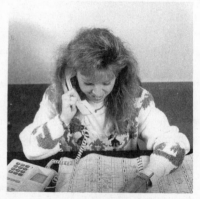

23.3 – Booking appointments

TELEPHONE TECHNIQUES FOR THE BARBER-STYLING SHOP

An ever-increasing part of shop business is handled over the telephone. Good telephone habits and techniques make it possible for the shop owner and barber-stylist to increase business. With each call the opportunity is provided to build up the shop's reputation.

The telephone serves many useful purposes in the barber-styling shop, such as:

1. To make or change appointments.
2. To go after new business, or strayed or infrequent clients.
3. To remind clients of needed services.
4. To answer questions and render friendly service.
5. To adjust complaints and satisfy clients.
6. To receive messages.
7. To order equipment and supplies.

Certain fundamental principles allow the telephone to be used as a successful business tool.

It is important to place the phone in a convenient and quiet place. A comfortable seat should be provided. An appointment book should be readily accessible, along with a pencil or ball-point pen and a pad of paper. Have an up-to-date list of commonly called telephone numbers and a recent telephone directory.

The shop's telephone number should be prominently displayed on stationery, advertising circulars, and in newspaper ads. Business cards should be available in the waiting area. They save clients the trouble of looking up the shop's phone number, thus making it easier to call.

Good telephone etiquette requires the application of a few basic principles that add up to common sense and common courtesy. Any barber-stylist should be able to learn the following four basic rules and to follow them:

1. Display an interested, helpful attitude, as revealed by the tone of voice and what is said.
2. Be prompt. Answer all calls as quickly as possible.
3. Give all information necessary to the caller. This means identifying yourself and the shop when making or receiving a call. If the requested information is not readily available, ask the client to hold on while you get it.
4. Be tactful. Avoid saying or doing anything that may offend or irritate the caller.

a) Inquire who is calling by saying, "Who is calling, please?"
b) Address people by their last names. Use polite expressions such as *thank you, I'm sorry,* or *I beg your pardon.*
c) Avoid making side remarks during a call.
d) Let the caller end the conversation. Do not hang up loudly at the end of a call.

Every time you call someone, you make a definite impression—your voice, what you say, and how you say it reveal you to others. A good telephone personality includes:

1. Clear speech
2. Correct speech
3. Pleasing tone of voice

As a general rule, the most effective speech is that which is correct and at the same time, natural. A cheerful, alert, and enthusiastic voice most often comes from a person who has these same personal qualities.

To make a good impression over the phone, assume good posture; relax and draw a deep breath before answering the phone. Pronounce the words distinctly, use a low-pitched, natural voice, and speak at a moderate pace. Clear voices carry better than loud voices over the phone.

If your listeners sometimes break in with such remarks as "What was that?" or "I'm sorry, I didn't get that," it usually means that your voice is not doing its job well. Try to find out what is wrong and correct it. It is possible that:

1. You are speaking too loudly or too softly.
2. Your lips are too close or too far away from the mouthpiece.
3. The pitch of your voice is too low or too high.
4. Your pronunciation is not precise.

The telephone, when properly used, is a valuable aid for obtaining business and making appointments. Every time the telephone is used, it affords an opportunity to render service and spread good will for the barber-styling shop.

Booking Appointments by Phone

1. When booking appointments, be familiar with all services and products available in the shop and their costs.

2. Be fair when making assignments. Do not schedule six appointments for one barber-stylist and two for another unless, of course, a client requests a particular individual.

3. If someone calls asking for an appointment with a specific barber-stylist on a particular day, at a particular time and that technician is not available, then there are several ways to handle the situation:

    a) If the client uses one barber-stylist regularly, suggest other times the barber-stylist is available.

    b) If the client cannot come in at any of those times, suggest another barber-stylist.

    c) If the client is unwilling to try another barber-stylist, offer to call the client if there is a cancellation at the desired time.

Handling Complaints by Telephone

Handling complaints, particularly over the phone, is a difficult task. The caller is probably upset and short-tempered. Try to use self-control, tact, and courtesy, no matter how trying the circumstances may be.

Remember that the tone of voice must be sympathetic and reassuring. Your manner of speaking should make the caller believe that you are really concerned about the complaint. Do not interrupt the caller. Listen to the entire problem. After hearing the complaint in full, try to resolve the situation quickly and effectively. The following are suggestions for dealing with some problems. If other problems arise, follow the policy of the shop or check with the owner/manager for advice.

1. Tell the unhappy client that you are sorry for what happened and explain the reason for the difficulty. Tell the client that the problem will not happen again.

2. Sympathize with the client by saying that you understand and that you regret the inconvenience suffered. Express thanks that the person called this matter to your attention.

3. Ask the client how the shop can remedy the situation. If the request is fair and reasonable, check with the owner or manager for approval.

4. If the client is dissatisfied with the results of a service, suggest a visit to the shop to see what can be done to remedy the problem.

5. If a client is dissatisfied with the behavior of a barber-stylist call the owner or manager to the phone.

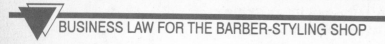

BUSINESS LAW FOR THE BARBER-STYLING SHOP

Before Buying or Selling a Barber-Styling Shop

1. A written purchase and sale agreement should be formulated in order to prevent any misunderstandings or errors between the contracting parties.
2. For safe keeping and enforcement, the written agreement should be placed in the hands of an impartial third person who is to deliver the agreement to the grantee (one to whom the property is transferred) upon the fulfillment of the specified contract.
3. The buyer or seller should take and sign a complete statement of inventory (goods, fixtures, etc.) and the value of each article.
4. If there is a transfer of chattel mortgage, notes, lease, and bill of sale, an investigation should be made to determine any default in the payment of debts.
5. Consult a lawyer for additional guidance.

A buyer should check equipment prices against costs of new equipment to avoid overpayments for used equipment.

An agreement to buy an established barber-styling shop should include:

1. Correct identity of owner.
2. True representations concerning the value and inducements offered to buy the shop.
3. Use of shop's name and reputation for a definite period of time.
4. A written agreement; understanding that the seller will not compete with the prospective owner within a reasonable distance from the present location.

Protection in Making a Lease

1. Secure exemption of fixtures or appliances that may be attached to the store or loft, so that they can be removed without violating the lease.

2. Insert into the lease an agreement relative to necessary renovations, such as painting, plumbing, fixtures, and electrical installation.

3. Secure an option from the landlord to assign the lease to another person in the event of the sale of the shop.

Protection Against Fire, Theft, and Lawsuits

1. Employ honest and able employees and keep the premises securely locked.

2. Follow safety precautions to prevent fire, injury, and lawsuits. Liability, fire, and burglary insurance should be obtained.

3. Do not violate the medical practice law of your state by attempting to diagnose, treat, or cure disease.

4. Become thoroughly familiar with the laws and sanitary code of your city and state.

5. Keep accurate records of the number of workers, salaries, length of employment, and social security numbers for various state and federal laws affecting the social welfare of employees.

NOTE: Ignorance of the law is no excuse for its violation.

CAUTION: Do not have business transactions with a total stranger, and never pay a stranger cash. Never make out a check to an individual who is working for a firm; make check payable to the firm.

THINGS TO CONSIDER WHEN GOING INTO BUSINESS

CAPITAL
Amount available
Amount required
ORGANIZATION
Individual
Partnership
Corporation
BANKING
Opening a bank account

Deposits
Drawing checks
Monthly statements
Notes and Drafts
SELECTING A LOCATION
Population
Transportation facilities
Quality of area
Trade possibilities

THINGS TO CONSIDER WHEN GOING INTO BUSINESS

(Continued)

Space required
Zoning ordinances

DECORATING and FLOOR PLAN

Selection of furniture
Floor covering
Installing telephone
Interior decorating
Exterior decorating
  Window displays
  Electric signs

EQUIPMENT and SUPPLIES

Selecting equipment
Comparative values
Installation
Labor-saving steps

ADVERTISING

Planning
Direct mail
Local house organs
Newspaper
Radio
Television

LEGAL

Lease
Contracts
Claims and lawsuits

BOOKKEEPING SYSTEM

Installation
Record of appointments
Receipts
Disbursements
Petty cash
Profit and loss
Inventory

COST OF OPERATION

Rent, light
Salaries
Supplies
Depreciation
Linen service

Sundries
Taxes

MANAGEMENT

Methods of building good will
Analysis of materials and labor
  in relation to service charges
Greeting clients
Adjusting complaints
Handling employees
Selling merchandise

OFFICE ADMINISTRATION

Stationery and office supplies
Inventory

INSURANCE

Liability and malpractice
Compensation
Unemployment
Social Security
Fire, theft and burglary

METHODS OF PAYMENT

In advance
C.O.D.
Open account
Time payments

COMPLIANCE WITH LABOR LAWS

Minimum wage and hour law
Hours of employment
Minors

ETHICS

Courtesy
Observation of trade practices

COMPLIANCE WITH STATE LAWS

Concerning equipment
Size and placement of barber-
  styling chairs and lavatories

LICENSING

Of barber-styling shop managers and barber-stylists

1. Name 10 essential functions performed by a barber-styling shop owner or manager.
2. List three important shop policies that should be explained to new employees.
3. Name three forms of ownership.
4. What is the best location for a barber-styling shop?
5. Of what protection is a lease for a barber-styling shop?
6. What is the best form of advertising?
7. Of what value are records in the barber-styling shop?
8. Name at least seven uses for a telephone in the barber-styling shop.
9. What are four basic rules to follow when using a telephone?

24

Licensing Laws

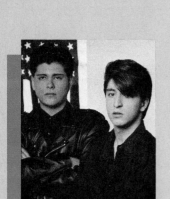

Learning Objectives

After completing this chapter, you should be able to:

1. *Discuss the responsibilities of the State Barber Board.*
2. *Identify the primary objective of barber-styling licensing laws.*
3. *Explain the purpose of the state board inspectors.*
4. *Discuss the state board rules and regulations of your state.*

Courtesy of: Hair: Indola of North America. Photo: Jack Cutler.

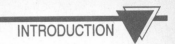

Although state board rules and barber-styling license laws may vary from state to state, the basic licensing law concepts of professional regulatory boards remain the same.

LICENSE LAW REVIEW QUESTIONS

The following questions and answers are designed to review general licensing law concepts:

1. What government body is responsible for the efficient and orderly administration of the barber-styling license law?
   The State Barber Board.
2. Where does the authority to conduct disciplinary hearings rest?
   With the State Barber Board.
3. What additional authority is given to the State Barber Board in order to properly administer the barber-styling license law?
   The power to issue rules and regulations.
4. What is the primary objective of the barber-styling license law?
   To protect the health, safety, and welfare of the public.
5. What is the objective of the barber-styling license examination?
   To evaluate a license applicant's competency.
6. How may the state board abuse the intent of the barber-styling license law?
   By using the law to limit the number of licenses.
7. What is one of the important personal requirements of an applicant for a barber-styling license?
   That the applicant be of good moral character.
8. Under what circumstances should a barber-stylist be forbidden to perform services upon clients?
   When the stylist is suffering from a communicable disease.
9. How may the state board discipline a barber-stylist?
   By revocation or suspension of an operator's license.
10. What protection does the licensee have against unlawful action of the state board?
    The barber-stylist is protected by the laws of the state.
11. What action must be taken by the state board before it can revoke or suspend a license?
    It must grant the licensee a hearing.
12. What can be done to a licensee who violates the provisions of the barber-styling license law?
    The licensee can be cited for disciplinary action.
13. If a person acts as a barber-stylist without obtaining a license, of what is

that person guilty?

Of practicing in an unlawful manner.

14. What recourse is available to a barber-stylist whose license has been suspended or revoked?

    The right to appeal to the courts.

15. Of what crime is a person guilty when convicted of violating any of the provisions of the license law?

    A misdemeanor.

16. What purpose is served by the periodic inspection of barber-styling shops?

    To be certain that they are complying with sanitary requirements.

17. Of what is a barber-stylist guilty who willfully fails to display a license or certificate?

    Guilty of violation of the barber-styling law.

18. What does the law require be done with a barber-stylist's license that has been suspended or revoked?

    It must be surrendered to the State Barber Board.

19. How may the state board punish a barber-stylist who is guilty of immoral behavior?

    It may suspend or revoke that person's license.

20. How may a barber-stylist guilty of gross malpractice be punished by the state board?

    By suspension or revocation of the license.

21. Who is responsible for posting the barber-styling law and/or the state board rules and regulations in the barber-styling shop?

    The shop owner.

22. Who practices barber-styling under the constant and direct supervision of a licensed barber-stylist?

    An apprentice.

NOTE: State board examinations include questions pertaining to the licensing laws of that state. In preparation for your state board examinations your instructor(s) should furnish you with the licensing rules and regulations of your state.

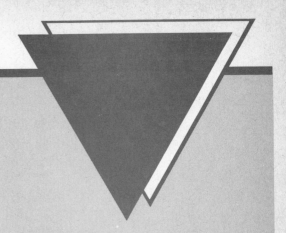

Answers

History of Barbering

1. The word barber is derived from the Latin word *barba*, meaning beard.
2. As a sign of wisdom, strength, and manhood or for religious reasons.
3. Ancient Egypt and China.
4. About 400 years B.C. (before the birth of Christ).
5. About 296 B.C.
6. About 500 B.C.
7. Barbers who assisted the clergy in the practice of surgery and medicine.
8. During the Middle Ages (after the birth of Christ).
9. Besides barbering, they did blood-letting, performed operations, pulled teeth, and dressed wounds.
10. A striped pole, from which was suspended a basin. The white band around the pole indicated the ribbon for bandaging the arm, the red band indicated the bleeding, and the basin was intended to receive blood.
11. It started in the days when the barber-surgeons bled their patients when treating diseases.
12. A trade guild or society formed for the protection of barber-surgeons.
13. During the thirteenth century.

14. In 1371.
15. The early Dutch and Swedish settlers.
16. Master-barber organizations.
17. Journeymen-barber organizations.
18. 1887.
19. 1893.
20. 1897.
21. Shop and salon owners/managers.
22. To standardize barber training and upgrade the profession.
23. To standardize the operation of barber schools.
24. To standardize the qualifications of barber examination applicants and the methods of evaluation to be used.
25. 1929.
26. Maintaining high standards of education and training.
27. Maintains the standards of the profession; protects barber-stylists' rights; protects the health and welfare of the public.
28. The implementation of regulatory and educational standards. The improved practice of sanitation in the shop. The use of better professional implements and tools. The use of electrical appliances in the shop. The study of anatomy dealing with those parts of the body (head, face, and neck) that are serviced by the barber-stylist. The study of products and preparations used in connection with facial, scalp, and hair treatments.

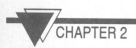

CHAPTER 2

Your Professional Image

1. Personality, personal hygiene, good grooming, general health, posture, attitude, moral character, professional ethics, and technical ability.
2. The branch of science that is concerned with healthful living; the daily maintenance of cleanliness and healthfulness.
3. Personal hygiene, rest, exercise, relaxation, nutrition, healthy lifestyle, healthy thoughts, and good posture.
4. The outward reflection of your inner feelings, thoughts, attitudes, and values; listening skills, voice, speech, manner of speaking, and conversational skills; the psychology of getting along well with others.
5. By self-esteem, confidence, and the respect shown to others.
6. The study of standards of conduct and moral judgment.

Bacteriology

1. Bacteriology is necessary to protect individual and public health.

2. Bacteriology is the science that deals with the study of micro-organisms called bacteria.

3. Bacteria are minute, one-celled vegetable micro-organisms found nearly everywhere.

4. Bacteria can exist almost anywhere, for example, on the skin, in water, air, decayed matter, secretions of body openings, on clothing, and beneath the nails.

5. a) Non-pathogenic bacteria—helpful, harmless, perform useful functions such as decomposing refuse. b) Pathogenic bacteria—harmful, produce disease when they invade plant or animal tissue.

6. a) Parasites are harmful pathogenic bacteria that require living matter for their growth. b) Saprophytes are helpful non-pathogenic bacteria that live on dead matter and do not produce disease.

7. a) Cocci are round-shaped organisms that appear singly. b) Bacilli are rod-shaped organisms. They are the most common bacteria and produce diseases. c) Spirilla are curved or corkscrew-shaped organisms.

8. a) Staphylococci are pus-forming organisms that grow in bunches or clusters. They cause abscesses, pustules, and boils. b) Streptococci are pus-forming organisms that grow in chains. They cause infections such as strep throat. c) Diplococci grow in pairs and cause pneumonia.

9. Bacteria grow and reproduce under favorable conditions with sufficient food. When they reach their largest size, they divide into two new cells by a process called mitosis.

10. During the active or vegetative stage, bacteria grow and reproduce. During the inactive, spore-forming stage, no growth or reproduction occurs.

11. By hairlike projections called flagella or cilia.

12. a) A local infection is indicated by a boil or pimple that contains pus. b) A general infection results when the bloodstream carries the bacteria to all parts of the body, as in syphilis.

13. One that can spread from one person to another by contact.

14. Infections can be prevented and controlled through personal hygiene and public sanitation.

15. a) Plant parasites can produce contagious diseases, such as ringworm and favus, a skin disease of the scalp. b) Animal parasites can produce contagious diseases, such as scabies, and infection of the scalp by lice called pediculosis.
16. Immunity is the ability of the body to destroy bacteria that have gained entrance, and thus to resist infection. The two types are natural immunity and acquired immunity.
17. Bacteria can be destroyed by disinfectants and by intense heat.

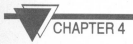
CHAPTER 4

Sterilization and Sanitation

1. The process of making an object germ-free by destroying all kinds of bacteria, whether harmful or beneficial.
2. chemical.
3. Ultraviolet rays and vapors keep objects clean after they have been sanitized.
4. Pathogenic bacteria.
5. Infectious diseases may be spread from one person to another.
6. Asepsis—free from disease germs.
   Sterile—free from all germs.
   Sepsis—poisoning due to germs.
7. hot
8. formalin.
9. A chemical agent that may kill or retard the growth of bacteria.
10. A chemical agent that destroys bacteria.
11. A vapor used to keep clean objects in a sanitary condition until ready for use.
12. a) Quats—1 to 5 minutes.
    b) 25 percent formalin—10 minutes.
    c) 10 percent formalin—20 minutes.
13. A receptacle containing a disinfectant solution. By immersing clean implements into it for the required time.
14. Thoroughly wash each object with soap and water and place into a suitable disinfectant solution for the required time.
15. Convenient to prepare, quick acting, non-corrosive, non-irritating to skin, odorless, and economical.

16. Rinse them in clean water, dry with a clean towel, and place in a dry or cabinet sanitizer until ready for use.

17. Wrap them in individual paper envelopes or place them in a cabinet sanitizer or ultraviolet ray cabinet until ready for use.

18. A closed, airtight cabinet containing an active fumigant (formaldehyde gas).

19. Place one tablespoon of borax and one tablespoon of formalin solution on a small tray or blotter on the bottom of cabinet sanitizer.

20. 37 percent to 40 percent solution of formaldehyde gas in water.

21. Rub the surface and sharp edges with a cotton pad dampened with 70 percent alcohol.

22. Gently rub exposed surface with a cotton pad dampened with 70 percent alcohol.

23. infections.

24. a) 25 percent
    b) 5 percent

25. a) Short disinfection time, odorless, non-toxic, and stable.
    b) 1:1000 solution

26. Purchase chemicals in small quantities and store in cool, dry place. Measure carefully. Label all containers. Keep under lock and key. Avoid spilling.

Public Sanitation

1. The application of measures designed to promote public health and prevent spread of infectious disease.

2. Contact with a person having an infectious disease; unclean hands; use of unsanitized instruments; common use of towels, combs, brushes, drinking cups, shaving mugs, or styptic pencils.

3. Wash hands with tincture of green soap and water and apply 60 percent alcohol or rinse hands in an antiseptic solution.

4. Keep the shop well ventilated and lighted. Keep the walls, curtains, and floor coverings in a clean condition. Have a continuous supply of running hot and cold water. Thoroughly cleanse hands before and after serving a client. Keep all waste materials in closed containers and have them removed regularly.

5. Cover the headrest with a clean towel or paper tissue and change it for each client.
6. To prevent shaving cloth or chair cloth from touching the client's neck.
7. Keep them in closed, clean containers.
8. With a sanitized spatula.
9. In closed, clean cabinet.
10. In closed containers, separate from the clean towels.
11. Neck strip, headrest covering, and towels.
12. To prevent spread of infection.
13. Sanitize it before using on a client.
14. To help prevent disease.
15. Keep them in covered receptacles and remove regularly.
16. It is one of the most common means of transmitting disease.

Safe Work Practices and First Aid

1. To be conscientious in the performance of duties, and maintain sanitation, efficiency, and safety in the workplace.
2. Sanitize tools and implements; be observant; try to prevent accidents; and use common sense.
3. A thorough technical knowledge of products; safe and efficient work practices; and common sense.
4. Inform the client.
5. Honest and conscientious.

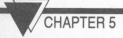

CHAPTER 5

Implements, Tools, and Equipment

1. Comb, shears, clipper, trimmer, razor, brush, and blow-dryer.
2. High quality, good workmanship, guarantee, and reliability of the manufacturer.
3. The type of service to be performed and the barber-stylist's preference.
4. All-purpose comb.
5. For mustache trims and for blending around the ear areas.
6. Wide tooth comb.
7. For sectioning long hair and for making partings to wrap on perm rods.
8. Moving point, moving blade, still point, still blade, two cutting edges, pivot screw, two shanks, finger grip, thumb grip, and finger brace.

9. The German type has no finger brace. The French type has a brace for the small finger.
10. Shears are usually measured by half inches. 7 and 7 ½ inch lengths are mostly used.
11. The plain grind and the corrugated grind. The plain grind is mostly used.
12. Smooth, medium, and coarse. The medium finish is preferred.
13. Measure the shear against the length of the base of the palm to the tip of the middle finger.
14. To remove excess bulk in the hair or to create texturing effects.
15. Hand clipper and electric clipper.
16. Magnetic type and motor driven.
17. Cutting blade, still blade, heel, switch, set screw, and conducting cord.
18. Edger or outliner.
19. #0000.
20. Conventional straight razor and the changeable blade razor.
21. Their various parts, styles, widths, balance, lengths, tempers, grinds, and finishes.
22. Head, back, shoulder, pivot, blade, point, edge, heel, shank, tang, and handle.
23. After it is used, strop and dry the razor and then apply a little castor oil over the blade.
24. A solid block containing an abrasive for sharpening razors.
25. Natural hone, synthetic hone, and combination hone.
26. Water hone and Belgian hone.
27. Those made from canvas, cowhide, horsehide, and imitation leather.
28. Remove excess hair and dirt, wash in hot water, soap, and rinse; place into a disinfectant solution for 20 minutes, rinse, wipe dry, and place in dry sanitizer until needed.
29. With 70 percent ethyl alcohol.

Honing and Stropping

1. By consistent practice and experience.
2. The razor acquires a perfect cutting edge.
3. Hold the razor at an angle and use smooth, even strokes and pressure on both sides of the blade.
4. Stroke the razor blade to the left diagonally across the hone, from heel to point toward the edge.

5. Turn the razor over on its back and stroke the blade to the right diagonally across the hone, from the heel to the point toward the edge.

6. The abrasive material on the hone makes small cuts in the sides of the razor's edge.

7. To determine if the razor edge is blunt, keen, coarse, or rough.

8. It has five teeth and tends to dig into the nail with a smooth, steady grip.

9. It passes over the nail smoothly, without any cutting power.

10. It tends to dig into the nail with a jerky feeling.

11. It has large teeth that stick to the nail and give a harsh, grating sound.

12. Follow manufacturer's directions. After using, wipe clean and keep covered.

13. To smooth the razor's edge.

14. The stroking of the razor blade in stropping is just the reverse of honing.

15. The leather strop.

16. Grasp the end of the strop with the left hand and hold it firmly.

17. Hold the razor in the right hand with the fingers wrapped around the handle and shank at the pivot.

18. Start at the top edge of the strop closest to the hydraulic chair.

19. Place the razor flat against the strop with the back toward the barber-stylist. Draw the razor toward the barber-stylist. Turn the razor over on its back with the fingers. Draw the razor away from the barber-stylist. Repeat these movements until razor is properly stropped.

20. The thumb and next two fingers of the right hand.

21. Use normal pressure at the point and heel for both sides of the razor.

22. Touch the razor edge lightly over the cushion part of the thumb.

23. It produces a keen drawing sensation, and the razor does not slide over the thumb.

24. It produces no drawing sensation, sliding freely over the thumb.

25. Apply lather or soap to it, and then wipe it clean to remove accumulated grit.

26. To smooth and shape the edge of the razor into a keen cutting implement.

27. Either suspended, attached to a swivel, or laid flat.
28. A good quality strop dressing.

CHAPTER 6 ▼

The Skin and Scalp

1. It is slightly moist, soft, and flexible; slightly acid in reaction; free from any disorder or disease.
2. Soft, smooth, and with a healthy color.
3. The epidermis and dermis.
4. It is the outermost layer of the skin and is the outer protective covering of the body.
5. Stratum corneum (horny layer); stratum lucidum (clear layer); stratum granulosum (granular layer); stratum germinativum (germinative layer).
6. Stratum corneum.
7. In the deepest layer of the stratum germinativum of the epidermis and the papillary layer of the dermis.
8. It consists of an elastic network of cells containing blood and lymph vessels, nerve endings, sweat glands, oil glands, and hair follicles.
9. Papillary and reticular layers.
10. The elastic fibers in the dermis.
11. Hair, nails, and sweat and oil glands.
12. By blood and lymph.
13. Motor, sensory, and secretory.
14. The fingertips.
15. To muscles attached to hair follicles.
16. Heat, cold, touch, pressure, and pain.
17. They regulate the excretion of perspiration from sweat glands and control the flow of sebum to the surface of the skin.
18. Blood circulation through the skin and evaporation of sweat.
19. Sense of vibration.
20. A combination of nerve endings.
21. After expansion, such as swelling, the skin regains its former shape almost immediately.
22. Its loss of elasticity.
23. The coloring matter (melanin) in the skin, and the blood supply.
24. Lanolin cream.

25. Protection, heat regulation, secretion, excretion, sensation, and absorption.

Sweat and Oil Glands

1. An organ that removes certain materials from the blood and forms new substances. Sudoriferous, or sweat glands; sebaceous, or oil glands.
2. They consist of a coiled base and a tube-like duct which forms a pore at the surface of the skin.
3. Practically all parts of body, but more numerous on the palms, soles, forehead, and in armpits.
4. Help to eliminate waste products from the body in the form of sweat and regulate body temperature.
5. Heat, exercise, emotions, and certain drugs.
6. They consist of small sacs whose ducts open into the hair follicles.
7. Sebum, an oily substance.
8. It lubricates the skin and hair, keeping them soft and pliable.
9. On all parts of the body, with the exception of the palms and soles.

The Hair

1. To understand the proper hair care and treatment beneficial to clients.
2. Trichology.
3. A slender thread-like outgrowth of the skin and scalp of the human body.
4. The coloring matter in hair.
5. Keratin.
6. Each layer is laced together to form coiled strands.
7. Harmful cosmetic applications or faulty hair treatments.
8. They cause intense swelling of the hair and breakage of the bonds.
9. Hair root and hair shaft.
10. That portion of the hair that extends beyond the skin.
11. That portion of the hair structure found beneath the skin surface.
12. A tube-like depression or pocket in the skin.
13. Arrector pili muscle and sebaceous gland.

14. A club-shaped structure forming the lower part of the hair root. It fits over and covers the papilla.
15. A small cone-shaped elevation at the bottom of the hair follicle that fits into the hair bulb.
16. From rich blood and nerve supply in the papilla.
17. The papilla produces hair cells during hair growth.
18. The direction of the natural flow of hair on the scalp.
19. a) A cowlick is a tuft of hair standing up. b) A whorl is an area of the scalp where the hair forms in a swirl effect, such as in the crown area.
20. germs
21. Fear or cold, which causes the arrector pili muscles to contract.
22. Oil glands secrete sebum, an oily substance, which keeps the hair and scalp in a soft and pliable condition.
23. Diet, blood circulation, emotional disturbances, stimulation of endocrine glands, and drugs.
24. The shape and size of the hair follicle.
25. Straight hair, which is usually round. Wavy hair, which is usually oval. Curly hair, which is usually flat.
26. Medulla, cortex, and cuticle.
27. The medulla.
28. The cortex.
29. The cuticle.
30. Palms, soles, lips, and eyelids.
31. Lanugo hair is fine, soft, and downy and is usually found on all areas of the body.
32. It helps in the evaporation of perspiration.
33. The new hair is formed by cell division from the growing point at the root of the hair around the papilla.
34. Growth, fall, and replacement of hair.
35. About 1/2" per month.
36. About 120 square inches.
37. Moisture in the air deepens the natural wave. Cold air will cause hair to contract. Heat will cause hair to expand and absorb moisture.
38. Between 50 and 80.
39. From two to four years.
40. The loss of natural pigment and the presence of air spaces in the hair.
41. A person who is born with white hair and without pigment to color the skin or iris of the eyes.
42. Sight, touch, hearing, and smell.

43. Texture, porosity, elasticity, and condition of the hair.
44. Touch and sight.
45. Degree of coarseness or fineness of the hair.
46. a) Blond—140,000. b) Black—108,000. c) Brown—110,000.
47. Ability of hair to absorb moisture.
48. Ability of hair to stretch and return to its original form without breakage.
49. Normal hair can be stretched about one-fifth its length; wet hair can be stretched from 40–50 percent its length.
50. The cortical layer.

Disorders of the Skin, Scalp, and Hair

1. To prevent their spread and avoid more serious conditions.
2. To safeguard his/her own and the public's health.
3. To be able to recognize the various infectious diseases and suggest proper measures to be taken to prevent more serious consequences.
4. Any departure from a normal state of health.
5. A structural change in the tissues caused by injury or disease.
6. Macule, papule, wheal, tubercle, tumor, vesicle, bulla, and pustule.
7. An objective lesion can be seen, as pimples. A subjective lesion can be felt, as itching.
8. Scale, crust, abrasion, fissure, ulcer, scar, and skin stain.
9. a) Dry or greasy epidermal flakes. b) Dandruff.
10. Milia, acne, comedones, and seborrhea.
11. Acne is a chronic inflammatory disease of the sebaceous (oil) glands.
12. a) Blackheads. b) Whiteheads.
13. Bromidrosis refers to foul-smelling perspiration. Anidrosis is lack of perspiration. Hyperidrosis is excessive perspiration.
14. A worm-like mass of hardened sebum obstructing the duct of the oil glands.
15. Pityriasis capitis simplex (dry dandruff) and pityriasis steatoides (greasy or waxy type of dandruff).
16. Poor circulation, lack of nerve stimulation, improper diet, uncleanliness, infection, and injury.
17. An inflammatory condition of the skin.
18. The lesions are round, dry patches covered with coarse, silvery scales.

19. On the scalp, elbows, knees, chest, and low back.
20. Alopecia is the technical term for any form of abnormal loss of hair.
21. Ringworm.
22. Vegetable parasites.
23. A small, reddened patch of little blisters, which spread outward and heal in the middle with scaling.
24. It is the technical term for gray hair.
25. Congenital—exists at or before birth and occurs in albinos and occasionally in persons with normal hair. Acquired—may be due to old age or premature, as in early adult life.
26. Split hair ends.
27. Hirsuties and hypertrichosis.
28. Acne simplex and acne vulgaris.
29. Furuncle.
30. Staphylococci.
31. Head louse.
32. Abnormal white patches in the skin or the hair.
33. A congenital absence of pigment in the body including the skin, hair, and eyes.
34. Birthmark.
35. Verruca.
36. A small, brownish spot or blemish on the skin.

CHAPTER 7

Draping

1. To protect the client's skin and clothing.
2. Consideration for the client.
3. To prevent contact of the cape with the client's skin.
4. Prepare materials and supplies; sanitize hands; ask client to remove jewelry; remove objects from hair; turn client's collar to the inside.
5. Plastic.
6. Nylon or cotton, because it sheds wet hair better.

Shampoo Chemistry

1. Head and tail.
2. a) The tail of the molecule attracts dirt, debris, grease, oil, etc. b) The head has an attraction for water.
3. The shampoo is applied and worked into the hair. The dirt is attracted to the tails of the molecules and becomes firmly

attached to them. During the rinsing, the heads are attracted to the water and are carried from the hair, taking the tails with attached dirt with them.

4. An alkali mixed with an oil or fat.
5. Soap, soapless, and cream.
6. A cleansing or surface active agent that describes organic compounds brought together by chemical synthesis to create wetting, dispersing, emulsifying, solubilizing, foaming, or washing agents.
7. The base surfactant or combination of surfactants.
8. Anionic, cationic, nonionic, and ampholytic.
9. Sodium lauryl sulfate and sodium laureth sulfate.
10. Anionic—harsh cleanser that produces a rich foam, rinses easily from hair; cationic—has an anti-bacterial action; nonionic—versatile, stable, ability to resist shrinkage, mild cleansing action, low incidence of irritation to human tissues; ampholytic—can behave as an anionic or a cationic depending on pH of solution, clings to the hair, conducive to hair manageability, germicidal properties, does not sting the eyes.

Water

1. A solvent; has the ability to dissolve another substance.
2. Oil and wax.

pH

1. A value used to indicate acidity or alkalinity of water-based solutions; expresses the hydrogen-ion concentration of a solution.
2. Through the use of meters and indicators.
3. Because it influences how that product will affect various layers of the hair and skin.
4. Shrink, constrict, and harden; soften, swell, and expand.
5. Anything below 7.0 to 0; anything above 7.0 to 14.
6. Water—7; hair and skin—4.5 to 5.5; shampoo—4.5 to 7.5; conditioners—3.0 to 5.5; lemon juice—2.

Shampooing

1. To keep hair and scalp in a clean and healthy condition.
2. As often as necessary.
3. Plain liquid soap or a detergent-based product.
4. Proper preparation of client; selection of a good shampoo; proper application of shampoo and water; sufficient scalp massage to stimulate scalp; thorough rinsing to remove dirt and lather; drying and combing the hair.
5. After lathering, stand behind the client. Place fingertips at the back of the head just below the ears. Apply rotary movements from the ears to the temples up to the forehead, then over the top of the head down to the neck. Repeat these movements for several minutes.

Hair Rinses

1. It cleanses the hair and scalp; brings out hair luster; conditions the hair and scalp; adds highlights and color to the hair.
2. Water, acid, dandruff, and bluing rinses.
3. Acid rinse.
4. It eliminates yellow tinge in gray hair and brightens black hair.

Conditioners and Hair Conditioning

1. Dry, brittle, or damaged.
2. To restore some natural oils, proteins, and moisture to the hair.
3. Protein or moisturizers.
4. Cream and liquid.
5. Lanolin, moisturizers, fatty acids, quats, vegetable oils, proteins, or herbs.
6. shampooed or towel dried.
7. Instant, protein penetrating, neutralizing, and moisturizing.
8. Texture and condition of hair.
9. One to five minutes.
10. Slightly increases hair diameter by a coating action and gives it body.

11. Hydrolized protein; penetrate into the cortex and replace lost keratin; texture, elasticity, and equalize porosity.
12. Neutralizing conditioners neutralize alkaline conditions; acid pH; one to five minutes.
13. Draw moisture into the hair, and seal moisture inside damp hair by coating the cuticle.
14. Severely damaged hair.
15. A pretreatment for chemical services designed to neutralize metallic elements in or on the hair.

Scalp Treatments

1. To maintain a healthy scalp and hair and to combat such disorders as dandruff and excessive hair loss.
2. The blood flow is increased, while the nerves are rested and soothed.
3. To keep the scalp and hair clean and healthy, to promote hair growth, and to try to prevent excessive hair loss.
4. It stimulates the blood supply to the scalp.
5. If there is a deficiency of natural oil in the scalp and hair.
6. Leading an indoor life; frequent washing of hair; continued use of drying lotions, tonics, and shampoos.
7. Excessive intake of fatty foods in the diet, resulting in over-activity of the oil glands.
8. The appearance of white scales on the scalp and hair accompanied by itching scalp.
9. Poor circulation of blood to the scalp; improper diet; uncleanliness; infection.
10. Poor blood circulation; lack of proper stimulation; improper nourishment; certain infectious scalp diseases, such as ringworm; constitutional disorders.
11. Stimulating the blood supply to the hair papillae encourages the growth and replacement of hair.

Hair Tonics

1. Cosmetic solutions used on the hair.
2. The steaming of the scalp by means of steaming towels or a scalp steamer, usually followed by the application of a hair tonic.

CHAPTER 8

Muscles

1. Fibrous tissues.
2. Ability to stretch, contract, and produce all movements of the body.
3. Origin, insertion, and belly.
4. a) Part that does not move; b) Part that does move.
5. Massage, electric current, light rays, heat rays, moist heat, nerve impulses, and chemicals.
6. Voluntary muscles.
7. Epicranius; frontalis and occipitalis.
8. Draws the scalp forward, elevates eyebrows, and wrinkles skin of forehead.
9. Orbicularis oculi.
10. Orbicularis oris.
11. Trapezius.
12. Sternocleidomastoid.

Nerves

1. Long, white fibrous cords originating on the brain and spinal column.
2. Message carriers to and from all parts of the body.
3. Contract and expand.
4. Relaxation; contraction.
5. Chemicals, massage, electric current, light rays, heat rays, and moist heat.
6. There are 12 pairs of cranial nerves.
7. The fifth or trifacial nerve; the seventh or facial nerve; the eleventh or accessory nerve.
8. The fifth cranial nerve.
9. It is the chief sensory nerve of the face and the motor nerve of the muscles of mastication.
10. The seventh cranial nerve.
11. a) The optic nerve. b) The olfactory nerve. c) The auditory nerve.
12. The scalp at the back part of the head, as far up as the top of the head.
13. The spinal portion of the eleventh cranial nerve.
14. a) Supra-orbital. b) Nasal. c) Infra-orbital. d) Mental. e) Auriculo-temporal. f) Zygomatic.

15. a) Temporal. b) Mandibular. c) Cervical. d) Posterior auricular. e) Buccal. f) Zygomatic.

Arteries

1. Common carotid arteries.
2. Internal common carotid artery and external common carotid artery.
3. Internal branch of the common carotid artery.
4. External branches of the common carotid arteries.
5. Facial artery.
6. Submental artery.
7. Frontal artery.
8. The back of the head up to the crown.
9. Parietal artery—the crown and side of the head. Frontal artery—the forehead.
10. Posterior auricular artery.
11. The infra-orbital artery.
12. Internal jugular and external jugular.

Theory of Massage

1. A system of manipulations applied with the hands or with the aid of electrical devices.
2. The head, face, and neck.
3. Effleurage, or stroking movements; petrissage, or kneading movements; friction, or deep rubbing movements; percussion (tapotement), or tapping, slapping, or hacking movements; vibration, or shaking movements.
4. The skin and all its structures are nourished.
5. It is increased.

Facial Treatments

1. They cleanse the skin; increase circulation; activate glandular activity; relax tense nerves; maintain muscle tone; strengthen weak muscle tissue; correct certain skin disorders; help prevent the formation of wrinkles and aging lines; improve skin texture and complexion; help reduce fatty tissues.
2. Hot and cold water, towels, vibrator, therapeutic lamp and various preparations, such as facial creams, ointments, lotions, oils, packs, masks, and powders.

3. In order to select the proper cream for each type of skin and be able to apply the proper massage manipulations.

4. Make client comfortable and give a facial as restful and refreshing as possible.

5. To avoid inhaling each other's breath or smelling each other's body odor.

6. Arrange all necessary supplies. Wash hands. Adjust linens and towels. Protect client's hair by fastening a towel around his/her head. Recline the client.

7. Apply cleansing cream over the face, using stroking and rotary movements. Remove cleansing cream with a smooth, warm, damp towel. Steam face mildly with three towels. Apply tissue cream to the skin with fingertips. Gently massage the face, using continuous and rhythmic movements. Wipe off excess cream with a hot towel. Steam the face with hot towels. Remove hot towels and follow with a cool towel. Pat an astringent or face lotion over the face and dry. Apply powder over the face and remove excess powder. Raise hydraulic chair. Comb hair to desired style.

8. Have client thoroughly relaxed. Provide quiet atmosphere. Maintain clean, orderly arrangement of supplies. Follow systematic procedure. Give facial massage properly.

9. Harming or scratching the skin; excessive or rough massage; getting facial cream into eyes; using towels that are too hot; breathing into the client's face; not being careful or sanitary; not showing interest in the client's skin problems; carelessness in removing cream, by leaving a greasy film behind the ears, under the chin, and in other areas; not permitting the client to relax, either by talking or being tense while giving facial manipulations; leaving chair to get materials or supplies; heavy, rough, or cold hands.

10. To stimulate the activity of the oil glands and to replenish a deficiency of natural oil in the skin.

11. Excessive intake of starchy and oily foods, and faulty hygienic habits.

12. Sanitized comedone extractor.

13. It has a mild tonic effect that helps prevent undue wrinkling of the skin.

14. Acne facial.

15. Clay pack, acne facial, and hot oil mask.

16. Oily skin facials and acne facials.

17. Extremely dry, parched, and scaly skin.

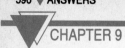

CHAPTER 9

Shaving

1. Sensitivity of skin, texture of hair, and grain of beard.
2. Properly sanitized razor, hands, and towels; properly honed and stropped razor; well-lathered beard; properly heated and applied towels; smoothly cut beard; lather completely removed; properly applied astringent or face lotion; thoroughly dried face; evenly applied powder.
3. Arrange chair cloth. Change headrest paper and adjust headrest to proper level. Recline chair to comfortable position. Tuck in towel.
4. Apply lather to face. Apply steam towel over lather. Remove lather with steam towel. Re-lather beard.
5. Use clean hands, sanitized razor, sanitary receptacle for shaving soap, sanitary tissue to wipe lather from razor, and clean linen.
6. Use the cushion tips of fingers in a rotary movement.
7. It softens the hair and lubricates the skin and beard.
8. The heat softens the outer layer of the hair and stimulates the flow of oil from the skin glands. The added lubrication helps the razor to glide over the face.
9. If the face is very sensitive, irritated, chapped, or blistered.
10. Free hand, back hand, reverse free hand, and reverse back hand.
11. Hold the razor in a free-hand position. Use a gliding stroke toward the point of the razor in a forward sawing movement.
12. Hold the razor in a back-hand position and stroke it in a forward sawing movement away from you toward the point of the razor.
13. The razor is held similarly to the free-hand position. The stroke is performed with a slight rotation of the wrist, forming a small upward arc.
14. With the grain of the hair.
15. To make the left sideburn outline and for shaving the left side behind the ear.
16. 14.
17. The right side is shaved first. The free-hand stroke is the first stroke.
18. When performing each of the 14 shaving steps, a few more

strokes across the grain may be taken, thereby assuring a complete and even shave, with a single lathering.

19. The sides below the ears.
20. Comb the hair neatly. Wipe off excess powder and any loose hair.
21. Just before beginning the final steps in face shaving.
22. Just before combing the hair.
23. Dull or rough razors; unclean hands, towels, and chair cloth; cold fingers; heavy touch of hand; poorly heated towels; too cold or too hot lather; glaring overhead lights; unshaven hair patches; scraping of skin and close shaving.
24. By shaving the beard against the grain of the hair during the second time over.
25. It may irritate the skin and cause ingrown hairs or infection.

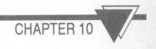

CHAPTER 10

Haircutting Principles

1. The precise designing, cutting, and shaping of hair.
2. the foundation of good hairstyles.
3. By producing a precise and professional haircut.
4. Accentuate client's good points; minimize poor features.
5. Head shape, facial contour, neckline, and hair texture.
6. Envisioning.
7. Front, top, crown, back, nape, right temporal, right side, right sideburn, left temporal, left side, left sideburn.
8. The basic laws of haircutting.
9. Design line, guide, parting, degree, elevation, 0-degree, 45-degree, 90-degree, uniform, layering, tapering, weight line, texturing, outlining, thinning, hairstyling.
10. 90-degree angle.
11. Finger and shear, razor, shear over comb, and clipper.
12. Clean and damp.

Men's Haircutting

1. Finish one vertical strip at a time before proceeding with the next strip to the left. Working from right to left gives a better view of the work.
2. The comb is held parallel to the shears.
3. It shortens the hair evenly and helps to reduce any ridges that may appear in the haircut.

Basic Principles of Men's Hairstyling

1. Study the client's features in order to suggest the most suitable hairstyle.
2. To be able to give the proper styling advice.
3. The oval.

Haircutting Techniques

1. On the left side of the head and carried around to the right side. Some barber-stylists prefer to start clipper work on the right side of head and proceed to the left side. Each procedure is correct.
2. Gradually tilt the blade so that the clipper rides on the heel of the bottom blade.
3. The comb is held parallel to the shears.
4. Finish one vertical strip or area at a time before proceeding with the next strip or area to the left. Working from right to left gives a better view of the work.
5. Depending on the desired hairstyle, shave the sideburns, around the ears, and the sides and back of the neck.
6. a) Use a free-hand stroke. b) Use a reverse back-hand stroke.
7. Wipe off loose hair from client's neck. Remove towel and chair cloth from client. Make out check for client. Thank client as you hand him/her the check.

Men's Razor Haircutting

1. The client's wishes, features, head shape, facial contour, and hair texture.
2. To thin and shorten hair; taper and blend hair; make resistant hair more manageable.
3. Guarded and straight open-blade razors.
4. Free hand and straight handle positions.
5. Light taper-blending, heavier taper-blending, terminal blending.
6. Light taper-blending.
7. With continuous movements, the hair is cut with the razor and removed with the comb. At the same time, the hair is re-combed for the next stroking.
8. a) Use more strokes and heavier tapering. b) Use fewer strokes and lighter pressure.

9. To detect any unusual condition, such as the presence of any growths, scars, disorders, or thinning areas.
10. Tapering too close to the hair part; thinning hair too close to the scalp; over-tapering the hair.
11. The beginner should use a razor with a guard. Avoid annoyance or distraction while cutting the hair. Keep sharp implements in a closed case.

Women's Haircutting

1. Haircutting shears, razor, thinning shears, combs, and clipper.
2. It removes excess bulk without shortening length of hair.
3. If coarse hair is thinned too close to the scalp the short, stubby hair ends will protrude through the top layer, while fine hair, being softer and more pliable, will lay flatter on the head.
4. a) Fine hair—from one-half to one inch. b) Medium hair—from one to one and a half inches. c) Coarse hair—from one and a half to two inches.
5. Hairline at the nape of the neck (ear to ear); at the side of the head (above ears); around facial hairline; and in hair part.
6. The cut ends would be seen in the finished hairstyle.
7. It is impossible to correct a haircut when too much hair has been removed during the thinning process.
8. In order to avoid pulling the hair and prevent dulling the razor.
9. Combing the short hair of the strand toward the scalp.
10. Thinning and tapering the hair at the same time by using regular haircutting shears.

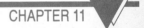

CHAPTER 11

Air-Waving

1. The temporary reshaping of the client's hair with the aid of a styling dryer, comb, brush, and special cosmetics.
2. Blow-waving, wind-waving, and air-jet waving.
3. Styling dryer (air-waver), combs (metal and/or hard rubber), and styling brushes.
4. Styling dryer without attachments and styling dryer with attachments.
5. By adjusting a dial on the side of the dryer.
6. Cutting, shampooing, and towel drying of the hair.

7. In a moist or damp condition.
8. Styling lotion.
9. Styling gel.
10. Along the side of the ridge, in a back-and-forth movement.
11. Each ridge and wave should match evenly without a break in the ridge or the wave.
12. Brush the hair toward the back and with a twist of the wrist, turn and push the brush forward, creating a lift. The hair is held in this position until it is dried with hot air from the blower.
13. To keep the finished hairstyle in place.
14. Dry and brittle hair.
15. In a rotating or back-and-forth movement, directed to the hair.
16. A metal comb retains heat and if permitted to touch the scalp it may cause a burn.

Curling Iron Techniques

1. The technique of styling hair with the aid of curling irons and without styling or setting creams or lotions.
2. The rod and shell.
3. Less heat than for normal hair.
4. On a tissue neck strip.
5. In a position that is comfortable and permits complete control.
6. Metal combs.
7. To create volume or lift in finished hairstyle.

Finger Waving Men's Hair

1. The technique of creating hairstyles in wet hair by means of the fingers and a comb.
2. By proper draping with a clean towel and shampoo cape.
3. By placing a styling hair net over the hair.
4. Naturally wavy hair and permanently waved hair.
5. It should harmonize with client's head shape and facial features.
6. Because they do not contain harmful ingredients.
7. To protect the client from excessive heat of the pedestal type of hair dryer.

CHAPTER 12

Mustache and Beard Design

1. For personal adornment.
2. In accordance with the facial features of the wearer.
3. It should correspond with the size of the client's facial features.
4. Drape client; consult with client; thin mustache with comb and shears; trim length and check corners of mouth area for evenness; shape or outline mustache with trimmer or razor.
5. Clipper, trimmer, shears, and comb.
6. Trim excess hair with shears and comb; draw or envision beard design; trim from front center to side areas, taper and blend the beard; return client to sitting position; outline cheek and upper areas blending with sideburns; trim and blend mustache; check and retouch beard; recomb hairstyle.
7. Clipper comb attachment.
8. To better balance the beard with the hairstyle.

CHAPTER 13

Permanent Waving

1. A procedure involving physical and chemical actions on the hair.
2. rods.
3. neutralization.
4. Waving solution and neutralizer or fixative.
5. Softens the hair to the shape of the curling rods.
6. Stops the action of the waving lotion and rehardens the hair into a new position.
7. A correct analysis of the client's scalp and hair condition.
8. Scalp condition, hair porosity, hair texture, hair elasticity, hair density, and hair length.
9. The elasticity and texture of the hair.
10. To permit better saturation and action of the waving solution and neutralizer.
11. Follow your teacher's instructions or the manufacturer's directions.
12. The size of the rod, the blocking (subsectioning), hair texture, and hair elasticity.
13. To determine in advance how the client's hair will react to the permanent waving process.
14. Immediately after the last rod is secured; following the rewet application of lotion; every 30 seconds thereafter.

15. When the wave forms a firm letter *S*.
16. Weak or fine hair.
17. To protect the client.
18. It is very curly when wet, frizzy when dry, and is difficult to comb into a wave pattern.
19. If a tint is given first, the waving solution will lighten the hair and may cause an uneven color. If the permanent wave is given first, the tint may distort or weaken the wave pattern.
20. It may disturb the wave pattern.
21. Hair porosity, texture, and elasticity.
22. When the waving solution remains on the skin or scalp too long.
23. Absorb the solution with pledgets saturated with cold water or neutralizer.
24. Apply a milder waving solution to those hair sections that are too curly. Retain it on the hair until the curl has relaxed sufficiently. Then, thoroughly neutralize the hair.
25. A mild strength waving solution.
26. To protect dry, brittle, and damaged hair.
27. Diameter of the rod and density and texture of the hair.
28. The length of the blockings.
29. The texture and porosity of the hair.
30. Without elasticity, the hair will not hold the curl or wave.
31. a) Strong curl patterns, fast processing time, room-temperature processing; b) when perming resistant hair, when a strong, tight curl is desired, or when the client has a history of early curl relaxation.
32. a) Softer curl patterns, slower, more controllable processing time, gentler treatment for delicate hair types; b) when perming delicate, fragile hair, when soft, natural curl or wave is desired, and when style support rather than strong curl is desired.
33. When only a section of a whole head of hair is permed.
34. Apply a heavy cream conditioner to hair not being permed.

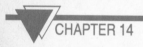

CHAPTER 14

Chemical Hair Relaxing and Soft Curl Permanent

1. It has a softening and swelling action on the hair.
2. To determine the true condition of the client's hair in order to give a correct hair relaxing treatment.

3. Porosity, texture, elasticity, and any possible hair damage.
4. The stabilizer. Fixative.
5. Hair strand test.
6. After the hair has received a series of reconditioning treatments and it has returned to a healthy condition.
7. To determine the degree of porosity, to determine the elasticity, and to determine the results to be expected.
8. Because the chemical hair relaxer may cause serious infection if any scalp eruptions or abrasions are present.
9. It serves as a guide for return treatments.
10. To help protect against lawsuits.
11. Hair previously treated with hot irons or severely damaged hair.
12. To protect the scalp and hairline from irritation caused by the chemical hair relaxer.
13. The chemical in the hair relaxer may be very harmful to the skin.
14. To help stop the action of the chemical relaxer by removing most of it from the hair.
15. To avoid irritation to the scalp by the teeth of the comb, which may cause infection.
16. The cream shampoo will readily stick to the hair and help to prevent tangling.
17. The hair is very fragile due to the action of the relaxer and tangled ends can be broken easily.
18. In order to remove all chemicals from the hair. Any chemical left in the hair will cause continuous processing and breakage.
19. It stops the softening action of the relaxer on the hair shaft and rehardens the hair into its new shape.
20. The hair is ready for combing when the stabilizer has rehardened the hair.
21. It is given in the same manner as for a regular chemical relaxing treatment except that the relaxer is applied to the new growth only.
22. The shampoo is given prior to the application of the relaxer.
23. By a three-step rinsing process: a) Rinse out half of the cream with warm water. b) Comb the hair, with the balance of the relaxer, for five minutes. c) Rinse balance of cream from the hair.
24. By combing the hair away from direction of the natural growth.

25. Faster, provides thorough coverage, and underneath hairs are covered.
26. Wide-tooth combs.
27. To restore some of the natural oils that have been removed by the chemical relaxer.
28. A color rinse.
29. The heat applied over relaxed hair would cause damage to the hair.
30. The reaction of the chemical in the relaxer would damage the hair.
31. A method of permanently waving over-curly hair.

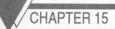

CHAPTER 15   Hair Coloring

1. The science and art of changing color of hair.
2. To restore gray hair to its natural color; to change the shade of hair because he/she feels present shade is a handicap to business; to maintain a youthful appearance.
3. The general structure of hair and scalp; proper selection and application of hair tints and lighteners; chemical reactions following their applications.
4. One that has had no previous lightening or tinting treatment.
5. Temporary, semi-permanent, and permanent.
6. Color rinses, highlighting color shampoos, and crayons.
7. To color the hair for a period of four to six weeks.
8. Aniline derivative tints, pure vegetable tints, metallic or mineral dyes, and compound dyes.
9. Hair colorings with a base derived from aniline, a coal tar product.
10. It is required by federal law, and to determine whether or not the client is allergic to the tint.
11. When mixed with peroxide, they penetrate the cuticle layer of the hair shaft and deposit the coloring in the cortical layer of the hair.
12. Wash a spot behind the ear or on the inner fold of the elbow with mild soap and water. Blot the area dry. Mix a capful of 20–volume peroxide and a capful of the tint to be used. Cover the area with the mixture. Do not disturb for 24 hours. After 24 hours, check for irritation.
13. In the preparation of the tint. The semi-permanent tint is applied to the patch test area without mixing with hydrogen peroxide.

14. By the presence of redness, swelling, burning, itching, blisters, or eruptions.
15. Client's age and skin tones.
16. To determine the actual color and condition of client's hair.
17. Signs of a positive skin test; scalp sores or eruptions; contagious scalp or hair disease; presence of either a metallic or a compound dye.
18. To use as a guide for future hair coloring treatments.
19. A single-application tint.
20. Save time by eliminating pre-shampooing, or pre-lightening. The hair may be colored lighter or darker than client's natural color. Leave no line of demarcation.
21. A patch test is required. Pre-lightening is necessary if hair color is to be made lighter. Pre-softening is necessary when hair is resistant.
22. They cleanse the hair and highlight its natural color in a single operation.
23. When using a double-application tint and if the client desires a complete color change to a lighter shade.
24. When gray hair is resistant to color or before toner is applied.
25. To avoid irritation to the scalp.
26. The metallic and compound dyes.
27. Color is self-penetrating. Color is applied the same way each time. Retouching is eliminated. Color does not rub off.
28. To bring out highlights and to temporarily restore faded hair to its natural shade.
29. With soap and water. For difficult stains, apply pledget of cotton dipped in leftover tint in a circular motion or use prepared tint stain remover.
30. Applied only to the new growth of the hair.

Hair Lightening

1. Hair lightening is the partial or total removal of the natural pigment or artificial color from the hair.
2. Oil lighteners, cream lighteners, and powder or paste lighteners.
3. Hydrogen peroxide.
4. 20–volume strength.
5. It speeds the liberation of oxygen gas which hastens the lightening (bleaching) action.

6. It softens the cuticle of the hair and makes it more receptive to the penetrating action of an aniline derivative tint.
7. To judge the length of time required to leave mixture on the hair and to find out in what condition the hair is for lightening.
8. Because a toner contains an aniline derivative product.
9. Use of a strong lightening formula, over-lapping, or retaining the lightener too long on the hair.
10. Only to the new growth of the hair.
11. To prevent hair breakage and/or scalp irritation.
12. They make the hair porous and lighter in color.
13. Toners are aniline derivative tints of a pale and delicate color.
14. In the same manner as double-application tints.
15. To make it porous enough to accept the toner.
16. Frosting—strands of hair are lightened over various parts of the head. Tipping—wisps of hair are lightened in various areas of the head. Streaking—lightened strand, usually at front hairline.

Miscellaneous

1. Since lightened hair is over-porous, it requires corrective treatments to help prevent it from breaking.
2. They recondition lightened, tinted, or otherwise damaged hair.
3. Conditioner and color fillers.
4. If hair is in a damaged condition and if there is doubt that finished color will be an even shade.
5. A color filler treatment.
6. Lightening and dye solvent methods.
7. individual
8. To prevent its chemical action from continuing on the hair.
9. Check the natural color of the hair at the scalp area. Make two or more test strands. Select the appropriate color filler shade.
10. a) An agent that deposits a basic color and gives uniform porosity to the hair. b) Accumulation of residue on the outside of the hair shaft. c) A method of removing tint from the hair by means of a dye solvent, commercial product, or lightening treatment. d) A chemical reaction that takes place when peroxide and a tinting solution are mixed.

Coloring Mustaches and Beards

1. An aniline derivative tint. It may cause serious irritation or damage to the delicate membranes in the nostrils or to the lips.
2. Crayons, pomades in tubes, and two-bottle set solutions.

CHAPTER 16

Men's Hairpieces

1. Wanting or needing to cover thinning or balding areas of the head.
2. Human, animal, and synthetic.
3. By using a tape measure and by making a pattern.
4. So that the manufacturer can match the ordered hairpiece with the client's hair.
5. Without front lace and with front lace.
6. Hard, soft, net, plastic, combination.
7. Two-sided tape.
8. Spirit gum.
9. Remove all old tape from the foundation. Swish the hairpiece back and forth in a cleaner in an open bowl. Gently press out cleaner or allow it to drip into the bowl. Fasten hairpiece on covered head mold and allow to dry naturally.
10. How to sell, measure, fit, cut, style, service, and recondition them.
11. Because the products in the bleach tend to damage the foundation.
12. To prevent dryness or brittleness of the hair and to liven up the appearance of the hairpiece.
13. A wide-tooth comb.
14. Word-of-mouth advertising; window display; before and after pictures of men wearing hairpieces; barber-stylists wearing hairpieces; listing in the telephone directory.
15. Stock and custom.

CHAPTER 17

Nails, Nail Disorders, and Manicures

1. Horny protective coverings at the tips of the fingers and toes.
2. It is firm and flexible, and exhibits a slightly pinkish color. Its surface is smooth, curved and unspotted, without any hollows or wavy ridges.

3. Keratin.

4. a) The nail root is at the base of the nail, underneath the skin. b) The nail body is the visible portion of the nail resting upon the nail bed. c) The free edge is that portion of the nail which extends over the fingertip. d) The nail bed is the part of the skin upon which the nail rests.

5. Nutrition and general good health.

6. General poor health, disease of the nails, and injury to the matrix.

7. The matrix.

8. In the matrix.

9. From the matrix, which contains nerves, lymph, and blood vessels.

10. About one-eighth inch per month.

11. A nail disorder is a condition caused by injury to the nail, disease, or an imbalance in the body.

12. The golden rule states that if the nail or skin to be worked on is infected, inflamed, broken, or swollen, a nail technician should refer the client to a doctor.

13. Five nail disorders that can be serviced by a nail technician are: a) hangnails; b) discolored nails; c) eggshell nails; d) furrows; e) leuconychia; f) onychatrophia or atrophy; g) onychauxis; h) onychophagy; i)onychorrhexis; j) ptergium; k) saleronychia. (Only five are needed.)

14. Five nail disorders that cannot be serviced by a nail technician are: a) mold; b) onychia; c) onychogryposis; d) onycholysis; e) onychoptosis; f) paronychia; g) pyrogenic granuloma. (Only five are needed.)

15. Equipment used in nail technology are: a) manicure table with an adjustable lamp; b) client's chair and nail technician's chair or stool; c) finger bowl; d) wet sanitizer; e) client's cushion; f) sanitized cotton container; g) supply tray; h) electric nail dryer. (Only three are needed.)
Implements needed for a manicure include: a) orangewood stick; b) steel pusher; c) metal nail file; d) emery board; e) cuticle nipper. (Only three are needed.)
Materials needed for a manicure include: a) disposable towels or terry towels; b) cotton or cotton balls; c) plastic bags; d) 70 percent ethyl alcohol; e) powder alum or styptic powder. (Only three are needed.)
Nail cosmetics include: a) polish remover; b) cuticle cream; c) cuticle oil; d) cuticle solvent; e) nail bleach; f) nail whitener; g) dry nail polish; h) colored polish; i) liquid enamel

or lacquer; j) base coat; k) nail strengthener; l) top coat or sealer; m) liquid nail dry; n) hand cream or lotion. (Only three are needed.)

16. Two reasons for having a manicure table that is sanitary and properly equipped are: a) anything needed during a service will be at your fingertips; b) having an orderly table will give you and your client confidence during the manicure.

17. Four basic nail shapes are: a) rectangular or square; b) round; c) oval; d) pointed.

18. The six steps in the basic manicure pre-service are: a) pre-service sanitation procedure; b) set up standard manicuring table; c) greet client; d) have client wash hands with an antibacterial soap; e) do client consultation; f) begin working with the hand that is not the client's favored hand.

19. The basic manicure procedure is as follows: a) remove polish; b) shape nails; c) soften cuticles; d) clean nails; e) dry hand; f) apply cuticle remover; g) loosen cuticles; h) nip cuticles; i) clean under free edge; j) repeat steps d–i on other hand; k) bleach nails (optional); l) buff with chamois buffer (optional); m) apply cuticle oil; n) bevel nails; o) apply hand lotion and massage hand and arm; p) remove traces of oil; q) choose color; r) apply polish.

20. Five types of polish applications are: 1) full coverage; 2) free edge; 3) hairline tip; 4) half moon or lunula; 5) slimline or free walls.

21. The five steps in the basic manicure post-service are: 1) make another appointment; 2) sell retail products; 3) clean up around your table; 4) discard used materials; 5) sanitize table and implements.

22. A man's manicure is the same as a woman's except that a colored polish is not used in a man's manicure.

23. A manicure that is given at the styling chair while the client is receiving a hair service.

24. Five hand massage techniques are: a) relaxer movement; b) joint movement on fingers; c) circular movement in palm; d) circular movement on wrist; e) circular movement on back of hand and fingers. Five arm massage techniques are: a) distribute cream or lotion; b) effleurage on arms; c) wringing movements on arm-friction massage movement; d) kneading movement on arm; e) rotation of elbow-friction massage movement.

CHAPTER 18

Electricity

1. A form of energy capable of producing magnetic, chemical, or heat effects.
2. A substance that readily carries an electric current. Most metals are used as conductors.
3. A substance that resists the passage of an electric current. Examples: rubber and silk.
4. They serve as points of contact when applying electricity to the body.
5. A constant and even-flowing current, traveling in one direction.
6. A rapid interrupted current, flowing first in one direction and then in the opposite direction.
7. A converter.
8. A rectifier.
9. A unit of electrical pressure.
10. A unit of electrical strength.
11. A unit of electrical resistance.
12. The negative or positive state of electric current.
13. The process by which chemical solutions are introduced into tissues through the skin by galvanic current.
14. Galvanic, faradic, sinusoidal, and high-frequency currents.

High-Frequency or Violet Ray

1. A current having a high rate of vibration.
2. Tesla current.
3. Either stimulating or soothing, depending on the method of application.
4. Facial electrode, scalp electrode, and metal electrode.
5. Direct surface application, indirect application, and general electrification.
6. The barber-stylist holds the electrode and applies it directly over client's skin.
7. While the client holds a metal or glass electrode, the barber-stylist massages the surface being treated.
8. The client holds the metal electrode in his/her hand, thereby charging the body with electricity.
9. General electrification.
10. By lifting the electrode slightly from the area being treated and applying current through towel or clothing.
11. About five minutes.

12. Use high-frequency current first, followed by application of hair tonic.
13. Stimulates blood circulation. Increases glandular activity. Aids in elimination and absorption. Increases metabolism.
14. Falling hair, itchy scalp, tight scalp, dry and oily scalp, and skin conditions.

Light Therapy

1. Treatment by means of light rays.
2. Ultraviolet rays and infrared rays.
3. An electrical apparatus used in producing certain light rays.
4. Glass bulb lamp, hot quartz lamp, and cold quartz lamp.
5. Glass bulb lamp and hot quartz lamp.
6. Iron, vitamin D, red and white blood cells.
7. Increase the blood and lymph flow; restore nutrition; increase the elimination of waste products.
8. Acne, tinea, seborrhea, and dandruff.
9. They stimulate the growth of hair.
10. About 12 inches.
11. To prevent irritation and injury to the eyes.
12. About two or three minutes.
13. To seven or eight minutes.
14. It may cause severe sunburn and blisters.
15. The ultraviolet rays stimulate the production of pigment or coloring matter in the skin.
16. The slightest covering on the skin prevents these rays from reaching the skin.
17. Special glass bulbs.
18. Cover the eyes with pads dipped into boric acid or witch hazel solution.
19. About 30 inches from the skin.
20. To prevent constant exposure of the tissues.
21. Heat and relax the skin. Dilate blood vessels in the skin, thereby increasing blood flow. Increase metabolism and chemical changes within skin tissues. Increase the production of perspiration and oil on the skin. Relieve pain. Soothing to the nerves.
22. Dermal lights, with a tungsten or carbon filament in clear or colored bulbs.
23. To protect the eyes from the heat and glare of the light.
24. The heat relieves pain in congested areas.
25. Blue light.

26. It has a tonic effect on the bare skin and soothes the nerves.
27. Has a stimulating effect on the skin. Aids penetration of creams and ointments into skin. Softens and relaxes body tissue.

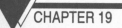

CHAPTER 19   Chemistry

1. For an intelligent understanding of the various products and cosmetics being used in the shop.
2. The branch of chemistry that deals with all substances containing carbon. Examples: plants, animals, petroleum, coal, natural gas.
3. Organic solvents. Examples: gasoline, benzine.
4. The branch of chemistry that deals with all substances that do not contain carbon. Examples: water, air, iron, lead, iodine, bones.
5. Anything that occupies space.
6. Solids, liquids, and gases.
7. The basic unit of all matter. 103.
8. An atom.
9. The smallest particle of an element or compound that possesses all the characteristics of that element or compound.
10. The tendency of its atoms to combine with other elements.
11. The chemical joining of two or more elements to form a new substance.
12. Oxides—compounds composed of any element combined with oxygen. Acids—compounds of hydrogen, a non-metal and, sometimes, oxygen. Bases (alkalis)—compounds of hydrogen, a metal, and oxygen. Salts—compounds formed by the reaction of acids and bases.
13. A physical combination of two or more elements that retain their individual identities.
14. Physical change—ice to water. Chemical change—soap formed from the chemical reaction of an alkaline substance and an oil.
15. An alteration of the properties without the formation of a new substance.
16. Where a new substance is formed, having properties different from the original substances.
17. Density, specific gravity, odor, color, and taste.
18. Potential hydrogen, or degree of acidity or alkalinity of a liquid.
19. Below 7.

20. Above 7.
21. Water.
22. Filtration and distillation.
23. Soft and hard water.
24. It contains mineral substances that curdle soap instead of permitting it to lather.
25. H_2O.

CHAPTER 20 ▼

Anatomy and Physiology

1. To have constructive knowledge of those parts receiving treatments.
2. The head, face, and neck.
3. The study of the gross structures of the body. Examples: muscles, bones, arteries, veins, and nerves.
4. The study of the functions or activities performed by the various parts of the body.
5. The study of the minute structures of the body. Examples: histology of skin, hair, sweat glands, and oil glands.

Cells

1. To understand anatomy and physiology.
2. The basic unit of all living matter.
3. It will contribute to an understanding of the skin, scalp, and hair and how they function.
4. Protoplasm.
5. Nucleus, cytoplasm, centrosome, and cell membrane.
6. Nucleus—affects reproduction of the cell. Cytoplasm—contains food materials for growth, reproduction, and repair of cell. Centrosome—also affects reproduction of the cell. Cell membrane—permits soluble substances to enter and leave the cell.
7. By direct or indirect division.
8. In the human body.
9. A complex chemical process whereby cells are nourished and supplied with energy to carry on their many activities.
10. Anabolism and catabolism.
11. The cell absorbs whatever food, water, and oxygen it needs.
12. The cell uses up whatever it has absorbed.
13. Groups of cells of the same kind performing a specific function.
14. Connective, muscular, nerve, epithelial, and liquid tissues.

15. It serves as a carrier of food, waste products, and hormones. Examples: blood and lymph.
16. A structure containing two or more different tissues combining to accomplish a definite function.
17. Brain, heart, lungs, kidneys, liver, stomach, and intestines.
18. Groups of organs that work together for the welfare of the entire body.
19. Skeletal, muscular, nervous, circulatory, endocrine, excretory, respiratory, digestive, and reproductive systems.

Skeletal System

1. Bone.
2. Give shape and strength to the body. Protect the organs from injury. Serve as attachments for muscles. Act as levers for all bodily movements.
3. The skeleton of the head.
4. Two parts. The cranium and the skeleton of the face.
5. Eight bones.
6. Occipital, two parietal, frontal, and two temporal.
7. Forms the lower back part of the cranium.
8. The sides and top of head.
9. The frontal bone.
10. Temporal bones.
11. Sphenoid bone.
12. 14 bones.
13. Two nasal bones, two zygomatic bones, two maxillae bones, and mandible bone.
14. The whole upper jaw.
15. The lower jaw.
16. Zygomatic bones.
17. In the front part of the throat.
18. It forms the top part of the spinal column and is located in the neck region.

Muscular System

1. It is a contractile, fibrous tissue upon which various movements of the body depend.
2. They cover, shape, and support the skeleton and produce all body movements.
3. Voluntary or striated muscle; involuntary or non-striated muscle; cardiac or heart muscle.

4. Voluntary muscles are controlled by the will. Involuntary muscles are not controlled by the will.
5. The skeletal and nervous systems.
6. a) Origin of a muscle refers to its more fixed attachment. b) Insertion of a muscle refers to its more movable attachment.

Nervous System

1. To understand how to administer scalp and facial treatments for the client's benefit and what effects these treatments have on the nerves in the skin and scalp and on the body as a whole.
2. The brain, spinal cord, and their nerves.
3. The cerebro-spinal, the peripheral, and the sympathetic nervous systems.
4. It controls consciousness, voluntary functions of the five senses, and voluntary muscle actions.
5. It consists of sensory and motor nerve fibers that carry messages to and from the cerebro-spinal nervous system.
6. Its functions are independent of the will. This system controls internal body functions, such as breathing, circulation, digestion, and glandular activities.
7. The structural unit of the nervous system.
8. A cell body and long and short fibers called cell processes.
9. Long, white cords made up of fibers, which carry messages to and from various parts of the body.
10. Sensory and motor nerves.
11. To carry messages regarding touch, heat, cold, sight, hearing, smell, taste, and pain to the nerve centers in the brain.
12. a) Sensory nerves—afferent nerves. b) Motor nerves—efferent nerves.
13. To carry impulses from the brain to the muscles, which produce movements of the body.
14. A quick removal of the hand from a hot object.

Circulatory System

1. Because the circulatory system supplies nourishment to the entire body as well as to the skin, hair, and nails.
2. It carries water, oxygen, food, and secretions to all cells of the body; carries away carbon dioxide and waste products for elimination; helps to equalize body temperature; aids in

protecting the body from harmful bacteria and infections through action of the white blood cells; clots the blood.
3. It keeps the blood moving within the circulatory system.
4. Arteries, veins, capillaries.
5. The arteries.
6. The veins.
7. They carry impure blood from various capillaries back to the heart.
8. Pulmonary system and general or systemic system.
9. It consists of plasma, red and white corpuscles, and blood platelets.
10. 98.6 degrees fahrenheit.
11. It is composed of about nine-tenths water and carries food elements, waste products, and other substances to and from cells.
12. To carry oxygen to the cells of the body.
13. To protect the body against disease.
14. Lymph is a colorless, watery fluid, circulating through the lymph-vascular system.
15. It acts as a middleman between blood and tissues; carries nourishment from blood to cells; removes waste materials from cells.
16. From the blood plasma.

Glands and Other Systems

1. Duct glands and ductless glands.
2. The kidneys, liver, skin, large intestine, and lungs.
3. With each cycle an exchange of gases takes place. During inhalation, oxygen is absorbed into the blood, while carbon dioxide is expelled during exhalation.
4. Mouth, pharynx, esophagus, stomach, and small intestine.

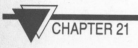

CHAPTER 21

The Job Search

1. Be realistic in expectations and goals; be cautious in business dealings; keep an open mind; be flexible in timing; believe in yourself.
2. Personality and attitude.
3. Trade shows and educational seminars; associations and organizations; student competitions; barber-styling school.

4. Receptionist; stylist's assistant; shampoo technician; manicurist.
5. The portfolio and the resumé.
6. Barber-styling school, instructors and classmates, suppliers, distributor classes, trade shows, newspapers, and telephone book.
7. Wage percentage, pay schedule, retail sales percentage, benefits, sick leave/vacation policies, dress code, equipment and supplies provided by the shop or salon, hours, new client policies.

CHAPTER 22 ▼

Selling in the Barber-Styling Shop

1. Establishing a clear, definite understanding of the client's needs and desires.
2. Improved appearance; improved social relationships; improved business and promotional opportunities; getting the most value for his/her money; improving his/her feeling of well being.
3. Atmosphere, sanitation, attitude.

CHAPTER 23 ▼

Barber-Styling Shop Management

1. Determine the services to be offered; create a business plan; determine mood, theme, and decor of premises; arrange for financing; find best location; purchase equipment, furniture, and fixtures; establish record keeping; establish shop policies; develop sales techniques; advertising.
2. Service requirements, employee duties, and shop procedures.
3. Individual ownership, partnership, and corporation.
4. A convenient location near other active businesses that attract people.
5. It protects against any possible increase in rent and defines the rights and responsibilities of the tenant.
6. A pleased client.
7. To determine income, expenses, profit and loss; to prove value of shop to a prospective buyer; to arrange for a bank loan; for government reports.

8. To make or change appointments; go after new business; remind clients of needed services; adjust complaints and satisfy clients; answer questions; receive messages; order equipment and supplies.
9. Display an interested, helpful attitude. Be prompt in answering the phone. Give all necessary information to the caller. Be tactful.

Page numbers in italic indicate information can be found in table(s) and/or figure(s).

Undertone, the underlying color that emerges during the lifting process of melanin, which contributes to the end result. When lightening hair, a residual warmth in tone always occurs, 421

Uniform, is used to denote a haircut that is cut at equal leng_ throughout the sections of the hair, 229

United States Pharmacopeia (U.S.P.), 515–17

Urea peroxide, a peroxide compound occasionally use_ases color. When added to an alkaline color mixture_ oxygen, 421

V

Vacuum, electric hair, 77

Vagus (VAY-gus) nerve, a sensory-motor n_ and sensation of the ear, pharynx_ esophagus, 168

Value. See Depth; Level

Vaporizer, facial treatment and, 18_id, greasy mass that is

Vascular (VAS-kyoo-lahr) syster

Vaseline, is a yellowish to w_rces, 421
almost insoluble in w_ade from various plants, such

Vegetable
color, a color derived_
tints, are hair colo_se, such as syphilis or gonorrhea,
as herbs and f_ commonly acquired by contact
Vein, cross sectio_on during sexual intercourse, 106,

Venereal (ve-N_wer, thick-walled chambers of the heart,
is a c_
with_ is the technical term for a wart. It is caused
120_ infectious, 109

Ventr_ is a blister with clear fluid in it, 108

_AY-shun), in massage the fingertips or vibrator
V_ransmit a trembling movement to the skin and its
_g structures, 177

_eatment and, 180
_treatment with, 153
_atory facial, 187–88

Vinegar (acid) rinse, 140

Virgin hair, natural hair that has not undergone any chemical or physical abuse, 422

Viruses, filterable (FIL-ter-a-bil), are living organisms so small that they can pass through a porcelain filter. They cause the common cold and other respiratory and gastrointestinal infections, 33

Viscosity, a term referring to the thickness of the solution, 422

Visible light, 493–94

Vitiligo (vit-i-LEYE-goh), is an acquired condition affecting skin or hair in which there are abnormal white patches. There is no treatment except the application of a matching cosmetic color, 107

Volt (V), is a unit for measuring the pressure that forces the electrical current forward, 484

_ume, the concentration of hydrogen peroxide in water solution. Expressed as volumes of oxygen liberated per volume of solution, 422

base curls, 297

Voluntary muscles, are controlled by will, such as those of the face, arms, and legs, 527

Vomer (VOH-mer) bone, is a single bone that forms part of the dividing wall of the nose, 525

W

Wart, is caused by a virus and is infectious, 109

Water,
chemistry of, 133, 505–6
hones, 67–68
purification of, 133–34
rinse, 140
shampooing and, 133

Water-in-oil (W/O) emulsions, emulsions that are formed with drops of water suspended in an oil base, 508

Watt (W), measures how much electric energy is being used in one second, 484

Waving. See type of waving

Waxy dandruff, 117

Weight line, refers to the heaviest perimeter area of a 0- or 45-degree cut, 230

Wet sanitizer, 37

Wheal (WHEEL), is an itchy, swollen lesion that lasts only a few hours, 108

White light, effects of, 493

Whiteheads, facial treatment and, 192

Wigs. See Hairpieces

Windings, permanent waves and, 324–27

Witch hazel, is a solution of alcohol, water, and powder ground from the leaves and twigs of the Hamamelis virginiana, 517
freshener lotions and, 513

Women,
clipper cut, 258–59
cutting hair of, 240–44
razor cut, 279–82

Work practices, safe, 44–46

Wrappings, permanent waves and, 324–27

Wrinkle treatments, 513

Wrist, is a flexible joint composed of eight small, irregular bones held together by ligaments, 526
circular movement massage, 479

Z

Zeolite tanks, 506

Zinc oxide, is a heavy white powder that is insoluble in _ 517

Zygomatic (zeye-goh-MAT-ik)
bones, form the prominence of the cheeks, 525
nerve, affects the skin of the temples, sides of the forehead, and upper part of the cheeks, 169, 170

Zygomaticus (zeye-goh-MAT-i-kus), muscle that extends from the zygomatic bone to the angle of the mouth. It elevates the lip, 166